THIRD EDITION

MEMORY LOSS, ALZHEIMER'S DISEASE, AND DEMENTIA

A PRACTICAL GUIDE FOR CLINICIANS

THIRD EDITION

MEMORY LOSS,
ALZHEIMER'S DISEASE, AND DEMENTIA
A PRACTICAL GUIDE FOR CLINICIANS

ANDREW E. BUDSON, MD
Neurology Service, Section of Cognitive &
   Behavioral Neurology,
Veterans Affairs Boston Healthcare System,
   Boston, MA;
Alzheimer's Disease Research Center &
   Department of Neurology,
Boston University School of Medicine,
   Boston, MA;
Harvard Medical School, Boston, MA;
The Boston Center for Memory, Newton, MA

PAUL R. SOLOMON, PhD
Department of Psychology, Program in
   Neuroscience,
Williams College, Williamstown, MA;
The Boston Center for Memory, Newton, MA

For additional online content visit expertconsult.com

ELSEVIER

Elsevier
1600 John F. Kennedy Blvd.
Ste 1800
Philadelphia, PA 19103-2899

MEMORY LOSS, ALZHEIMER'S DISEASE, AND DEMENTIA, THIRD EDITION   ISBN: 978-0-323795449

Previous editions copyrighted 2016 and 2011.
Library of Congress Control Number: 2021932129

Content Strategist: Melanie Tucker
Content Development Specialist: Dominque McPherson
Publishing Services Manager: Deepthi Unni
Project Manager: Radjan Lourde Selvanadin
Design Direction: Brian Salisbury

Printed in India

Last digit is the print number: 9 8 7 6 5 4 3

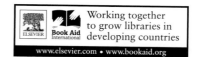

The cohesive text is an appealing blend of personal experience and clinical anecdotes, and is supported by a firm command of the rapidly changing clinical literature. The writing is crisp, lucid and, above all, practice-oriented … Budson and Solomon are especially adroit in identification of controversies, knowledge gaps, and areas in which diagnostic criteria are ill-defined or difficult to apply (e.g., fluctuating cognition in dementia with Lewy bodies). Readers are not abandoned without guidance; ambiguities are resolved by confident descriptions of personal approaches to specific situations … The book is an incredible compilation of practical advice.

Lancet Neurology,
March 2012

From the point of view of the busy clinician working in the trenches but looking for a practical and cutting-edge guide, Doraiswamy said he cannot think of a better book, noting, 'This is the clinical book of the year in our field.

Alzheimer's Research Forum review,
December 2011

Few books provide both a comprehensive review and a step-by-step guide. I strongly recommend this book to all those who treat patients with memory loss—physicians, social workers, psychologists, nurses—at every level of training and experience.

P. Murali Doraiswamy, MD
Professor & Head,
Division of Biological Psychiatry, Duke University,
and co-author of *The Alzheimer's Action Plan*

Memory Loss: A Practical Guide for Clinicians provides the assessment, diagnostic and therapeutic insights clinicians need to provide exemplary care to memory impaired patients. Don't go to the clinic without it.

Jeffrey L. Cummings, MD
Director, Cleveland Clinic Lou Ruvo
Center for Brain Health,
The Andrea L. and Joseph F. Hahn MD
Chair of Neurotherapeutics

Designed for easy reference to satisfy the real time needs of clinicians in hectic clinical settings, I'm sure this volume will be dog-eared in short order given its clear no-nonsense style.

Neil W. Kowall, MD
Professor of Neurology and Pathology,
Boston University School of Medicine,
Director, Boston University
Alzheimer's Disease Center,
Chief, Neurology Service,
Boston VA Healthcare System

This book summarizes complex material in a manner that benefits clinical practitioners at all levels. This is an excellent addition to the library of professionals serving older adults.

Maureen K. O'Connor, PsyD, ABCN,
Chief, Neuropsychology Service,
Edith Nourse Rogers Memorial
Veterans Hospital, Bedford, MA

This is a very good addition to the books on dementias. With this book, the authors provide a resource for clinicians who will be caring for the more than 5 million individuals with memory loss, whether their degree is in medicine, psychology, nursing, social work, or therapies. Primary care providers, nurses, psychologists, and students will find this book a very practical, clinically oriented guide that helps them know what to do when sitting in the office with a patient complaining of memory loss. Specialists will find this book a wealth of up-to-date information regarding the latest diagnostic tools and treatments for their patients with memory loss.

Eric Gausche, MD, University of Illinois
at Chicago College of Medicine
4 Star-Doody Rating, March 2013

PRAISE FOR THE SECOND EDITION

I do not know of any other publication that deals with memory loss and dementia in as comprehensive yet practical a manner.

Howard S. Kirshner, MD
Cognitive and Behavioral Neurology,
March 2016

This superb, anticipated second edition of an outstanding educational/training tool is essential reading for virtually all physicians on the diagnosis and treatment of this rapidly growing patient population. Written and edited by nationally recognized clinician-educators in the field, this update is a very welcome addition to the neurology and psychiatry literature.

Michael Joel Schrift, DO, MA
Northwestern University Feinberg School of
Medicine)
Doody's Score: 95—4 Stars!

CONTENTS

What an exciting—and challenging—time it is to be a clinician treating individuals with memory loss, Alzheimer's disease, and dementia. In the 5 years since the second edition of this book there have been myriad new developments. To help you understand these new developments and their implications, we have written three entirely new chapters in addition to updating and rewriting almost every other chapter, including:

- Chapter 2: Evaluating the Patient with Memory Loss or Dementia—*updated with FDA approved tau PET scans,*
- Chapter 3: Subjective Cognitive Decline, Mild Cognitive Impairment, and Dementia—*updated with subjective cognitive decline and the new National Institute on Aging-Alzheimer's Association (NIA-AA) Research Framework for syndromal staging of cognitive continuum,*
- Chapter 4: Alzheimer's disease—*updated with the new AT(N) (amyloid, tau, neurodegeneration) biomarker profile,*
- Chapter 5: Primary Age-Related Tauopathy—*new chapter,*
- Chapter 6: Limbic-predominant Age-related TDP-43 Encephalopathy—*new chapter,*
- Chapter 7: Vascular cognitive impairment and vascular dementia—*updated with new diagnostic criteria,*
- Chapter 8: Dementia with Lewy bodies—*updated with new diagnostic criteria, now including mild cognitive impairment with Lewy bodies,*
- Chapter 9: Primary Progressive Aphasia and Apraxia of Speech—*updated with new semantic variant videos,*
- Chapter 11: Posterior Cortical Atrophy—*new chapter,*
- Chapter 12: Progressive Supranuclear Palsy—*updated with new diagnostic criteria,*
- Chapter 14: Normal Pressure Hydrocephalus—*updated with the Evans index* and disproportionately enlarged subarachnoid space hydrocephalus,
- Chapter 16: Creutzfeldt-Jakob Disease—*updated with new diagnostic criteria,*
- Chapter 17: Other Disorders That Cause Memory Loss or Dementia—*updated with brain sagging syndrome,*
- Chapter 22: Nonpharmacological Treatment of Memory Loss, Alzheimer's Disease, and Dementia—*updated with new evidence for Mediterranean-style diets,*
- Chapter 23: Future Treatments of Memory Loss, Alzheimer's Disease, and Dementia—*updated with the latest therapies,* and
- Chapter 27: Pharmacological Treatment of the Behavioral and Psychological Symptoms of Dementia—*updated with pimavanserin (Nuplazid) and prazosin.*

Now, more than ever, frontline clinicians need a practical guide. We have worked to ensure that—despite the added complexity of the field—our book remains accessible to all clinicians who are and will be caring for the more than 44 million individuals throughout the world with memory loss, mild cognitive impairment, or dementia. Our book is written for generalists and specialists, students and experienced clinicians—whether their degrees are in medicine, psychology, nursing, social work, or the therapies. Primary care providers, nurses, social workers, therapists, psychologists, and students will find this book a very practical, clinically oriented guide that helps them know what to do when sitting in the office or by the bedside with a patient complaining of memory loss or exhibiting dementia behaviors. Specialists—including psychiatrists, neurologists, neuropsychologists, geriatricians, and others—will find in this book a wealth of up-to-date information regarding the latest diagnostic criteria, tools, and treatments for their patients with memory loss, mild cognitive impairment, and dementia.

Note that we have continued to take advantage of technology in using videos to illustrate various aspects of disorders that cannot easily be translated into words, such as tremors, speech and language difficulties, and gait problems. These videos can be viewed in the online, tablet, and smartphone versions of the book.

As was true for the prior editions, this book is based upon the most recent peer-reviewed published studies in the literature, combined with our opinions reflecting our experience in treating more than 5000 patients with memory loss and dementia over approximately 40,000 patient visits. Where our opinions are supported by the literature, we have provided appropriate references, and where our opinions differ from the literature, we have done our best to point this discrepancy out. There are, of course, large areas of clinical practice for which there are no randomized, double blind, placebo-controlled trials to guide one. It is here that our training and experience proves most valuable.

HOW TO USE THIS BOOK

Everyone should read *Chapters 1–8*, which cover the evaluation and the most common causes of memory loss and dementia. Other chapters can then be read when there are relevant issues, such as other diagnoses (*Section II, Chapters 9–17*), medications and other therapies for memory loss (*Section III, Chapters 18–23*), and the behavioral and psychological symptoms of dementia (*Section IV, Chapters 24–27*). Finally, *Section V* (*Chapters 28–30*) discusses driving, legal, financial, and other important issues. The web appendices provide additional useful information on cognitive tests and questionnaires (*Appendix A*), an expanded discussion on screening for memory loss (*Appendix B*), and a basic understanding of the different clinically relevant memory systems in the brain (*Appendix C*).

A note on abbreviations

Because we want this book to be accessible to a wide variety of audiences from diverse fields—each with their own standard jargon—we have endeavored to eliminate almost all abbreviations. Although this decision has made many sentences longer, we hope that these longer sentences will, on the whole, be more easily understood.

Andrew E. Budson, MD

Paul R. Solomon, PhD

This book is dedicated first to our patients and their caregivers; we are indebted for all that they have taught us. We also dedicate this third edition to those who supported, encouraged, and inspired us in more ways than we can list: Jessica and Todd Solomon; Danny, Leah, Sandra, and Richard Budson; and—of course—to Elizabeth Vassey and Amy Null. We thank you all.

Special thanks go to Thor Stein, MD, PhD and Ann C. McKee, MD, for providing the neuropathology figures, as well as Ana Vives-Rodriguez, MD and Chadrick E. Lane, MD for their invaluable reviews.

DISCLOSURES

Disclosures (current and/or during the past two years):

Dr. Budson receives grant support from the National Institute on Aging, National Institutes of Health (NIH), and from the Veterans Affairs Research & Development Service. He also receives or has received grant support from and/or has consulted for the following pharmaceutical companies: Acadia, Avanir, Biogen, EPI pharmaceuticals, Eisai, Eli Lilly, Cognito, and Cortexyme.

Dr. Solomon receives or has received grant support from Abbott, Acadia, AstraZeneca, Avanir, Biogen, Cognito, Cortexyme, Avid Radiopharmaceuticals, Eisai, EnVivo EPIX, Eli Lilly, Pfizer, TV Therapeutics, Sonexa, FORUM Pharmaceuticals, and Hoffmann-La Roche. He consults or has consulted for Abbott, Astellas, Avid, Biogen, Cognito, Eisai, EPIX, Pfizer, and Toyoma.

Note: The content of this book has been derived from the patients that Dr. Budson and Dr. Solomon have seen separately and together in the Boston Center for Memory, Newton, Massachusetts, and in The Memory Clinic in Bennington, Vermont, along with literature reviews conducted solely for the purpose of this book. These reviews and the writing of this book have been conducted during early mornings, late nights, weekends, and vacations. Dr. Budson's contribution to this book was conducted outside of both his VA tour of duty and his Boston University/NIH research time.

ABOUT THE AUTHORS

Dr. Budson received his bachelor's degree at Haverford College where he majored in both chemistry and philosophy. After graduating *cum laude* from Harvard Medical School, he was an intern in internal medicine at Brigham and Women's Hospital. He then attended the Harvard-Longwood Neurology Residency Program, for which he was chosen to be chief resident in his senior year. He next pursued a fellowship in behavioral neurology and dementia at Brigham and Women's Hospital, after which he joined the neurology department there. He participated in numerous clinical trials of new drugs to treat Alzheimer's disease in his role as the Associate Medical Director of Clinical Trials for Alzheimer's Disease at Brigham and Women's Hospital. Following his clinical training he spent 3 years studying memory as a post-doctoral fellow in experimental psychology and cognitive neuroscience at Harvard University under Professor Daniel Schacter. While continuing in the Neurology Department at Brigham and Women's Hospital, in 2000 he began work as Consultant Neurologist for The Memory Clinic in Bennington, Vermont. After 5 years as Assistant Professor of Neurology at Harvard Medical School, he joined the Boston University Alzheimer's Disease Center and the Geriatric Research Education Clinical Center (GRECC) at the Bedford Veterans Affairs Hospital. During his 5 years at the Bedford GRECC he served in several roles, including the Director of Outpatient Services, Associate Clinical Director, and later the overall GRECC Director. From March 2009 through February 2010 he served as Bedford's Acting Chief of Staff. In March 2010 he moved to Boston as the Deputy Chief of Staff of the Veterans Affairs Boston Healthcare System, where he is currently the Associate Chief of Staff for Education, Chief of the Section of Cognitive & Behavioral Neurology, and Director of the Center for Translational Cognitive Neuroscience. He is also the Director of Outreach, Recruitment, and Engagement at the Boston University Alzheimer's Disease Center, Professor of Neurology at Boston University School of Medicine, and Lecturer in Neurology at Harvard Medical School. Dr. Budson has had government research funding since 1998, receiving a National Research Service Award, a Career Development Award, a Research Project (R01) grant, and several VA Merit grants. He has given over 650 local, national, and international grand rounds and other academic talks, including at the Institute of Cognitive Neuroscience, Queen Square, London, UK; Berlin, Germany; and the University of Cambridge, England, UK. He has published over 100 papers in peer reviewed journals, including *The New England Journal of Medicine*, *Brain*, and *Cortex*, and is a reviewer for more than 50 journals. He was awarded the Norman Geschwind Prize in Behavioral Neurology in 2008 and the Research Award in Geriatric Neurology in 2009, both from the American Academy of Neurology. He serves on the medical scientific advisory board and board of directors for the Massachusetts/New Hampshire Chapter of the Alzheimer's Association. His current research uses the techniques of experimental psychology and cognitive neuroscience to understand memory and memory distortions in patients with Alzheimer's disease and other neurological disorders. In his Memory Disorders Clinic at the Veterans Affairs Boston Healthcare System he treats patients while teaching students, residents, and fellows, in addition to seeing patients at the Boston Center for Memory in Newton, Massachusetts.

Dr. Solomon received his PhD. in Psychology from the University of Massachusetts, Amherst. He was a postdoctoral fellow in the Laboratory of Richard F. Thompson in the Department of Psychobiology at the University of California at Irvine. He is currently Professor of Psychology and founding Chairman of the Neuroscience Program, Williams College. Dr. Solomon teaches in the areas of neuropsychology and behavioral neuroscience and conducts research on the neurobiology of memory disorders. He is particularly interested in the memory deficits associated with Alzheimer's disease. He is the author of 10 books, has also contributed chapters to 20 edited volumes, and has co-authored and presented more than 200 research papers. His work has been published in *Science*, *Scientific American*, *Journal of the American Medical Association*, and *The Lancet*. He has delivered more than 400 invited colloquia, symposia, grand rounds, lectures, and presentations. He has been the recipient of research grants from the National Science Foundation, the National Institute on Aging, the National Institute of Mental Health, and the United States Environmental Protection Agency, as well as private foundations and pharmaceutical research divisions. Dr. Solomon has received numerous awards, including a Distinguished Teaching Award from the University of Massachusetts, a National Research Service Award from the National Institutes of Health, a National Needs Postdoctoral Fellowship from the National Science Foundation, and a clinical research award from the American Association of Family Physicians. He has been elected a Fellow of the American Association for the Advancement of Science, the American Psychological Association and the American Psychological Society. He is listed in *Who's Who in America*, *American Men and Women of Science*, *Who's Who in Education*, and *Who's Who in Frontier Science and Technology*. Dr. Solomon has served on the editorial boards of several journals and serves as an external reviewer for numerous journals and granting agencies. He has lectured widely at colleges and universities on age-related memory disorders and at medical centers and hospitals on the diagnosis and treatment of Alzheimer's disease. He has also appeared frequently to discuss pharmacotherapy for Alzheimer's disease on national television, including *The Today Show*, *Good Morning America*, *The CBS Morning Show*, and *CBS*, *ABC*, and *NBC Evening News*. His work on screening for Alzheimer's disease has been featured on *Dateline NBC*. In addition to his academic undertakings, Dr. Solomon is a licensed psychologist in Massachusetts and Vermont. He is also founder and Clinical Director of the Memory Clinic in Bennington, Vermont, the Boston Center for Memory, and President of Clinical Neuroscience Research Associates. He has served as the first Director of Training for the Southwestern Vermont Psychology Consortium. He serves on the advisory board of the Massachusetts Alzheimer's Association and the Northeastern New York Alzheimer's Association.

VIDEO TABLE OF CONTENTS

1

Why Diagnose and Treat Memory Loss, Alzheimer's Disease, and Dementia?

QUICK START: WHY DIAGNOSE AND TREAT MEMORY LOSS, ALZHEIMER'S DISEASE, AND DEMENTIA?

- Current treatments can help improve or maintain the patient's cognitive and functional status by "turning back the clock" on memory loss.
- Families and other caregivers are helped by treatments that maintain or improve functional status and neuropsychiatric symptoms.
- Using current treatments saves money, as shown by pharmaco-economic studies.

- New, disease-modifying treatments are being developed and may be available soon.
- Accurate diagnosis helps define prognosis, facilitating future planning.
- Improving the quality (not quantity) of life is the goal.

A 72-year-old woman comes into the clinic at the urging of her son. She has noticed some difficulties finding words for the past 6 months, but denies problems with memory or other aspects of her thinking. Her son reports that his mother has had memory problems that began five years ago, and have been gradually worsening. He notes that his mother used to have an excellent memory, and would keep her calendar, grocery, and other lists in her head. Now she needs to write everything down or she is totally lost. She used to send out birthday cards to her grandchildren every year, but over the past two years has either forgotten to do this or sends them out at the wrong time. In addition to memory problems, he agrees that she also has word-finding difficulties, and often has trouble finishing sentences. From a functional standpoint, she is also having difficulty. She is living with her husband, and he has gradually been taking over household responsibilities that she used to do, such as going

to the grocery store. She continues to cook, but there are now just a few meals that she prepares, and these have become much simpler than they used to be.

The first question that needs to be addressed in this book is: What should be done about this 72-year-old woman? Why is it important to diagnose and treat memory loss? Although the answer to this question may seem obvious to some, in the current healthcare climate it is very reasonable. There are four basic answers to this question: (1) to help the patient, (2) to help the family and other caregivers, (3) to save money, and (4) to plan for the future.

HELPING THE PATIENT

Current pharmacologic treatments for Alzheimer's disease have been shown to be able to "turn the clock back" on memory loss for 6 to 12 months (Cummings,

2004). That is, although memory loss cannot be halted or reversed to where it was before their developing Alzheimer's disease, current treatments are able to improve patients' memory to where it was 6 to 12 months previously. Although to some this may not seem worthwhile, we believe that this level of improvement can make a significant difference in the lives of our patients. In addition, non-pharmacologic treatments have also been shown to be effective (Özbe, Graessel, Donath, & Pendergrass, 2019). When combined, pharmacologic and non-pharmacologic treatment can enable patients with very mild memory loss to take that last trip to Europe, attend and remember their grandchild's wedding, or finish writing their memoirs. For patients with mild memory loss, treatments allow them to continue independent activities, such as shopping for groceries and paying bills. For patients with moderate to severe memory loss, treatments may provide functional improvements in basic activities of daily living—such as dressing, bathing, and toileting—and reduce unwanted behaviors.

Additionally, many new treatments are being developed for patients with memory loss, some of which have the potential to dramatically slow down or even stop memory loss entirely. These so-called "disease-modifying" treatments will be specific to different diseases causing dementia, and thus accurate diagnosis will be critical.

HELPING THE FAMILY OR OTHER CAREGIVER

The majority of patients diagnosed with dementia live at home and are cared for by a family member. It follows logically that, if the patient is showing improvements, life for family members and other caregivers will also improve (Mossello & Ballini, 2012). If patients with mild memory loss can do their own shopping and pay their own bills, then no one has to spend time helping them with these chores. And, of course, if activities of daily living are improved, families and other caregivers will have more time for their own activities. One study found that treatment was associated with a saving of 68 minutes per day on average for caregivers (Sano et al., 2003). Moreover, once patients are diagnosed, caregivers can be provided with targeted interventions to improve

their own quality of life (Meichsner, Töpfer, Reder, Soellner, & Wilz, 2019).

SAVING MONEY

Several medications for memory loss are now generic, reducing the average cost of treatment per year from over $2000 for some name brands to as little as $180 for some generics. Are the beneficial effects for patients and caregivers worth the costs? Although certain aspects of this question cannot be readily answered, an easier question to answer is whether the dollars spent on medications to treat memory loss and to improve quality of life end up saving money. This issue has been studied and the results today are even clearer than before: treatment of memory loss does save money (da Silva et al., 2019; Touchon et al., 2014). When patients are treated for their memory loss, fewer medications to control behavior need be prescribed. There is less use of home health aids. Caregivers have more time to spend in the workplace bringing in revenue to the household. Additionally, placement in nursing homes can be delayed (Geldmacher et al., 2003; Lyseng-Williamson & Plosker, 2002).

PLANNING FOR THE FUTURE

Planning for the future is absolutely essential for any patient with progressive memory loss. Documents such as a power of attorney and healthcare proxy will need to be drawn up and signed. Banking, bill paying, and driving need to be addressed. The physical environment within the home will often need changes. Usually the patient will end up moving to a new residence. Some patients move in with a family member in a room, a separate suite, or an apartment in the house. Other patients move to senior housing, retirement communities, or assisted living. (See Chapters 28 and 29 for more on these important topics.) Understanding the patient's prognosis in as much detail as possible is invaluable when helping families to anticipate when some of these changes will likely take place, and which options to pursue. For example, we have had a number of families inform us that they are either adding an addition onto their house or are building a new house so the patient can live with them. Whether the construction will be completed in time to be of use to the patient will often depend upon the etiology of the memory loss.

QUALITY VERSUS QUANTITY

A word on the goal of treatment. We would argue that the goal of treating memory loss is not necessarily to prolong life, but is, rather, to improve the quality of life that the patient has available to him or her. For example, if a patient has 10 years between the time of diagnosis and death, the goal of treatment is to make those 10 years the very best they can be. Over time, memory loss progresses to dementia, and dementia progresses from mild to moderate to severe. At the end of life, the goal of therapy shifts to that of allowing the patient to die with dignity and comfort. At that point we would suggest it is appropriate to withdraw treatments for memory loss, and it is our observation that withdrawal of such treatments does allow the patient to die more quickly.

REFERENCES

Cummings, J. L. (2004). Alzheimer's disease. *The New England Journal of Medicine, 351*, 56–67.

da Silva, L. R., Vianna, C., Mosegui, G., Peregrino, A., Marinho, V., & Laks, J. (2019). Cost-effectiveness analysis of the treatment of mild and moderate Alzheimer's disease in Brazil. *Revista Brasileira de Psiquiatria (Sao Paulo, Brazil: 1999), 41*(3), 218–224.

Geldmacher, D. S., Provenzano, G., McRae, T., et al. (2003). Donepezil is associated with delayed nursing home placement in patients with Alzheimer's disease. *Journal of the American Geriatrics Society, 51*, 937–944.

Lyseng-Williamson, K. A., & Plosker, G. L. (2002). Galantamine: a pharmacoeconomic review of its use in Alzheimer's disease. *Pharmacoeconomics, 20*, 919–942.

Meichsner, F., Töpfer, N. F., Reder, M., Soellner, R., & Wilz, G. (2019). Telephone-based cognitive behavioral intervention improves dementia caregivers' quality of life. *American Journal of Alzheimer's Disease & Other Dementias, 34*(4), 236–246.

Mossello, E., & Ballini, E. (2012). Management of patients with Alzheimer's disease: pharmacological treatment and quality of life. *Therapeutic Advances in Chronic Disease, 3*, 183–193.

Özbe, D., Graessel, E., Donath, C., & Pendergrass, A. (2019). Immediate intervention effects of standardized multicomponent group interventions on people with cognitive impairment: A systematic review. *Journal of Alzheimer's Disease, 67*(2), 653–670.

Sano, M., Wilcock, G. K., van Baelen, B., et al. (2003). The effects of galantamine treatment on caregiver time in Alzheimer's disease. *International Journal of Geriatric Psychiatry, 18*, 942–950.

Touchon, J., Lachaine, J., Beauchemin, C., Granghaud, A., Rive, B., & Bineau, S. (2014). The impact of memantine in combination with acetylcholinesterase inhibitors on admission of patients with Alzheimer's disease to nursing homes: cost-effectiveness analysis in France. *The European Journal of Health Economics, 15*, 791–800.

2

Evaluating the Patient With Memory Loss or Dementia

QUICK START: EVALUATING THE PATIENT WITH MEMORY LOSS OR DEMENTIA

- Talking with the family (or other caregivers) is critical to obtaining an accurate history.
- Important elements of the history to investigate include:
  - Characterization of the onset and course of the disorder
  - Memory loss and memory distortions
  - Word-finding
  - Fluctuations in attention
  - Getting lost in a new or familiar environment
  - Problems with reasoning and judgment
  - Changes in behavior
  - Depression and anxiety
  - Loss of insight
  - Current functional status including basic and instrumental activities of daily living.
- Review of systems, past medical history, physical examination, and laboratory studies should evaluate for medical, neurological, and psychiatric problems that can impair cognition and memory, such as strokes, Parkinson's disease, and depression.

- Cognitive testing is essential, whether with brief tests in the office or a formal neuropsychological evaluation.
- Interpret current cognition and function in light of the patient's previous abilities.
- Routine screening for memory loss will allow patients to be diagnosed and treated earlier, which can help them to delay a decline in function and maintain quality of life.
- A brain CT or MRI scan is essential for evaluating possible strokes and other anatomic lesions.
- A functional imaging scan (technetium SPECT or fluorodeoxyglucose PET) can be helpful to confirm the diagnosis of an atypical dementia and to provide additional diagnostic information for young patients.
- A lumbar puncture, amyloid PET scan, or tau PET scan can confirm the diagnosis of Alzheimer's disease with a high degree of certainty.
- Beware of diagnosing dementia in the patient hospitalized for a medical issue!

In this chapter we will discuss how to evaluate a patient with memory loss and possible dementia, including the history, physical examination, cognitive testing, and laboratory and imaging studies. We will illustrate this evaluation by focusing on the most common cause of memory loss, Alzheimer's disease. Elements of the evaluation are similar to other medical assessments and should include:

1. a history of present illness
2. medical history
3. current and relevant past medications
4. allergies to medications

5. social history, including education, occupation, and any possible learning disabilities
6. family history, including a history of late-life memory problems even if considered normal for age at that time
7. physical and neurological examination
8. cognitive examination
9. laboratory studies
10. neuroimaging studies.

TALKING WITH THE FAMILY

One aspect of the evaluation that is both critically important and different from most other appointments is the need to speak with a family member or other caregiver. The family or caregiver must be interviewed to obtain an accurate history. Commonly, patients with memory loss truly do not remember the various instances in which they forget things. Or patients may remember at least some of these instances, but are reluctant to share them with the clinician. This reluctance may stem from a variety of issues. Often patients find it frightening to admit—even to themselves—that they have memory problems, because in our society the label of "Alzheimer's disease" has become tantamount to what cancer was 30 years ago: synonymous with a death sentence. Sometimes patients do not want to admit their memory problems to the clinician or their families, for fear that, at best, they will be condescended to and, at worst, they will be sent to a nursing home.

Ideally, family or other caregivers are interviewed separately from the patient. Family members are often reluctant to give a full, accurate, and detailed history to the clinician in the presence of the patient. Sometimes this reluctance is present because the history includes inappropriate sexual behavior, aggression, poor driving, or other sensitive subjects that families prefer to discuss in private. More often the reluctance is present because patients will often deny that they have memory problems for the reasons mentioned above. Some patients may become upset when confronted by what they view as accusations leveled against them by their family. Other patients may become visibly depressed. Even if family members begin to give an accurate history in front of the patient, they usually stop when they see their loved one becoming angry or depressed. In addition, family members quite correctly view it as impolite to discuss the patient in front of him or her as if they were not there. Lastly, talking in private can provide a comfortable atmosphere for the family or caregiver to discuss the patient candidly.

IN THE CLINIC

Setting Up the Appointment

There are many different ways to successfully set up a clinic appointment to evaluate the patient with memory loss. The part of the evaluation that is different from many others is the opportunity to speak with the family, preferably alone (Table 2.1). Because this takes time, the evaluation is often best divided into two or even three visits.

Another reason to divide the evaluation into separate visits is that time is necessary to build up a rapport with patients and families. When patients come to the clinic for an initial visit with laboratory studies and scans already completed and the diagnosis clear, it would seem logical to provide the diagnosis in that visit. However, we would not recommend doing this. It is our experience that many patients and families are

TABLE 2.1 Comparison Between a Typical Medical Evaluation and a Dementia Evaluation	
Medical Evaluation	**Dementia Evaluation**
Self-history important	Self-history can be unreliable
Family observations secondary	Family observations critical
Mental status examination can be deferred	Mental status examination critical
Laboratory studies often critical for diagnosis	Most laboratory studies are exclusionary, not diagnostic
Imaging studies may not be needed	Imaging studies critical

simply not prepared to hear a diagnosis of Alzheimer's or another dementia from a clinician they have just met. Although it will still be emotionally difficult for patients and families, it is better to invite the patient back to the clinic to discuss the diagnosis and treatment plan on another day. In the initial visit, the patients quite correctly perceive that they are seeing "a new doctor." Upon returning to the clinic on a later day, many patients will now feel that they are seeing "one of their doctors."

In our memory clinics we have the opportunity to have the patient perform cognitive testing with a member of the clinic staff, and it is during this time that we typically talk with the family alone. On occasions when the patient would not have testing with a member of the clinic staff, we will often simply ask the patient to sit in the waiting room for a few minutes while we speak with the family. There are, however, many other opportunities to speak with a family member alone. For example, in the busy internal medicine practice of one of our colleagues, when she is worried that a patient of hers is having memory problems, she will talk with the family member for a few minutes in a spare examination room while the patient is changing into a gown. Calling the family member on the phone at a different time is, of course, another option, and a necessary one if the family member did not accompany the patient. If a patient does not have a close family member (or one that they want contacted), talking with a close friend is a good substitute. For those patients who are still working, talking with an employer can sometimes be helpful, particularly if difficulties at work are the main issue. One must be careful, however, to maintain patient confidentiality when talking with any of these individuals, but particularly when talking with friends and employers.

Setting the Agenda

In all cases we believe it is important to begin by describing to the patient and the family what is going to happen in the appointment, and what the follow-up will be. Here is one example of a typical preamble that might be used by a clinician, in this case a neurologist:

Hi, Mr. Jones, I hear there are some concerns about your memory. Let me begin by telling you how I like to do my memory evaluations. I want to start by talking with you, to find out what problems you have

noticed, if any, with your thinking and memory. We will then go over your medical history, medications, family history, and other things like that. I am glad that you brought your family with you—I'm going to ask for their help when we go over your medical history, etc., so that I don't miss anything. We'll then do a physical and neurologic exam: listen to your heart and lungs, tap on your reflexes, that sort of thing. Next, we'll decide what blood work and CT or MRI scans need to be performed. Then you're going to spend some time with my assistant, who will give you some paper and pencil tests of your thinking and memory. While you're doing that, I'll spend a couple of minutes chatting with your family to get their perspective on your thinking and memory difficulties, if that is OK with you. That will be what we'll have time to do today, and then when I see you back in our next appointment we'll go over the results of all these tests, and make a plan of what to do to try to improve your memory. How does all that sound to you?

Here is another example, one that might better fit a busy internist's practice for an existing patient:

Hi, Mr. Jones, your wife is worried that you are having a bit of difficulty with your memory. While it may be part of normal aging, I don't want to miss any treatable diseases. To find out if there is anything going on—besides the fact that you're getting a bit older—I want to start by talking with you, to find out what problems you have noticed, if any, with your thinking and memory. We will then briefly review your medical history, medications, family history, and other things like that. We'll then do a physical exam. Next week I'd like you to come back to the office. At that visit I'll chat privately with your wife for a few minutes, if that is OK with you, to get her perspective on things. We'll also do a few minutes' pencil and paper tests to see how your thinking and memory are doing. Finally, we'll decide what blood work needs to be done, and we may get a CT or MRI scan to take a look at your brain. When I see you back next month we'll go over the results of all these tests, and see what we can do to improve your memory. How does all that sound to you?

AT THE BEDSIDE

Sometimes an evaluation of memory loss takes place in the inpatient setting of a hospital. Some things are much easier to accomplish in the hospital, and others are more difficult. It is usually easier to find time to speak with a family member, and it may also be easier to have laboratory and imaging studies completed in the hospital. It is more difficult, however, to see patients at their cognitive best. Often, the hospital setting alone will make a patient disoriented and confused, even aside from the illness or procedure that they are in the hospital for. Because of this, being in the hospital is a fine place to begin an evaluation of memory loss, but the evaluation must include an outpatient visit so that the clinician has the opportunity to see the patient at their cognitive best. Beware of diagnosing patients with memory loss or dementia having seen them only in the inpatient setting!

HISTORY

Location, Location, Location …

One of the keys to understanding the history of signs and symptoms in a patient with Alzheimer's disease is to understand the relative timing and distribution of Alzheimer's pathology in the brain. Alzheimer's pathology has a predilection for a number of particular regions of the brain (Fig. 2.1). These regions include the hippocampus and amygdala, as well as the parietal, temporal, and frontal lobes. Alzheimer's pathology also affects subcortical nuclei that project to the cortex, such as the basal forebrain cholinergic nuclei (which produce acetylcholine), the locus coeruleus (which produces norepinephrine), the raphe nuclei (which produce serotonin), and certain nuclei of the thalamus. Damage to particular regions leads to particular signs and symptoms (Box 2.1 and Table 2.2).

Memory Loss

The hippocampus and other medial temporal lobe structures are the earliest and most severely affected brain regions in Alzheimer's disease. The hippocampus is the brain structure that is most directly responsible for learning of new personal experiences, such as remembering a short story or what you had for dinner the previous night. This type of memory is usually referred to as *episodic memory* because it is memory for a specific episode of your life (see Appendix C). Thus impairment of episodic memory is usually one of the earliest signs of Alzheimer's disease.

Common symptoms of this memory loss include asking the same questions repeatedly, repeating the same stories, forgetting important appointments, and leaving the stove on. The memory disorder of Alzheimer's disease, like other disorders of episodic memory, follows a particular pattern identified by Ribot in 1881 (Ribot, 1881). Following Ribot's law, the patients show anterograde amnesia or difficulty learning new information. They also show retrograde amnesia or difficulty retrieving previously learned information. However, the patients typically demonstrate preserved memory for remote information. Thus a patient may report, "I've got short-term memory problems—I cannot remember what I did yesterday but I can still remember things from thirty years ago." Not understanding that this pattern is suggestive of the memory impairment common in Alzheimer's disease, family members may report that they feel confident that—whatever the patient's problem is—it "isn't Alzheimer's disease," because the patient can still remember what happened many years ago. The memory deficits experienced by patients with Alzheimer's disease are often referred to as *rapid forgetting* of information they have recently learned.

Memory Distortions

In addition to rapid forgetting, patients with Alzheimer's disease also experience distortions of memory and false memories (Turk et al., 2020). These distortions may include falsely remembering that they have already turned off the stove or taken their medications, leading patients to neglect performing these tasks. More dramatic distortions of memory may occur when patients substitute one person in a memory for another, combine two memories together, or think that an event that happened long ago occurred recently. Sometimes a false memory can be confused with a psychotic delusion or hallucination. For example, a patient may claim to have recently seen and spoken with a long-deceased family member. This patient is much more likely to be suffering from a memory distortion or a false memory than a true hallucination. The same is true for the patient who claims that people are breaking into the house and moving things around. That these symptoms likely represent memory distortions—rather than true hallucinations or delusions—has implications when the time comes for

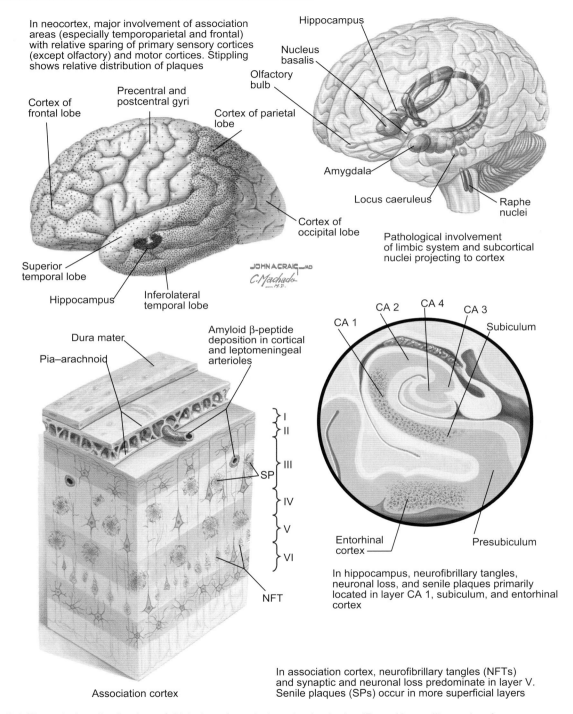

In neocortex, major involvement of association areas (especially temporoparietal and frontal) with relative sparing of primary sensory cortices (except olfactory) and motor cortices. Stippling shows relative distribution of plaques

Cortex of frontal lobe

Precentral and postcentral gyri

Cortex of parietal lobe

Superior temporal lobe

Hippocampus

Inferolateral temporal lobe

Cortex of occipital lobe

JOHN A CRAIG—AD
C. Machado —M.D.

Hippocampus

Nucleus basalis

Olfactory bulb

Amygdala

Locus caeruleus

Raphe nuclei

Pathological involvement of limbic system and subcortical nuclei projecting to cortex

Dura mater

Pia–arachnoid

Amyloid β-peptide deposition in cortical and leptomeningeal arterioles

I
II
III
IV
V
VI

SP

NFT

Association cortex

CA 1   CA 2   CA 4   CA 3

Subiculum

Entorhinal cortex

Presubiculum

In hippocampus, neurofibrillary tangles, neuronal loss, and senile plaques primarily located in layer CA 1, subiculum, and entorhinal cortex

In association cortex, neurofibrillary tangles (NFTs) and synaptic and neuronal loss predominate in layer V. Senile plaques (SPs) occur in more superficial layers

Fig. 2.1 The relative distribution of Alzheimer's pathology in the brain. (From Netter illustration from www.netterimages.com. Copyright Elsevier Inc. All rights reserved.)

BOX 2.1 Common Signs and Symptoms in Alzheimer's Disease

Memory
- Rapid forgetting
- Repeats questions and stories
- Loses items
- Puts items in wrong place
- Memory distortions

Language
- Word-finding difficulties
- Pauses in sentences
- Family members automatically filling in for missing words
- Word substitutions, either wrong word or a simpler word for a more complex one

Visuospatial
- Difficulty learning a new route
- Becomes confused or lost in familiar places

Reasoning and Judgment (Executive Function)
- Makes poor decisions
- Difficulty planning and/or carrying out activities such as a simple repair or preparing a meal

Behavioral and Psychiatric Symptoms
- Apathy
- Depression
- Anxiety
- Irritability
- Delusions such as people are in the house or stealing money

treatment, as memory distortions are best treated with memory-enhancing medications (such as cholinesterase inhibitors) rather than antipsychotic medications. (A true hallucination, on the other hand, may suggest dementia with Lewy bodies rather than Alzheimer's disease; see Chapter 8.)

Word-Finding

After memory loss, difficulty finding words (often referred to as an anomia) is one of the most common symptoms of Alzheimer's disease. There are several areas of the brain that are critical for word-finding, the majority of which are affected by Alzheimer's disease. There is evidence to suggest that the lower, lateral portion of the temporal lobes is involved in the representations of words and their meanings (Damasio et al., 1996; Mesulam et al., 2015). This part of the brain is involved in our general store of conceptual and factual knowledge, such as the color of a lion or the first president of the United States, which is not related to any specific memory (see the section on semantic memory in Appendix C). The frontal lobes, by contrast, are thought to be involved in the selection or choice of the particular word that is searched for (Faulkner & Wilshire, 2020). Both the inferolateral temporal lobes and the frontal lobes are affected by the pathology of Alzheimer's disease (Price & Morris, 1999) (see Fig. 2.1).

Word-finding difficulties manifest in several different ways in patients with Alzheimer's disease. Frequently, patients will substitute a simpler word for a more complex one or they may be unable to complete sentences. Sometimes there will be circumlocutions, in which patients will describe the word because they cannot retrieve it. For example, the patient may say, "He went to the place where they sell the food," referring to the grocery store. Some patients will refer to missing words by using generic terms, such as "Bring me the whatchamacallit" or "use the thing if you're going to do that." Family members become accustomed to filling in missing words. As the disease progresses, word substitutions (often referred to as paraphasic errors) occur. These word substitutions are typically not random, but instead are usually related to the word by meaning (often referred to as semantic paraphasic errors) or sound (often referred to as phonemic paraphasic errors). For example, the patient who meant to say "Are we going in the boat?" may instead say either "Are we going in the car?" or "Are we going in the coat?" Sometimes the speech is fluent, but is relatively uninformative (often called *empty speech*). For example, when asked what he or she did before retiring, the patient may respond, "I worked at my job," rather than mentioning a specific company or occupation. As the disease progresses, speech may remain fluent, but almost devoid of content. For example, a patient attempting to describe what they did yesterday might say, "I went with them to the thing over there."

Getting Lost

The parietal lobe is another region of the brain affected very early by Alzheimer's disease. The parietal lobe is involved in spatial function, and is particularly

TABLE 2.2   Neurocognitive Domains

Cognitive Domain	Examples of Symptoms or Observations	Examples of Assessments
Complex attention (sustained attention, divided attention, selective attention, processing speed)	*Major:* Has increased difficulty in environments with multiple stimuli (TV, radio, conversation); is easily distracted by competing events in the environment. Is unable to attend unless input is restricted and simplified. Has difficulty holding new information in mind, such as recalling phone numbers or addresses just given, or reporting what was just said. Is unable to perform mental calculations. All thinking takes longer than usual, and components to be processed must be simplified to one or a few. *Mild:* Normal tasks take longer than previously. Begins to find errors in routine tasks; finds work needs more double-checking than previously. Thinking is easier when not competing with other things (radio, TV, other conversations, cell phone, driving).	*Sustained attention:* Maintenance of attention over time (e.g., pressing a button every time a tone is heard, and over a period of time). *Selective attention:* Maintenance of attention despite competing stimuli and/or distractors: hearing numbers and letters read and asked to count only letters. *Divided attention:* Attending to two tasks within the same time period: rapidly tapping while learning a story being read. Processing speed can be quantified on any task by timing it (e.g., time to put together a design of blocks; time to match symbols with numbers; speed in responding, such as counting speed or serial 3 speed).
Executive function (planning, decision making, working memory, responding to feedback/error correction, overriding habits/inhibition, mental flexibility)	*Major:* Abandons complex projects. Needs to focus on one task at a time. Needs to rely on others to plan instrumental activities of daily living or make decisions. *Mild:* Increased effort required to complete multistage projects. Has increased difficulty multitasking or difficulty resuming a task interrupted by a visitor or phone call. May complain of increased fatigue from the extra effort required to organize, plan, and make decisions. May report that large social gatherings are more taxing or less enjoyable because of increased effort required to follow shifting conversations.	*Planning:* Ability to find the exit to a maze; interpret a sequential picture or object arrangement. *Decision making:* Performance of tasks that assess process of deciding in the face of competing alternatives (e.g., simulated gambling). *Working memory:* Ability to hold information for a brief period and to manipulate it (e.g., adding up a list of numbers or repeating a series of numbers or words backward). *Feedback/error utilization:* Ability to benefit from feedback to infer the rules for solving a problem. *Overriding habits/inhibition:* Ability to choose a more complex and effortful solution to be correct (e.g., looking away from the direction indicated by an arrow; naming the color of a word's font rather than naming the word). *Mental/cognitive flexibility:* Ability to shift between two concepts, tasks, or response rules (e.g., from number to letter, from verbal to key-press response, from adding numbers to ordering numbers, from ordering objects by size to ordering by color).

(Continued)

TABLE 2.2   Neurocognitive Domains (*Continued*)

Cognitive Domain	Examples of Symptoms or Observations	Examples of Assessments
Learning and memory (immediate memory, recent memory [including free recall, cued recall, and recognition memory], very-long-term memory [semantic; autobiographical], implicit learning)	*Major:* Repeats self in conversation, often within the same conversation. Cannot keep track of short list of items when shopping or of plans for the day. Requires frequent reminders to orient to task at hand. *Mild:* Has difficulty recalling recent events, and relies increasingly on list making or calendar. Needs occasional reminders or re-reading to keep track of characters in a movie or novel. Occasionally may repeat self over a few weeks to the same person. Loses track of whether bills have already been paid. Note: Except in severe forms of major neurocognitive disorder, semantic, autobiographical, and implicit memory are relatively preserved, compared with recent memory.	*Immediate memory span:* Ability to repeat a list of words or digits. Note: Immediate memory is sometimes subsumed under "working memory" (see "Executive Function"). *Recent memory:* Assesses the process of encoding new information (e.g., word lists, a short story, or diagrams). The aspects of recent memory that can be tested include (1) free recall (the person is asked to recall as many words, diagrams, or elements of a story as possible); (2) cued recall (examiner aids recall by providing semantic cues such as "List all the food items on the list" or "Name all of the children from the story"); and (3) recognition memory (examiner asks about specific items—e.g., "Was 'apple' on the list?" or "Did you see this diagram or figure?"). Other aspects of memory that can be assessed include semantic memory (memory for facts), autobiographical memory (memory for personal events or people), and implicit (procedural) learning (unconscious learning of skills).
Language (expressive language [including naming, word-finding, fluency, and grammar and syntax] and receptive language)	*Major:* Has significant difficulties with expressive or receptive language. Often uses general-use phrases such as "that thing" and "you know what I mean," and prefers general pronouns rather than names. With severe impairment, may not even recall names of closer friends and family. Idiosyncratic word usage, grammatical errors, and spontaneity of output and economy of utterances occur. Stereotypy of speech occurs; echolalia and automatic speech typically precede mutism. *Mild:* Has noticeable word-finding difficulty. May substitute general for specific terms. May avoid use of specific names of acquaintances. Grammatical errors involve subtle omission or incorrect use of articles, prepositions, auxiliary verbs, etc.	*Expressive language:* Confrontational naming (identification of objects or pictures); fluency (e.g., name as many items as possible in a semantic [e.g., animals] or phonemic [e.g., words starting with "f"] category in 1 minute). *Grammar and syntax (e.g., omission or incorrect use of articles, prepositions, auxiliary verbs):* Errors observed during naming and fluency tests are compared with norms to assess frequency of errors and compare with normal slips of the tongue. *Receptive language:* Comprehension (word definition and object-pointing tasks involving animate and inanimate stimuli): performance of actions/activities according to verbal command.

(Continued)

TABLE 2.2   Neurocognitive Domains (*Continued*)

Cognitive Domain	Examples of Symptoms or Observations	Examples of Assessments
Perceptual-motor (includes abilities subsumed under the terms *visual perception, visuoconstructional, perceptual-motor, praxis,* and *gnosis*)	*Major:* Has significant difficulties with previously familiar activities (using tools, driving motor vehicle), navigating in familiar environments; is often more confused at dusk, when shadows and lowering levels of light change perceptions. *Mild:* May need to rely more on maps or others for directions. Uses notes and follows others to get to a new place. May find self lost or turned around when not concentrating on task. Is less precise in parking. Needs to expend greater effort for spatial tasks such as carpentry, assembly, sewing, or knitting.	*Visual perception:* Line bisection tasks can be used to detect basic visual defect or attentional neglect. Motor-free perceptual tasks (including facial recognition) require the identification and/or matching of figures best when tasks cannot be verbally mediated (e.g., figures are not objects); some require the decision of whether a figure can be "real" or not based on dimensionality. *Visuoconstructional:* Assembly of items requiring hand-eye coordination, such as drawing, copying, and block assembly. *Perceptual-motor:* Integrating perception with purposeful movement (e.g., inserting blocks into a form board without visual cues; rapidly inserting pegs into a slotted board). *Praxis:* Integrity of learned movements, such as ability to imitate gestures (wave goodbye) or pantomime use of objects to command ("Show me how you would use a hammer") *Gnosis:* Perceptual integrity of awareness and recognition, such as recognition of faces and colors.
Social cognition (recognition of emotions, theory of mind)	*Major:* Behavior clearly out of acceptable social range; shows insensitivity to social standards of modesty in dress or of political, religious, or sexual topics of conversation. Focuses excessively on a topic despite group's disinterest or direct feedback. Behavioral intention without regard to family or friends. Makes decisions without regard to safety (e.g., inappropriate clothing for weather or social setting). Typically, has little insight into these changes. *Mild:* Has subtle changes in behavior or attitude, often described as a change in personality, such as less ability to recognize social cues or read facial expressions, decreased empathy, increased extroversion or introversion, decreased inhibition, or subtle or episodic apathy or restlessness.	*Recognition of emotions:* Identification of emotion in images of faces representing a variety of both positive and negative emotions. *Theory of mind:* Ability to consider another person's mental state (thoughts, desires, intentions) or experience story cards with questions to elicit information about the mental state of the individuals portrayed, such as "Where will the girl look for the lost bag?" or "Why is the boy sad?"

From American Psychiatric Association. (2013). *Diagnostic and statistical manual of mental disorders* (5th ed., pp. 593–595). Washington, DC: APA.

important for real-time spatial navigation, such as when walking or driving (DiSalvio et al., 2020). It is, in part, because of the parietal involvement in Alzheimer's disease that patients with the disorder often make wrong turns and become lost or confused. These difficulties occur even when traveling familiar routes, and patients with Alzheimer's disease have great difficulty planning new routes. Families often report that they suspected something was wrong when the patient became lost in an airport, couldn't find the way to a new place, or had to search the restaurant to find the right table after using the restroom. Later, the patient may become lost when going to a familiar location. For example, a patient we have cared for was trying to go to her doctor's office, a location that she had been to frequently for many years. Although it was only 20 minutes away in a neighboring town, she spent over 7 hours trying to find the office, driving through many towns that were far from the office. She ultimately gave up and went home.

Reasoning and Judgment

Alzheimer's disease affects the frontal lobes, specifically the prefrontal cortex. This part of the frontal lobes is involved in many aspects of brain functioning, including problem solving, abstraction, reasoning, and judgment. These cognitive abilities are sometimes collectively referred to as *executive function*. The frontal lobes are also critical for attention, concentration, and working memory—the ability to temporarily maintain and manipulate information (see Appendix C for details).

Patients with Alzheimer's disease manifest difficulties in these areas in several different ways. Difficulties with complex tasks such as paying bills and balancing a checkbook occur frequently. They may be unable to perform tasks requiring even simple reasoning that would have been easy for them previously. For example, an electrical engineer may be unable to connect a DVD player to a television, and a gourmet cook may be unable to make anything but the simplest meals. They may also have difficulty planning and organizing a task, such as a household repair or Thanksgiving dinner.

Behavior Issues

In addition to reasoning, judgment, and attention, the frontal lobes are involved in the control of behavior, as well as personality and affect. The amygdala, a small brain structure in the anterior medial temporal lobe, is affected by Alzheimer's pathology early in the course of the disease and is involved in regulation of behavior and affect. Over 80% of individuals diagnosed with Alzheimer's disease experience a change in behavior and affect at some point in the disease; these changes often occur early in the disease course and progress with the disease. Although how these changes manifest is somewhat variable; apathy is the most common behavioral change early in the disease, followed by irritability. As the disease progresses, many patients show an exacerbation of their previous personality characteristics. A person who was always competitive may become aggressive, whereas a person who was a wallflower may stop initiating conversation entirely. Sometimes patients exhibit more dramatic changes in personality, as when someone who was previously aggressive becomes passive, or vice versa. In general, however, the personality changes in Alzheimer's disease are relatively mild. Although the patient may be acting in a more aggressive or more passive manner than usual, family members still think of the patient as their "father" or "husband" acting differently, rather than as a completely different person (in contrast to many patients with behavioral variant frontotemporal dementia, see Chapter 10). Often these mild personality changes will not be apparent during the formal office evaluation or even in brief social settings. One good rule of thumb is that the patient with mild Alzheimer's disease can appear normal at a cocktail party for 5 minutes, and can "pull it together" in a doctor's office and behave normally during an evaluation. Because of this fact, it is important to discuss changes in behavior and personality during the interview with a family member or friend.

Several symptoms often result from the combination of frontal lobe dysfunction in conjunction with cognitive loss. Apathy and disinterest are two such symptoms. For example, an avid reader may not be able to remember enough of a book to enjoy it. A builder of model ships may no longer possess the attention, spatial, and problem-solving skills necessary to put together a model consisting of several hundred parts. Suspiciousness and paranoia are two other common symptoms that may result from frontal lobe dysfunction in conjunction with cognitive dysfunction. The usual scenario is that the patient puts their valuables away in a safe place so that they cannot be stolen, forgets where they put them, and then is certain that they have been stolen—only to be found later.

Depression and Anxiety

Depression and anxiety are extremely common in the earliest stages of Alzheimer's disease (Li et al., 2001; Tonga et al., 2020). These symptoms are understandable, because there are few things as depressing and anxiety-provoking as realizing that one has memory loss or worrying that one has Alzheimer's disease. It has long been thought that depression is a common cause of memory problems. Although it is true that individuals with depression will often complain of memory problems, it has been our experience that it is more likely that patients with memory complaints in addition to depression or anxiety will have an underlying primary memory disorder, such as Alzheimer's disease. We discuss the relationship between depression and Alzheimer's disease in Chapter 17.

Insight

An older rule of thumb that some clinicians have used is that if the patient complains of memory problems then he or she does not have a memory disorder; it is the patient who denies memory problems who has Alzheimer's disease or another dementia. This rule of thumb brings up the issue of insight. Commonly, patients in the very early stages of Alzheimer's disease—particularly those with the pre-dementia stage of mild cognitive impairment (MCI) (see Chapters 3 and 4 for details)—show insight into their memory deficits (Hanseeuw et al., 2020). Occasionally, even patients with moderate Alzheimer's disease dementia demonstrate some preserved insight. In our experience younger patients, regardless of their disease stage, are more likely than older patients to demonstrate insight into their difficulties. Presumably this is attributable to younger patients having better preserved frontal lobe function than older patients. Thus many patients in the very earliest stage of Alzheimer's disease are aware of and complain about their memory difficulties.

Function

Understanding the patient's ability to function is critical in any evaluation of memory loss or dementia. Part of the definition of dementia is that the patient has had a noticeable decline from their prior level of functioning. For mildly affected patients, we often ask about their ability to organize and prepare meals (both simple and more involved for holiday gatherings), do volunteer or

---

> ### BOX 2.2   Activities of Daily Living and Instrumental Activities of Daily Living
>
> Knowing if a patient has difficulties with instrumental and/or basic activities of daily living is one way to quickly understand how much function the patient does and does not have. (See the section below in this chapter, *Evaluating Function*, for additional information.)
>
> **Activities of Daily Living**
> - Bathing
> - Dressing and undressing
> - Eating
> - Transferring from bed to chair and back
> - Walking
> - Control of bowel and bladder
> - Using the toilet
>
> **Instrumental Activities of Daily Living**
> - Light housework
> - Preparing meals
> - Taking medications
> - Shopping for groceries and clothes
> - Using the telephone
> - Managing money and paying bills

---

other work, pay bills, balance their checkbook, and go grocery shopping. For the more impaired patients we often ask about being able to take their medications independently, whether there is any wandering from the house, and whether there are any difficulties with bathing, dressing, and toileting. One good method of evaluating patients' level of function is to determine how they are doing in their basic and instrumental activities of daily living (Box 2.2).

REVIEW OF SYSTEMS

As with any disorder, it is important that the clinician conducts a review of systems that includes signs and symptoms of disorders in the differential diagnosis of memory loss. Ask about whether the following have ever occurred:

- A significant brain infection, such as meningitis or encephalitis
- A significant head injury in which the patient lost consciousness
- Repetitive mild head injuries from football, other sports, or other causes

- A stroke or a transient ischemic attack
- A seizure
- Fluctuating levels of alertness or periods of being relatively unresponsive
- Visual hallucinations of people or animals
- A disturbance of gait
- Falls
- A tremor
- Rigidity and other signs of parkinsonism
- A dramatic change in personality such that the patient seems like a different person
- Any major psychiatric problems earlier in life, such as major depression or bipolar disease
- Any weakness or numbness in the face or of an arm or a leg
- Problems with fevers, chills, or night sweats
- Problems with nausea, vomiting, or diarrhea
- Problems with chest pain or shortness of breath
- Any incontinence of bowel or bladder
- Problems going to sleep (insomnia), staying asleep, or early morning awakening; any naps?
- Acting out dreams during sleep or other abnormal movements while sleeping
- Difficulty distinguishing dreams from reality when transitioning to and from sleep.

The significance of these signs and symptoms will be made clearer in Section II: *Differential Diagnosis of Memory Loss and Dementia.*

MEDICAL HISTORY

In addition to obtaining a general medical history, it is worthwhile asking specifically about disorders that can predispose an individual to memory loss. These include the following, which are mainly related to cerebrovascular disease (note that disorders covered in the review of systems have not been repeated):

- hypertension
- hypercholesterolemia
- coronary artery disease
- atrial fibrillation and other cardiac arrhythmias
- obstructive sleep apnea.

ALLERGIES TO MEDICATIONS

When eliciting a history of allergies, it is worthwhile to be attuned to two particular kinds of reactions to medications.

First, are there medications that caused significant confusion or agitation when administered? Susceptibility to confusion from medications may be present before the clinical onset of Alzheimer's disease or other dementia. Such medications may include narcotics, such as Percocet or Darvocet, benzodiazepines, such as diazepam and lorazepam, antihistamines, such as Benadryl and Tylenol PM, and anticholinergic medications, such as scopolamine and meclizine.

Second, are there reactions to medications used to treat Alzheimer's disease? If so, are these true allergic reactions to the medications, common side effects, or rare and unusual problems? If side effects to potential treatment medication are present (such as nausea to a cholinesterase inhibitor), these should be carefully noted. Discussions regarding how to best deal with side effects to treatment medications are discussed in Section III: *Treatment of Memory Loss, Alzheimer's Disease, and Dementia.*

SOCIAL HISTORY

Several elements of the social history are important when diagnosing memory loss.

Habits

Cigarette smoking, whether past or present, is of course a risk factor for cerebrovascular disease. Current smoking also poses a significant risk of fires, as the patient with memory loss may forget and leave their lit cigarette or cigar in a place where it may start a fire.

Alcohol use is important to ascertain for two reasons. First, when alcohol use is severe, it can cause memory loss from Wernicke–Korsakoff syndrome (see Chapter 17), and even more mild chronic alcohol use can cause frontal/executive dysfunction. Second, many patients with mild memory loss experience an exacerbation of their memory difficulties while drinking, and remember very little during the time that the alcohol is in their system. Some patients may become outright confused with as little as two glasses of wine. Patients may also not remember how many drinks they have had, and end up drinking too much. Lastly, patients with Alzheimer's disease may also be self-medicating for anxiety and/or depression.

Use or abuse of prescription medications and other drugs should also be elicited. Benzodiazepines and narcotics are all too commonly abused, and can present as an apparent dementia, particularly when fluctuations in mood, behavior, and cognition are present.

Education and Occupation

When making a diagnosis of memory loss, other cognitive impairment, or dementia—particularly when symptoms are very mild—it is critical to take into account the patient's education and previous occupation. We expect, of course, that a college professor with a PhD would score better on most standard cognitive tests than an individual with a high school education. Taking education and occupation into account is particularly important when interpreting standard cognitive tests. For example, scoring 28 out of 30 on the Mini-Mental State Examination (MMSE) (Folstein et al., 1975) or 27 out of 30 on the MoCA (the Montreal Cognitive Assessment; www.mocatest.org) may be normal for the 65-year-old factory worker with a high school education, but would be very concerning for a retired physician of the same age with 20 years of education.

Does the patient have any longstanding prior problems with attention, memory, or other cognitive function? Do they have dyslexia, another learning disability, or attention-deficit hyperactivity disorder? Has she always had a poor memory for names? Did he always become lost when trying to find a new place? Understanding the patient's baseline memory and other cognitive abilities can help you interpret the current symptoms and the results of the cognitive tests appropriately.

Social Supports

Patients with memory loss need the support of others. Support can be present in many forms, including emotional, financial, and assistance with daily function at many levels. Knowing what supports the patient has will help to guide treatment options, such as whether prescribed medications can be complicated or need to be simple, and whether options such as day programs, moving in with a family member, or moving to an assisted living facility are available.

FAMILY HISTORY

Studies have shown that having a first-, second-, or third-degree relative with Alzheimer's disease all increase the risk of developing the disorder (Cannon-Albright et al., 2019). Thus a family history of Alzheimer's disease can be a clue in a patient who presents with memory loss.

Additionally, the family history may point to a disorder other than Alzheimer's disease, such as vascular disease, Parkinson's disease, or frontotemporal dementia.

We have found that it is best to not only ask for a history of Alzheimer's disease, but also to ask whether there is a history of memory loss, senility, or dementia late in life. Most of the time the correct diagnoses of these family members is Alzheimer's disease based upon what can be inferred from the history. Even a putative diagnosis of vascular or multi-infarct dementia or "hardening of the arteries" in the era before the advent of computed tomography (CT) and magnetic resonance imaging (MRI) was often Alzheimer's disease in reality. Similarly, the history of a parent or grandparent with a late-onset psychosis is much more likely to be a dementia (most commonly due to Alzheimer's disease, frontotemporal dementia, or dementia with Lewy bodies) than a true primary psychotic disorder presenting for the first time in old age.

PHYSICAL EXAMINATION

General Physical Examination

In evaluating memory loss, it is important to perform a thorough general physical examination. Many medical problems can contribute to memory difficulties, including congestive heart failure, pneumonia, and the like. Listening at the neck is useful because a carotid bruit, if found, may suggest cerebrovascular disease. (See Box 2.3).

Neurological Examination

There are three main types of abnormalities to look for on the neurological examination: signs of focal brain lesions, signs neurodegenerative disorders, and frontal release signs. Although an anatomical brain lesion should be detectable on an imaging study, it is still worthwhile to look for signs of brain pathology, such as focal weakness, brisk or asymmetric reflexes, and Babinski's sign. These focal signs may indicate a stroke, tumor, multiple sclerosis lesion, or other pathology. See Videos 2.1 and 2.2 for examples of selected elements of the neurological exam.

More important is to look for signs suggestive of neurodegenerative diseases, because these will not typically show up on imaging or laboratory studies. For example, Parkinson's disease may present with a tremor, rigidity

---

BOX 2.3 Relevant Elements of the Neurological Examination

Focal Signs Suggesting Possible Cerebrovascular Disease or Other Cause of Brain Injury
- Neck auscultation (? carotid bruit)
- Focal weakness
- Asymmetric reflexes
- Extensor plantar (Babinski's sign)
- Focal sensory loss
- Visual field deficits
- Incoordination

Signs of Possible Extrapyramidal Disease
- Tremor
- Rigidity
- Gait disorder

Signs of Possible Dementia
- Snout
- Grasp
- Palmomental reflex
- Apraxia (see Chapter 13)

Unusual Signs
- Alien limb (see Chapter 13)
- Eye movement abnormalities (see Chapter 12)

---

of the limbs, shuffling gait, a tendency to fall backwards, or all of these signs. Progressive supranuclear palsy (see Chapter 12) often presents with frequent falls, rigidity of the neck and spine, swallowing difficulty, and impaired voluntary gaze (i.e., difficulty moving the eyes to command, particularly up and down; see Video 2.3).

In our experience, so-called "frontal release signs" are often more sensitive to the overall degree of bilateral brain pathology, and are not specific for frontal lobe dysfunction. These signs are discussed more below.

Tremor

The most common etiology of tremor is "essential" tremor, a hereditary tremor, about 6 to 8 Hz, unrelated to other conditions (think of Katharine Hepburn in her later years). Another common cause is an enhanced physiological tremor. Everyone has a small amplitude, fast, physiological tremor, about 8 to 9 Hz, that can be noticeable when one is nervous or carrying something heavy. Physiological tremor can also be enhanced by medications, such as stimulants. A parkinsonian tremor is slow,

about 4 to 6 Hz, often present at rest (though can be with action), and is typically described as a "pill-rolling" tremor in the hands. Some patients have what is often described as a coarse tremor of the hands but is actually a combination of asterixis and myoclonus, common in corticobasal degeneration (see Chapter 13). See Videos 2.4 and 2.5 for examples of some of these different tremors.

Rigidity

There are two main types of rigidity: one that primarily affects the limbs (appendicular rigidity) and one that primarily affects the neck and trunk (axial rigidity). Appendicular rigidity can often be brought out by using enhancement/distraction techniques such as drawing a circle in the air with the opposite hand. Parkinsonian rigidity is often described as "cogwheeling" when tremor is present and "lead pipe" when it is not. Axial rigidity is commonly tested by gently flexing the patient's neck.

Gait

Gait disorders are very common in the elderly, often multifactorial, and sometimes inscrutable. Relevant for memory disorders are parkinsonian and frontal gait disorders. A parkinsonian gait consists of slow, shuffling steps, which increase in speed after initiation. There is a tendency to retropulse and fall backwards. A frontal gait is sometimes described as a magnetic gait or (in French) a *marche à petits pas*, the walk of little steps. In a frontal gait disorder, the feet look like they are stuck to the floor, which is usually caused by bilateral frontal lobe subcortical white matter pathology. The etiology of this bilateral frontal subcortical white matter pathology may, in turn, be attributed to small vessel ischemic vascular disease (as in a vascular dementia), normal pressure hydrocephalus, multiple sclerosis, traumatic brain injury, or other etiology.

Frontal Release Signs

Frontal release signs are so named because of the theory that these are reflexes present in infants that are inhibited once frontal lobes become myelinated; when the frontal lobes degenerate these infantile reflexes then become "released." In our experience these signs are more likely to be present with significant bilateral brain dysfunction, not necessarily confined to the frontal lobes. Frontal release signs are of little clinical importance in isolation, but can be helpful, supportive evidence of a dementia when a patient presents with memory loss. Three of the more reliable frontal release signs are the snout, grasp, and palmomental reflexes (see Video 2.6).

Snout. The snout is commonly elicited by very gently tapping the broad aspect of the reflex hammer against the lips. It is a good idea to warn the patient that you are going to tap gently on their lips, and to make sure that the mouth is closed. If the lips protrude outward when they are tapped, this is an abnormal response (see Video 2.6). The snout is thought to be related to the rooting response observed in infants. Sometimes the lips and mouth open as the hammer approaches; this may indicate a visual suck response—another frontal release sign that is typically present in the more advanced dementia.

Grasp. A grasp response may be elicited in several different ways. One is to have the patient put their hands in a prone, palm down, relaxed position, and then to use your fingertips to stroke gently upwards as you move from palm to fingertips. The abnormal response is for the patient to close down and grasp your fingers (see Video 2.6). Sometimes the normal patient may not be clear what you are doing or what you want them to do and may grab your hand as well. For this reason, if the patient grasps your hands, repeat the action while instructing the patient not to hold your hand. If the grasp reflex is strongly present, it will be apparent even when you tell the patient not to hold your hand, and also with different types of contact across the palm. The grasp is thought to be related to the reflex that is common in infants when they tightly hold your finger in their hand.

Palmomental reflex. When the palmomental reflex is present, the mentalis muscle of the chin below the lower lip contracts when the palm is stroked (see Video 2.7). The stroke in the palm may be performed by gently flicking the thumbnail from lower ulnar surface of the palm, up and across the palm to the base of the index finger. You must be watching the mentalis muscle as you do this, as it occurs quickly, if present. The reflex often rapidly habituates, so that it may only be present the first time it is performed in a several minute interval. There is one palmomental reflex on each side (left and right).

COGNITIVE TESTS AND QUESTIONNAIRES

Although the interview with the patient and informant(s) provides a wealth of information and may be sufficient to make a preliminary diagnosis, supplementing the history with the results of cognitive tests and questionnaires is crucial. Our general approach is to both conduct an interview and perform cognitive tests. Cognitive tests can be performed by the clinician or an assistant in the office; it may also be part of a formal neuropsychological evaluation by a neuropsychologist.

Cognitive instruments can be used for a variety of purposes. First, they may be used to screen for subtle cognitive dysfunction. For example, some primary care practices are now using cognitive tests and questionnaires to screen for mild memory loss that could be attributed to Alzheimer's disease. A second purpose is to determine the degree of cognitive impairment. For example, we might use a test to classify an Alzheimer's disease dementia patient as mild, moderate, or severe. A third purpose of cognitive testing is to help with diagnosis, because certain test result patterns are suggestive of different causes of dementing illness (Alzheimer's disease versus vascular dementia, for example). In general, using cognitive tests for differential diagnosis will not be carried out in primary care practices, but rather in the context of referral to specialists including behavioral neurologists, geriatric psychiatrists and neuropsychiatrists, and neuropsychologists. Lastly, cognitive tests can be used to follow a patient's degree of impairment over time.

There are numerous brief measures of cognition that can be helpful to the clinician. Several of these are discussed briefly below; see Appendix B for more detail. The MMSE (Folstein et al., 1975) is often used for initial screening for cognitive dysfunction and is also for staging patients (mild, moderate, or severe dementia) based upon the score. The Blessed Information, Memory, Concentration (BIMC) test (Blessed, Tomlinson, & Roth, 1968) is an older test that is still used for screening in day-to-day practice. Both of these instruments briefly and quickly evaluate cognitive domains that can be affected by dementia including orientation, memory, attention, and concentration. A newer overall mental status test, the MoCA (www.mocatest.org), has become the new standard. Rather than advocating for a particular test, we believe it is most important that clinicians become comfortable with a test that is helpful for differentiating normal versus impaired cognition in their patient population. See Appendix A for details on the use and administration of these and other cognitive tests.

Mental Status Screening Tests
The Mini-Mental State Examination

The MMSE is one of the most widely used tests in clinical medicine for assessing a patient's overall cognitive function (Folstein et al., 1975). A revised version is now available, published by Psychological Assessment Resources, Inc. (Lutz, Florida); more information about it is available online at www.minimental.com.

The MMSE evaluates orientation to time and place, recent memory, attention/concentration, praxis, and language. It is scored on a 30-point scale, with 30 as a perfect score. A rule of thumb is that patients with Alzheimer's disease who are untreated decline at a rate of about 2 or 3 points each year.

The advantages of the MMSE include that it is well known, easy to administer in about 5 to 10 minutes, samples a number of cognitive functions, and has test–retest and inter-rater reliability. A limitation is that only three words are to be remembered on the recall test, making the MMSE insensitive for patients with mild but clinically relevant memory problems. Another limitation is that the interval between registration and recall is not standard; instead, it is dependent upon the time it takes for the patient to perform the attention and calculation section. Thus patients who take a long time to complete the attention and calculation section will end up with a more difficult memory test than those who complete the attention and calculation section more quickly. Lastly, the MMSE is not sensitive in detecting frontal/executive dysfunction.

Numerous studies have evaluated the MMSE in the last 40 years. When using the MMSE as a screening instrument for cognitive dysfunction, we favor flexible cut-offs with the understanding that a result below this number does not definitively indicate dementia or other cognitive impairment, but suggests that a more thorough evaluation is warranted. Scores that warrant concern are those below 29 for adults younger than 50 years old, below 28 for those aged 50 to 79 years, and below 26 for those aged 80 to 89 years (Bleecker et al., 1988). In addition to age, lower levels of education are also associated with lower scores in the absence of cognitive impairment (Crum et al., 1993).

When reporting the results of the MMSE, we encourage clinicians to report which items were missed in addition to the total score. The implications of scoring 26 out of 30 may be very different depending upon which items are missed. For example, a patient who misses all three of the recall items and the date shows evidence of episodic memory dysfunction, whereas the patient who misses only four points on the attention and calculation section does not.

The Blessed Dementia Scale

The BIMC test is similar to the MMSE in that it measures orientation for time and place, recent memory, and attention and concentration. It also measures orientation for person, as well as personal information (autobiographical memory). It is often paired with the Blessed Dementia Scale, a brief caregiver questionnaire.

Note that the number of impaired responses (or errors) is commonly reported for the Blessed, rather than the number of correct responses. Thus the most severely demented patient would score 28 on the caregiver scale and 37 on the Blessed test. For the caregiver scale, scoring less than 4 suggests that the patient is unimpaired; a score from 4 to 9 suggests mild impairment; scores higher that 10 suggest moderate to severe impairment (Eastwood et al., 1983). For the BIMC test, fewer than 4 errors suggests no impairment, 4 to 10 errors suggests mild impairment, 11 to 16 errors suggests moderate impairment, and more than 16 errors suggests severe impairment (Locascio, Growdon, & Corkin, 1995). Untreated patients decline approximately 3 or 4 points per year.

The Montreal Cognitive Assessment

The MoCA evaluates orientation, memory, attention, language (naming), executive function, and visuospatial function. In head-to-head studies with the MMSE the MoCA appears more sensitive in detecting patients with mild cognitive impairment (MCI) (18% for the MMSE vs. 90% for the MoCA) and mild Alzheimer's disease dementia (78% for the MMSE vs. 100% for the MoCA). Specificity was 100% for the MMSE and 87% for the MoCA (Nasreddine et al., 2005). See Videos 2.8–2.13 for examples of two patients performing different sections of the MoCA.

The MoCA has a number of advantages as a screening test for memory loss and dementia. First, the test and instructions are available on a website, www.mocatest.org. Second, it has clear instructions and scoring. Third, it has been translated into more than 60 languages, many with alternate versions and versions specifically for blind patients. Fourth, it covers a variety of cognitive domains. Its main limitation is that it requires online training, which costs a fee. Nonetheless, it is rapidly becoming the standard mental status screening test of many clinics.

Single Neuropsychological Tests
Clock Drawing Test

There are multiple versions of the clock drawing test, which all ask the patient to draw the face of a clock and then to draw the hands to indicate a particular time. This single test may be sensitive to dementia because it involves many cognitive areas that can be affected by dementia, including executive function, visuospatial abilities, motor programming, and attention and concentration. Many of our patients have difficulty with analogue watches in the early stages of a dementing illness (we often address this problem by suggesting they wear a digital watch).

There are many versions of the clock drawing test, in terms of both administration procedures and scoring. We have used and validated a relatively straightforward system that is easy to administer and accurate as part of a larger cognitive battery. (See Appendix A for details.)

The main downside of the clock drawing test is that it is insensitive to mild cognitive impairment. For this reason, we do not recommend its routine use in isolation as a screening test. Note that the MoCA includes the clock drawing test.

Category Fluency

The category fluency test requires that the subject names as many members of a semantic category as possible in a fixed period of time—typically 1 minute. This type of test has been shown to be sensitive to Alzheimer's disease. One easily and quickly administered version of the category fluency test is animal naming (see Video 2.14). Patients are simply asked to name all the animals they can in 60 seconds. The total number of animals they name produces the score. A quick rule of thumb for determining performance on the category fluency test is that the individual should name approximately the number of animals that equals their number of years of education (e.g., a high school graduate has 12 years) plus 4. (See Appendix A for details.)

Delayed Word Recall

This test was initially described by Knopman and Ryberg (1989) and takes advantage of the finding that healthy elderly individuals benefit from mnemonic strategies that facilitate the storage and retrieval of information, whereas patients with dementia show substantially less benefit from some strategies. Knopman and colleagues showed a list of 10 words to patients with Alzheimer's disease (and healthy elderly controls) and asked that they make up a sentence using each word. The rationale was that, by asking the subjects to make up a sentence, they were assuring that each individual was paying attention to the word and relating it to other words and concepts with which they were familiar. After a 5-minute delay, they asked the participants to recall as many of the 10 words as possible in any order. Patients with Alzheimer's disease typically recalled four or fewer words, while healthy elderly subjects typically recalled five or more.

Trailmaking A and B

These are two parts of a well-established neuropsychological test that was developed during World War II. "Trails" is generally sensitive to brain damage and is particularly sensitive to executive dysfunction. It consists of two parts (trails A and B) and takes five minutes to administer. In trails A, the patient is given a single sheet of paper that contains 25 small circles consecutively numbered from 1 to 25. The circles are placed in a seemingly random distribution on the page. The patient is asked to draw lines to join the consecutively numbered circles. In trails B, half the circles contain numbers and half letters, and the patient's job is to connect alternating consecutive numbers and letters (e.g., 1, A, 2, B, 3, etc.). Scoring is simply the time it takes to complete the task. If a subject makes a mistake, the administrator points out the mistake and asks the subject to correct it before proceeding (imposing a time penalty).

Trails A requires attention, visual search, and psychomotor speed, and trails B adds sequencing, working memory, response inhibition, and set shifting, which are all sensitive to executive/frontal lobe functioning. We have found this test particularly useful when we suspect frontal lobe dementias, and patients with Alzheimer's disease often show impairment as well.

Screening Instruments That Combine Single Tests
The Mini-Cog

Developed in 2000, the Mini-Cog consists simply of three words that must be memorized and then recalled after the drawing of a clock with the hands at 10 minutes after 11 o'clock; the circle is provided (Borson et al., 2005). As a screening tool for dementia, the test is considered negative (i.e., no dementia) if either all three words are recalled or at least one word is recalled with a normal clock; the test is considered positive (i.e., suggestive of dementia) if no words are recalled or if fewer than three words are recalled with an abnormal clock. The Mini-Cog is relatively insensitive to level of education and it has been shown to be accurate in multicultural settings, primarily because it relies minimally on language abilities. We agree that, when the Mini-Cog is positive (suggesting dementia), the patient likely has cognitive impairment. However, the criteria for a negative test are too insensitive to make the Mini-Cog a good instrument for screening. We would therefore be cautious in using the Mini-Cog.

The 7 Minute Screen

The 7 Minute Screen was specifically developed for use as a screening assessment for dementia. It consists of four subtests: orientation (month, date, year, day, time), memory (16 items, four at a time, cued and uncued), clock drawing, and verbal fluency (naming animals in 1 minute) (Solomon et al., 1998). Unlike most tests, however, the interpretation is performed automatically by entering the results of the four subtests into a special calculator or website (http://memorydoc.org/7minute-screen), leading to a high or low probability that the patient has Alzheimer's disease dementia. (The calculated formula is based upon the results of a logistic regression comparing 60 patients with Alzheimer's disease dementia and 60 healthy control subjects.) The 7 Minute Screen demonstrates sensitivity, specificity, test–retest reliability, and inter-rater reliability all greater than 90%. The test has been validated in the primary care setting as a screening tool for patients over the age of 60 (Solomon et al., 2000), and it has also been validated in other languages (Meulen et al., 2004; Tsolaki et al., 2002).

Advantages of this test include that it is sensitive, reliable, easy to administer, takes little time, and the interpretation is performed automatically. The main limitation is that an online calculator is needed for interpretation. If the result from the calculator reads "HI," the patient has a high probability of dementia characteristic of Alzheimer's disease, and it is suggested that the patient undergoes a full diagnostic evaluation. The test instructions caution (and we agree) that it is inappropriate to

diagnose Alzheimer's disease dementia based only on the results of the 7 Minute Screen. If the calculator reads "LO," the patient has a low probability of dementia characteristic of Alzheimer's disease; in this circumstance, the patient may or may not need further evaluation depending upon the history and clinical setting. In less than 5% of cases the calculator may also indicate that the data are insufficient to make a judgment; in this situation, either using other evaluation measures or rescreening the patient in 6 to 9 months would be appropriate.

Caregiver-Completed Questionnaires

Informant-based questionnaires may be preferable to other screening methods because: (1) they require no time from medical professionals; (2) they do not require the cooperation of the patient; (3) they can potentially be completed via telephone, mail, or Internet; and (4) they can be completed by the informant confidentially. It is for these reasons that the most recent trend in screening for cognitive dysfunction is a questionnaire completed by the caregiver. In general, these questionnaires ask someone who knows the patient well to answer a series of questions about the patient's memory and other cognitive functions. Because they are typically completed in the waiting room, the results can be made available to clinicians before they see the patient.

IQCODE

The IQCODE (the Informant Questionnaire on Cognitive Decline in the Elderly) is a 26-item questionnaire in which informants are asked to rate the degree of change in the patient's memory and intelligence over a 10-year period (Jorm & Jacomb, 1989). This rating is done on a five-point scale: much improved, a bit improved, not much change, a bit worse, much worse. Subsequent research has shown that a shortened 16-item version is just as accurate as the 26-item questionnaire (Jorm, 1994). Research has shown the IQCODE to be as sensitive as the MMSE in detecting patients with dementia (Jorm, 2004). The overall accuracy of the IQCODE ranged from 80% to 85% in detecting patients with dementia.

Alzheimer's Disease Caregiver Questionnaire

The Alzheimer's Disease Caregiver Questionnaire (ADCQ) is an 18-item yes/no questionnaire that can be completed by a caregiver in 5 to 10 minutes. It asks questions regarding multiple aspects of cognition, including memory, language, executive function, visuo-spatial abilities, and praxis. It also asks questions regarding functional abilities, mood, and behavior, as well as progression of symptoms. Validation studies have indicated that the instrument approaches 90% accuracy in determining which patients have symptoms of dementia suggestive of Alzheimer's disease (Solomon & Murphy, 2008; Solomon et al., 2003). (See Appendix A for additional information.)

AD8 Dementia Screening Interview

The AD8 Dementia Screening Interview (AD8) is an eight-item questionnaire that can be completed by the caregiver. For each question, the caregiver indicates "Yes" there has been a change in the patient's ability, "No" there has not been a change in the patient's ability, or "N/A, don't know" if they are unable to rate the item (Galvin et al., 2005, 2007). The score is simply the number of endorsed "Yes" items. The authors state that it is preferable for the questionnaire to be answered by the informant, but suggest that the patient can also complete it. A score of 0 or 1 suggests normal cognition and a score of 2 or greater suggests that cognitive impairment is likely to be present. When administered to either the informant or the patient, the sensitivity is greater than 84% and the specificity greater than 80% (see Appendix A for additional information).

SCREENING IN THE CLINIC

When and Who to Screen

As with any other disease, there is debate about who to screen and how often to screen. The U.S. Preventive Services Task Force and the American Academy of Family Physicians concluded that there is insufficient evidence to recommend cognitive screening (Falk, Cole, & Meredith, 2018), whereas the Canadian Task Force on Preventive Health Care recommended against screening in asymptomatic individuals for fear of false positives (Canadian Task Force on Preventive Health Care et al., 2016). Nonetheless a set of guidelines has previously been suggested (Solomon & Murphy, 2005) and these have been adopted by several groups. These guidelines suggest that screening should be routine for people over 65 or those who have memory complaints, raised by either the patient or family, and that the frequency of screening be increased as individuals age and the

TABLE 2.3 Recommendations for Screening for Alzheimer's Disease in Primary Care Practice		
Age Range	Prevalence of Dementia	Recommendation
65–74	3%	Discretionary, based on risk factors including family history and cognitive complaints from either patients or family
75–84	19%	Every two years or sooner if there are cognitive complaints from either patients or family
>85	47%	Annually

From Solomon, P. R., Murphy, C. A. (2005). Should we screen for Alzheimer's disease? A review of the evidence for and against screening Alzheimer's disease in primary care practice. *Geriatrics, 60,* 26–31.

probability of a dementing illness increases. Table 2.3 summarizes these guidelines.

Recommendations for In-Office Screening

As we have discussed, there are many potentially useful screening instruments. We recommend that you routinely use one or two so that you gain comfort and familiarity with administering and interpreting those instruments. In terms of specific suggestions, we generally try to use both a clinician-administered instrument and a caregiver-completed instrument. Below are two recommended combinations that you may find helpful.

The 7 Minute Screen and the Alzheimer's Disease Caregiver Questionnaire

We routinely use these two instruments that were developed in our centers. We find that input from both the patient and caregiver is useful. In some instances, the patient comes alone and, of course, in these cases we use the 7 Minute Screen in the office and have a member of the clinic staff administer the ADCQ to a family member over the phone.

The Montreal Cognitive Assessment and the AD8 Dementia Screening Interview

A second combination of instruments that are being widely used are the MoCA, a clinician-administered instrument, and the AD8, a caregiver questionnaire.

Both are easily administered and accurate. The published data from each and our experience to date indicate that they may be appropriate for in-office screening.

How to Interpret a Screen (Table 2.4)
Positive Screens

As is the case for screening instruments for all diseases, a positive memory screen should not be used to make a diagnosis of Alzheimer's disease or other dementia. Instead, a positive screen provides the opportunity to discuss the results with the patient and family and encourages patients to undergo a full diagnostic evaluation. We always emphasize that this measure is only a screen and does not mean that the person has Alzheimer's disease or another dementia. Rather it just means that we should carry out a more complete evaluation. We find that using the analogy of false positives for mammography for breast cancer often helps the patient and family understand the process. In our experience, most patients and caregivers readily agree to an evaluation.

Negative Screens

A negative screen provides the opportunity to reassure the patient and family that, although there are changes in memory that occur as people age, they are most likely a normal part of the aging process. Again, in most cases, the patients are accepting of this and indeed often relieved. Occasionally, a caregiver will tell us that, despite what the screen indicates, this is not the same person they knew a year ago and would like a more comprehensive evaluation. In these cases we proceed with a full diagnostic evaluation.

Neuropsychological Evaluation

In most cases, comprehensive neuropsychological evaluation is not necessary to make a diagnosis of Alzheimer's disease dementia. A careful taking of history combined with office-based cognitive screening will usually provide the necessary information for making a diagnosis. In some cases, however, formal neuropsychological testing may be helpful. A neuropsychological evaluation consists of standardized tests that evaluate multiple cognitive areas, including: memory; executive function including reasoning, judgment, and problem-solving;

TABLE 2.4	Summary of Characteristics of Various Screening Instruments			
Instrument	Administration Time	Level of Clinical Judgment/Training to Administer/Score	Sensitivity	Specificity
Clinician-Administered Instruments				
Mini-Mental State Examination	5–10 min	Moderate	MCI 18% Mild AD 78%	Up to 100%
Montreal Cognitive Assessment	5–10 min	Moderate	MCI 90% Mild AD 100%	87%
7 Minute Screen	5–10 min	Moderate	>90%	>90%
Clock drawing	Not reported	Moderate	80%–90%	80%–90%
Mini-Cog	<5 min	Moderate	>90%	>90%
Informant-Completed Instruments				
Informant Questionnaire on Cognitive Decline in the Elderly	Not reported	Minimal	80%–90%	80%–90%
Alzheimer's Disease Caregiver Questionnaire	Not reported	Minimal	80%–90%	80%–90%
AD8	<5 min	Minimal	>84%	>80%

AD, Alzheimer's disease; *MCI*, mild cognitive impairment.

language; visuospatial functioning; praxis; and attention. Additionally, the neuropsychologist will screen for mood (e.g., anxiety and depression) and functional deficits (e.g., activities of daily living). They will also obtain a complete history of cognitive complaints. A typical neuropsychological evaluation takes 2 to 6 hours and is generally conducted in a single day.

In our experience, neuropsychological evaluation can be beneficial:

- when family members continue to be concerned, even in the presence of normal office-based cognitive screening
- when the patient has high premorbid intellectual functioning resulting in performing in the "normal" range on office-based screening instruments at the same time the family is reporting cognitive decline
- when a preexisting cognitive problem is present such as traumatic brain injury or mental retardation attributed to, for example, Down's syndrome
- when a coexisting major psychiatric condition is present
- to help with differential diagnosis, for example, Lewy body dementia versus Alzheimer's disease or frontal lobe dementia versus Alzheimer's disease.

Screening for Depression

Depression is common in the elderly and even more common in patients with mild cognitive impairment and Alzheimer's disease. Major depressive disorder occurs in between 4% and 9% of community-dwelling elderly (Sjöberg et al., 2017) and almost 40% of cognitively intact elderly patients in nursing home settings (Hu et al., 2018). In Alzheimer's disease patients, the prevalence of depression is nearly 50% at some point in the disease (Novais & Starkstein, 2015).

Because the symptoms of depression can overlap with the symptoms of dementia, the two diseases can be confused. Further complicating the picture is recent evidence suggesting that the late-life onset of depression signals the presence of Alzheimer's disease. As such, clinicians should be suspicious of an emerging dementia in elderly patients who exhibit new-onset depression.

In Chapter 17 we will discuss some strategies for discriminating between cognitive deficits caused by depression alone and those caused by Alzheimer's disease, with or without comorbid depression. For now, we would just note that any evaluation for memory loss, Alzheimer's disease, or dementia should include a screen for depression. There are several instruments that may be helpful. We have found the Geriatric Depression Scale (GDS; either the 5-, 10-, 15-, or 30-item version) and the somewhat longer Neuropsychiatric Inventory (NPI) to be useful in detecting depression and other psychiatric symptoms in the elderly.

The Geriatric Depression Scale

The GDS was designed specifically to screen for depression in geriatric populations. Therefore it taps the affective and behavioral symptoms of depression and excludes most symptoms that may be confused with somatic disease (e.g., slowness, insomnia, hyposexuality) or dementia.

The original GDS is a 30-item yes/no self-report questionnaire completed by the patient that is widely used to screen for depression in the elderly. The instrument is commonly used in primary care settings, geriatric clinics, and hospitals. The purpose of the scale is somewhat disguised to the patient by the title "Mood Assessment Scale." Shorter forms of the GDS have been developed and the 15-item and 10-item versions are the most commonly used. The 15-item version takes about 5 to 7 minutes to complete. Less is known about the 5-item version (Table 2.5) but data suggest that accuracy can approach that of the 15-item version (Rinaldi et al., 2003).

Neuropsychiatric Inventory

The Neuropsychiatric Inventory is a relatively brief interview with a family member or friend who knows the patient well and can evaluate 12 behavioral areas commonly affected in patients with dementia, including depression (Box 2.4). It is also routinely used to evaluate the effects of treatment on these symptoms. Evaluation in each of the 12 areas begins with a yes/no screening question. If the screening question is answered "Yes," the interviewer follows with additional questions.

A clinician generally administers the instrument in about 10 minutes. The scoring reflects not only the effect on the patient, but also the extent to which the symptom causes distress in the caregiver. There is also a brief version, the Neuropsychiatric Inventory Questionnaire (NPI-Q), that takes only five minutes to administer and may be more appropriate for primary care settings. See

TABLE 2.5   The 5-Item Geriatric Depression Scale

Question: Over the Past Week…	Positive Answer for Depression Screening
Are you basically satisfied with your life?	No
Do you often get bored?	Yes
Do you often feel helpless?	Yes
Do you prefer to stay home rather than going out and doing new things?	Yes
Do you feel pretty worthless the way you are now?	Yes

Depressed patients are likely to have >2 positive answers.

BOX 2.4   Neuropsychiatric Inventory

Description of the Neuropsychiatric Inventory (NPI)

The NPI consists of 12 behavioral areas or domains:
1. Delusions
2. Hallucinations
3. Agitation
4. Depression
5. Anxiety
6. Euphoria
7. Apathy
8. Disinhibition
9. Irritability
10. Aberrant motor behavior
11. Night-time behaviors
12. Appetite and eating disorders

Frequency is rated as:
1. Occasionally—less than once a week
2. Often—about once per week
3. Frequently—several times a week but less than every day
4. Very frequently—daily or essentially continuously present

Severity is rated as:
1. Mild—produces little distress in the patient
2. Moderate—more disturbing to the patient but can be redirected by the caregiver
3. Severe—very disturbing to the patient and difficult to redirect

Distress is scored as:
- 0—no distress
- 1—minimal
- 2—mild
- 3—moderate
- 4—moderately severe
- 5—very severe or extreme

For each domain there are four scores: frequency, severity, total (frequency × severity) and caregiver distress. The total possible score is 144 (i.e., a maximum of 4 in the frequency rating × 3 in the severity rating × 12 domains.)

Chapter 24 for more on evaluating the behavioral and psychological symptoms of dementia.

Evaluating Function

Often one of the first signs of cognitive decline is difficulty performing day-to-day activities, often called activities of daily living (ADLs) (Fig. 2.2 and Box 2.2). Validated scales that rate activities of daily living are helpful in initial diagnosis as well as tracking progression and determining the effectiveness of treatment. Because these scales are completed by the caregiver, they are appropriate for primary care practices.

Functional Activities Questionnaire

The Functional Activities Questionnaire (FAQ) evaluates ADLs such as preparing meals, writing checks, and participating in hobbies (Pfeffer et al., 1982). The FAQ is completed by a family member or friend who routinely observes the patient in his or her day-to-day activities. The informant rates the patient in 10 areas (Box 2.5) as: dependent (on others to complete the task) (3 points), requires assistance (2 points), has difficulty, but performs independently (1 point), or performs independently with no difficulty (0 points). Scores range from 0 to 30, with higher scores indicating more functional difficulty. Scores higher than 10 suggest reduced functional ability.

LABORATORY STUDIES

General Laboratory Studies

Although not causes of dementia, impairments in the function of almost any system of the body can impair cognition. Medical problems typically produce a

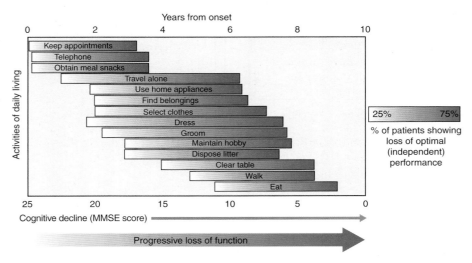

Fig. 2.2 Performance of daily activities declines as Alzheimer's disease worsens. *MMSE*, Mini-Mental State Examination. (From Galasko, D. (1998). An integrated approach to the management of Alzheimer's disease: assessing cognition, function, and behaviour. *European Journal of Neurology, 5*, S9–S17.)

BOX 2.5   Activities of Daily Living Rated in the Functional Assessment Questionnaire

1. Writing checks and maintaining other financial records
2. Assembling tax or business records
3. Shopping alone for clothes, household necessities, or groceries
4. Playing a game of skill or working on a hobby
5. Heating water for coffee or tea, turning off the stove
6. Preparing a balanced meal
7. Keeping track of current events
8. Paying attention to and understanding a TV show, book, or magazine
9. Remembering appointments, family occasions, holidays, or medications
10. Traveling out of the neighborhood (e.g., driving or arranging to take buses)

---

delirium (also referred to as an encephalopathy or acute confusional state), which impairs cognition by disrupting attention. We recommend obtaining general screening laboratory studies, including the electrolytes sodium (Na^+), potassium (K^+), chloride (Cl^-), and calcium (Ca^{2+}); measures of renal function, including blood urea nitrogen (BUN) and creatinine (Cr); measures of liver function, including aspartate aminotransferase (AST), alanine aminotransferase (ALT), and bilirubin; measures of blood cells, including red blood cell (RBC) count; possible signs of infection such as the white blood cell (WBC) count; and general measures of inflammation including erythrocyte sedimentation rate (ESR).

Causes of Reversible Cognitive Dysfunction

The two laboratory studies which are absolutely necessary to obtain are levels of vitamin B12 and thyroid-stimulating hormone (TSH), as abnormalities of both of these are common in the older adult and can impair cognition. Low levels of vitamin D have also been associated with impaired cognition, dementia, and Alzheimer's disease; levels of vitamin D should therefore either be checked or vitamin D supplementation recommended (Littlejohns et al., 2014; see Chapter 21). Other laboratory studies should be obtained if the clinician believes they would be helpful.

Vitamin B12 deficiency is very common in older adults, owing primarily to a loss of intrinsic factor, a hormone released in the stomach that is necessary for B12 to be absorbed. Thus B12 deficiency is typically not associated with diet, and oral vitamin supplementation may not correct the B12 loss. The exception is vegetarians because it is difficult to obtain adequate amounts of B12 through fruits and vegetables alone. B12 is stored in the liver, and the level can therefore be normal for some months after the time when the patient can no longer absorb it. B12 deficiency can present in many different ways, including as a macrocytic anemia, as hyper-reflexia and loss of posterior column function (loss of joint position and vibration senses) when it is often called subacute combined degeneration, as a peripheral neuropathy, and—most relevant for our evaluation—as a neuropsychiatric syndrome affecting mood and cognition. Fatigue, lethargy, sleepiness, and depression are the most prevalent symptoms, but loss of memory is also commonly reported. The treatment of B12 deficiency is either monthly parenteral injections of B12 (usually at a dose of 1000 micrograms), or nasal cyanocobalamin (Nascobal) taken weekly. Oral supplementation may not be effective because of the common inability to absorb B12. Once adequate stores have been built up in the liver, the frequency of injections can be reduced to every 2 to 4 months.

Thyroid disorders are also very common in older adults. In hypothyroidism, the usual cause of thyroid hormone deficiency is failure of the thyroid gland itself, and thus an elevation of the pituitary-derived TSH is the usual sign of hypothyroidism. Hypothyroidism may cause impaired memory, difficulty concentrating, slowed cognition, irritability, mood instability, and occasionally psychosis. Hyperthyroidism also presents with difficulty concentrating; here it is attributable to increased distractibility and restlessness. Hyperthyroidism may cause difficulty with memory as well as irritability, apathy, depression, and delirium.

Screening for *Lyme disease* should be considered in the appropriate clinical context by obtaining an enzyme immunoassay or immunofluorescent assay for IgG, with appropriate follow-up if positive with a western immunoblot for both IgG and IgM for confirmation. Lyme disease is common, endemic in many areas of the country, and has replaced syphilis as the "great mimicker," often presenting as other diseases. Cognitively, Lyme disease presents with a primary impairment in attention. Patients can become disorganized, easily distracted, and somnolent. We have diagnosed a number of patients with Lyme disease who presented clinically with memory loss.

Although screening for *neurosyphilis* by obtaining a rapid plasma reagent (RPR) is no longer routinely recommended, it is still worthwhile to consider, particularly if the patient is immunocompromised. For example, neurosyphilis is now most common in patients with HIV infection. Neurosyphilis causing dementia (also known as "general paresis of the insane") is extremely rare, but can present with personality changes, memory loss, and poor judgment, and can progress to depression, mania, and psychosis. Because it is a treatable disorder, the clinician should always think of it and, when uncertain, order the test.

Apolipoprotein E Testing

We advise caution when considering apolipoprotein E testing. See Chapter 4, for further discussion of this issue.

STRUCTURAL IMAGING STUDIES

A noncontrast, structural imaging study of the brain is essential in the work-up of memory loss. Strokes, tumors, hemorrhages, subdural hematomas and other fluid collections, normal pressure hydrocephalus, vascular dementia, and many other conditions may cause memory loss, and can only be accurately diagnosed with a structural imaging study. Additionally, most patients show some degree of small vessel ischemic strokes by the time they reach 70 years of age or older. It is our experience that, although this small vessel disease is unlikely to be the main cause of memory loss, it is often a contributing factor, making the underlying Alzheimer's disease present with more severe signs and symptoms than it otherwise would (Snowdon et al., 1997). Structural brain imaging allows a qualitative look at the contribution of this small vessel disease. CT and MRI are standard; each has advantages and disadvantages.

Magnetic Resonance Imaging Versus Computed Tomography

MRI scans have higher resolution than CT scans, and can use different sequences to highlight different tissues in the living brain (Figs. 2.3 and 2.4). For this reason, MRI scans provide an unparalleled view of the structure of the brain and almost any pathology. The one major exception is that MRI scans do not show an acute hemorrhage of almost any type as effectively as CT scans. Consequently, CT—and not MRI—is the modality of choice if an acute hemorrhage is suspected.

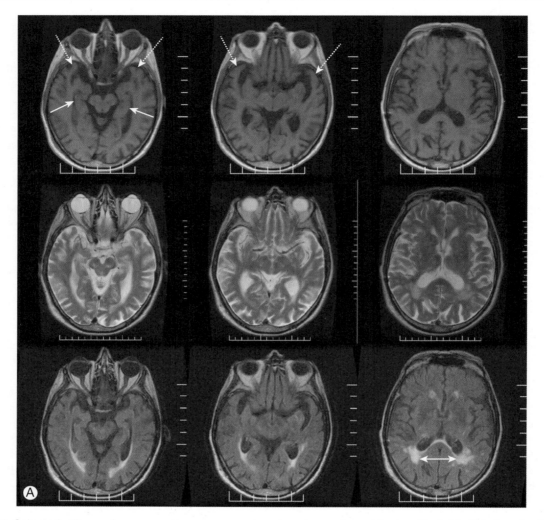

Fig. 2.3 Selected slices of a magnetic resonance imaging scan of a patient with mild Alzheimer's disease. Panels **(A)** and **(B)** show the same six axial slices of brain from T1 (*top*), T2 (*middle*), and fluid attenuated inversion recovery (FLAIR; *bottom*) sequences. Panel **(C)** shows five T1 coronal slices and one T1 sagittal slice. The T1 images provide the best anatomical resolution, showing mild atrophy of hippocampus (*thin solid arrows*), anterior temporal lobe (*thin dotted arrows*), and parietal cortex (*thick dotted arrows*). FLAIR images (in combination with T2) show vascular disease best (*double-headed arrow*). Note that the small vessel ischemic cerebrovascular disease shown here is average for an older adult.

Relative to CT, the MRI scan takes longer, is noisier, and involves going into a much narrower tube. If a patient is claustrophobic or agitated (as can often be the case in Alzheimer's disease dementia after the early stages), a CT scan is easier to obtain than an MRI scan. Thus CT scans are generally easier for the patient to tolerate than MRI scans. CT scans are fast and provide a completely adequate look at the structure of the brain. Both studies allow a look at the extent of small vessel ischemic disease, and can also evaluate for strokes, tumors, subdural fluid collections, normal pressure hydrocephalus, and many other conditions. Note that some findings on a CT scan, such as a mass, will prompt a subsequent MRI for additional characterization.

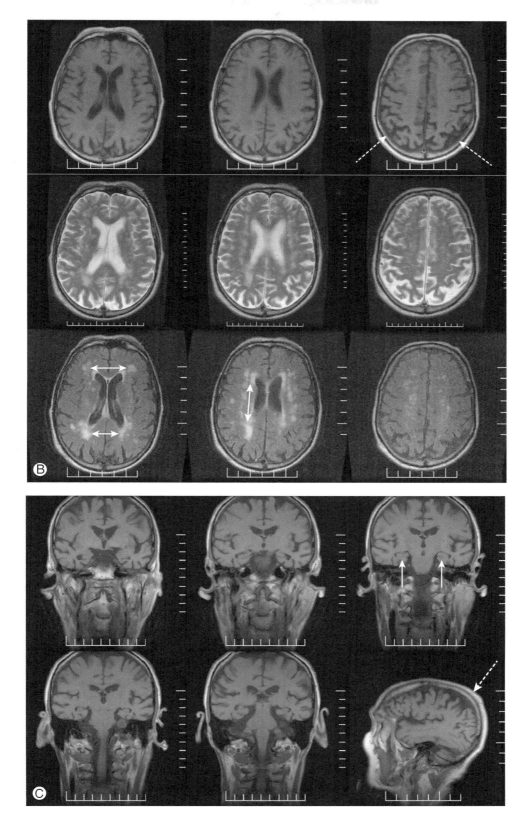

Fig. 2.3 (*Continued*)

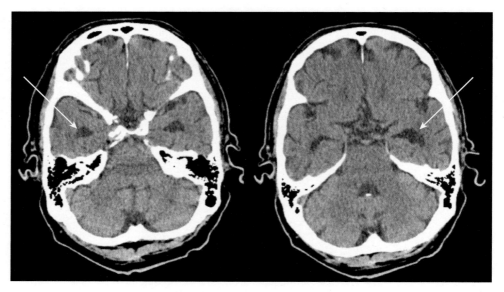

Fig. 2.4 Selected slices of a computed tomography scan of a patient with mild Alzheimer's disease. Note the prominent dilatation of the temporal horns of the lateral ventricles bilaterally (*arrows*). This so-called "ex-vacuo" dilatation (or enlargement caused by loss of tissue) of this part of the ventricles is as a result of underlying shrinkage of the hippocampi.

Questions for Structural Imaging Studies to Answer

Three questions should be answered when examining an imaging study of the brain in a patient with memory loss or dementia.

First, what is the pattern of atrophy (shrinkage of the brain) that is present? Is the atrophy more than is expected for age? Is it bilateral temporal and parietal with relative sparing of other brain regions, consistent with Alzheimer's disease? Is it predominantly frontal consistent with a frontotemporal dementia? Is there hippocampal atrophy consistent with memory loss? Is there no significant atrophy? In our experience, atrophy is almost never "global," that is, atrophy is almost never evenly distributed throughout the brain. Note that, although atrophy on a structural imaging study can be consistent with a neurodegenerative disease, it is never diagnostic or exclusionary of such a disease. In Alzheimer's disease there is typically atrophy of bilateral hippocampi, anterior temporal lobes, and parietal lobes—often asymmetric, for unknown reasons.

Second, how extensive is the small-vessel ischemic disease? Is the amount of these tiny, small-vessel strokes average for the patient's age, less, or more? Has the small-vessel disease affected critical areas of the brain such as the thalamus, where even a small stroke can cause memory loss? Note again that most patients aged 70 years or older have some small-vessel ischemic disease. As mentioned above it is often a minor contributing factor, sometimes a major contributing factor, and only very rarely is it the sole cause of the patient's memory loss.

Third, is there any other pathology present? Is there an old cortical stroke in the right frontal cortex? Is there loss of brain tissue (encephalomalacia) because of an old head injury? Is there a large cavum septum pellucidum? Are there subdural or epidural fluid collections? Is there a tumor? In brief, are there any "surprises" evident on the imaging study that may be a primary or contributing factor to the patient's memory loss?

FUNCTIONAL IMAGING STUDIES

In a routine case of memory loss, one in which the history, physical examination, cognitive testing, and structural imaging studies are all consistent with Alzheimer's disease, vascular dementia, dementia with Lewy bodies, or another etiology, a functional imaging study is not necessary. In a situation, however, in which one or more of the elements of the evaluation suggests that the patient has an atypical neurodegenerative disease, a functional imaging study that measures overall brain metabolism can be helpful.

We would also strongly recommend either a functional imaging study or a test that suggests Alzheimer's disease (see later) for a young person aged less than 66 years with dementia, even if the evaluation appears straightforward. The main reason to obtain a functional imaging study in a patient less than 66 years of age is simply that the prevalence of Alzheimer's disease causing memory loss relative to other etiologies is much less in the younger patient than in the older patient. For example, whereas the overall ratio of Alzheimer's disease to frontotemporal dementia may be 10:1 or even 100:1, this ratio drops to closer to 1:1 for individuals younger than 66 years (Brunnstrom et al., 2009).

Note that the sensitivity and specificity of functional imaging studies is not terribly high, which is one reason why they should not be conducted routinely. For example, a false-positive test suggesting dementia in the case of someone with only mild cognitive issues can be devastating to the patient and family. Thus these functional imaging studies are mainly helpful in distinguishing between different types of dementia in a patient who clearly has a dementia. They are not helpful in distinguishing between, for example, normal aging and MCI, or between depression and mild Alzheimer's disease.

Single Photon Emission Computed Tomography Versus Positron Emission Tomography

There are two main functional imaging technologies that measure overall brain metabolism used in clinical practice, SPECT (single photon emission computed tomography) and PET (positron emission tomography). In both cases a small amount of a radiolabeled dye (usually technetium-99 for SPECT and fluorodeoxyglucose [FDG] for PET) is injected into the patient's bloodstream and a collector outside the head records the amount of radioactivity detected in different areas of the brain. Areas that are more metabolically active show higher levels of radioactivity than areas that are less metabolically active.

Before an area of the brain becomes atrophic, it is likely that it first becomes metabolically less active. Thus functional imaging scans are typically more sensitive to early brain dysfunction than structural imaging scans. SPECT and PET imaging can vary widely from one institution to another, based upon the availability of the radiolabeled dye, quality of the SPECT and PET cameras detecting the radioactivity, and expertise of the radiologist interpreting the scans. Choosing between SPECT and PET imaging is thus dependent upon which technique is available in a given geographic area and, if both are available, which the radiologist feels is better for distinguishing between different neurodegenerative diseases. From a practical standpoint, both provide very similar information. The cost of these studies is covered by most insurance companies as well as Medicare.

Questions for Functional Imaging Studies to Answer

There is one question for a functional imaging study to answer. In a patient with cognitive impairment and a likely neurodegenerative disease, with which neurodegenerative disease is the pattern of impaired and preserved metabolism most consistent? In Alzheimer's disease the pattern is one of bilateral temporal and parietal hypometabolism (Fig. 2.5). As with structural imaging studies, for unknown reasons the hypometabolism is often asymmetric.

Note that these functional imaging studies are more likely than structural imaging studies to show significant changes over relatively brief periods of time, such as 6 to 12 months. Therefore if an evaluation of a patient is inconclusive at one time point and the patient continues to deteriorate, repeating the functional imaging study in 6 to 12 months is more likely to yield informative results than repeating the structural imaging study.

TESTS THAT SUGGEST ALZHEIMER'S DISEASE

There are two types of tests available that can suggest that the Alzheimer's disease pathophysiological process is present, helping to confirm either Alzheimer's disease dementia or mild cognitive impairment due to the Alzheimer's disease pathophysiologic process (Sperling et al., 2011). We do not recommend obtaining these tests

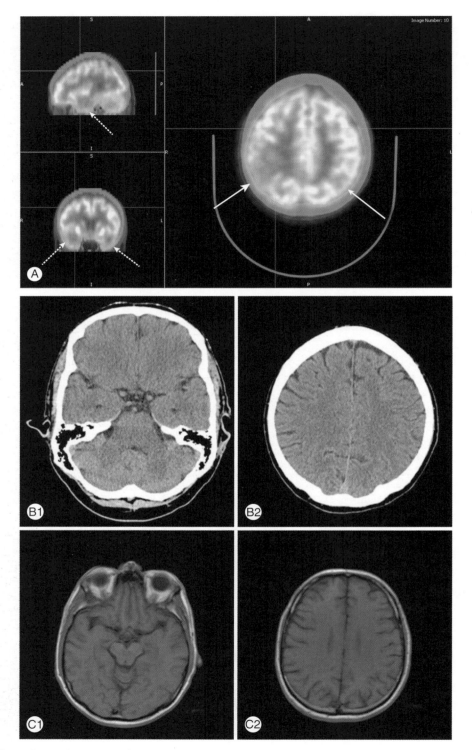

Fig. 2.5 Fluorodeoxyglucose positron emission tomography (PET) scan of a patient with mild Alzheimer's disease. Selected slices of a PET imaging study **(A)** of a patient with Alzheimer's disease demonstrating greatly reduced brain metabolism function in right parietal (*thick solid arrow*) and bilateral temporal (*dotted arrows*) regions, and more mild reduced metabolism in the left parietal (*thin solid arrow*) region. Note that both computed tomography **(B)** and magnetic resonance imaging **(C)** scans of this 67-year-old patient were essentially normal.

routinely, but they can be helpful whenever it is import-ant to more definitively determine (or rule out) if the patient has underlying Alzheimer's pathology present. In a routine case of memory loss or dementia, one in which the patient's age, history, physical examination, cognitive testing, and structural imaging studies are all consistent with Alzheimer's disease, these additional tests are usu-ally not necessary. We would recommend obtaining one of these tests, however, if the patient appears to have a straightforward case of Alzheimer's disease or mild cog-nitive impairment due to the Alzheimer's disease patho-physiologic process but is younger than 66 years old to confirm that this disorder is, in fact, present so that the work-up can be stopped. These tests can also be obtained in other circumstances where memory loss or dementia is thought to be because of Alzheimer's pathology and it is important to have additional diagnostic certainty. Whether to obtain the cerebrospinal fluid test versus an amyloid or tau PET scan depends on availability, cost/insurance coverage, and patient preference; there is not usually a reason to obtain both. Lastly, we would not recommend obtaining either of these tests in an asymp-tomatic patient because as there are currently no disease modifying therapies available outside of a clinical trial, it is not clear how a positive result could be helpful when caring for an asymptomatic patient.

Cerebrospinal Fluid Aβ and Tau

There are three biomarkers measured in the cerebral spinal fluid (CSF) that can be helpful in the diagno-sis of Alzheimer's disease: $A\beta_{42}$, total tau, and hyper-phosphorylated tau (p-tau). Initial studies using the ratio of low $A\beta_{42}$ and high total tau were able to differenti-ate between patients with Alzheimer's disease and controls with high sensitivity (85%) and specificity (86%), but were unable to separate patients with Alzheimer's disease from those with other forms of dementia (specificity 58%). Tau protein can by phosphorylated at several amino acids, forming different types of hyper-phosphorylated tau or "p-tau." Types of hyper-phosphorylated tau that have been studied include $p\text{-}tau_{231P}$, $p\text{-}tau_{181P}$, and $p\text{-}tau_{199P}$. Investigations have found that, when the biomarkers $A\beta_{42}$, total tau, and p-tau are combined, Alzheimer's dis-ease could be distinguished from other forms of demen-tia with sensitivity and specificity of 85% to 90%, and a

6-year study found that it was also possible to predict which patients with mild cognitive impairment would develop Alzheimer's disease with a sensitivity of 95% and specificity of 85% (Hansson et al., 2006; Hampel et al., 2008). Most insurance companies, as well as Medicare, cover the cost of these studies. Athena Diagnostics (www.athenadiagnostics.com) is one commercial labo-ratory that samples can be sent to.

Amyloid and Tau Positron Emission Tomography Scans

In April 2012 the U.S. Food and Drug Administration (FDA) approved the florbetapir (Amyvid) PET ligand, the first amyloid ligand for use in diagnosing patients with cognitive decline. Since then two additional ligands have been approved, flutemetamol (Vizamyl) and florbetaben (Neuraceq). These agents bind to β-amyloid plaques in the cortex, allowing the presence of cortical plaques (or their absence) to be detected (Fig. 2.6). When the results of 59 patients were com-pared to autopsy as the gold standard for detecting amy-loid plaques, the florbetapir PET scan had a sensitivity and specificity of 96% and 100% when the scan was obtained within one year of autopsy (Clark et al., 2012). The degree of florbetapir binding in the cortex has also been shown to correlate with cognitive performance (Saint-Aubert et al., 2013). One large study involving over 16,000 patients found that the use of amyloid PET scans was associated with changes in clinical manage-ment (Rabinovici et al., 2019). However, whether those management changes produced improved outcomes has yet to be determined.

In May 2020 the FDA approved flortaucipir (Tauvid), the first tau imaging ligand (Fig. 2.7). Although more studies need to be done, because this tau ligand is spe-cifically designed to detect tau tangles in Alzheimer's disease, when combined with clinical history it appears to be able to distinguish between Alzheimer's and other neurodegenerative diseases with a high degree of accu-racy (Hammes et al., 2020).

Amyloid and tau PET scans have the potential to radically change the diagnosis of Alzheimer's disease. At the time of going to press, however, Medicare and most insurance companies do not cover their cost.

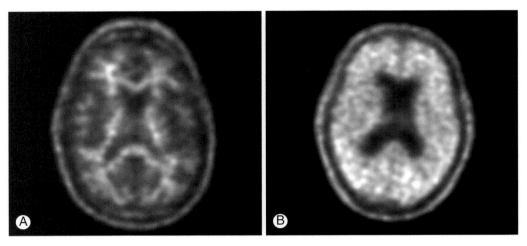

Fig. 2.6 Florbetapir positron emission tomography scans of an older adult without amyloid **(A)** and a patient with Alzheimer's disease **(B)**. Note that in the older adult without amyloid **(A)** the white matter (that takes up the tracer) can be clearly differentiated from the cortex (that does not take up the tracer) but in the patient with Alzheimer's disease **(B)** the white matter and the cortex cannot be differentiated, as both take up the tracer.

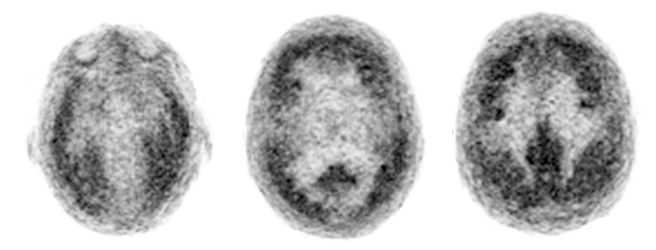

Fig. 2.7 Tau positron emission tomography scan of a patient with Alzheimer's disease.

SUMMARY

The key elements in an evaluation of memory loss include a history from both the patient and family to characterize the signs, symptoms, and current level of function; physical and neurological examinations; cognitive testing; and laboratory and brain imaging studies (Box 2.6). Additional elements of the evaluation can be included when required (Box 2.7).

BOX 2.6 Essential Elements in the Work-Up of Memory Loss

- History from the patient
- History from the caregiver, including at least a few minutes in private
- History should include whether there are problems with:
  - Memory
  - Word-finding
  - Getting lost
  - Reasoning and judgment
  - Mood
  - Behavior
  - Delusions, hallucinations, memory distortions
  - Activities of daily living
  - Instrumental activities of daily living
- Review of systems and past medical history including:
  - A significant brain infection such as meningitis or encephalitis
  - A significant head injury in which the patient lost consciousness
  - Repetitive mild head injuries from football, other sports, or other causes
  - A stroke or a transient ischemic attack
  - A seizure
  - Fluctuating levels of alertness or periods of being relatively unresponsive
  - Visual hallucinations of people or animals
  - A disturbance of gait
  - Falls
  - A tremor
- Rigidity and other signs of parkinsonism
- A dramatic change in personality such that the patient seems like a different person
- Any major psychiatric problems earlier in life, such as major depression or bipolar disease
- Any incontinence of bowel or bladder
- Problems going to sleep (insomnia), staying asleep, or early morning awakening. Any naps?
- Acting out dreams during sleep or other abnormal movements while sleeping
- Difficulty distinguishing dreams from reality when transitioning from sleep
- Habits including alcohol and smoking
- Previous education and occupation
- Family history of Alzheimer's disease, memory loss, or other neurological disorder
- Physical and neurological examination including:
  - Search for focal signs including weakness, abnormal reflexes, and Babinski's sign
  - Search for parkinsonism including tremor, rigidity, and gait disorder
  - Careful evaluation of eye movements
- Cognitive testing with brief cognitive screening instrument such as Mini-Mental State Examination (MMSE) or the Montreal Cognitive Assessment (MoCA)
- Laboratory studies including vitamin B12, vitamin D, and thyroid-stimulating hormone
- Structural imaging study, either magnetic resonance imaging or computed tomography (both noncontrast)

BOX 2.7 Additional Elements to Consider in the Work-Up of Memory Loss

- Consultations
  - Neuropsychology
  - Neurology
  - Psychiatry
- Laboratory studies
  - Rapid plasma reagent
  - Lyme titer
  - Erythrocyte sedimentation rate
  - Antibodies to detect limbic encephalitis and/or Hashimoto's thyroiditis
  - Cerebrospinal fluid evaluation for glucose, total protein, cells, $A\beta_{42}$, total tau, and p-tau
  - Apolipoprotein E4 testing
- Genetic testing for familial early-onset Alzheimer's disease
- Imaging studies
  - Magnetic resonance imaging with magnetic susceptibility (or other sequence looking for blood products)
  - technetium-99 SPECT
  - Fluorodeoxyglucose positron emission tomography (PET)
  - Amyloid PET
  - Tau PET
  - Dopamine transporter single photon emission computed tomography
- Electroencephalogram
- Sleep study

REFERENCES

Bleecker, M. L., Bolla-Wilson, K., Kawas, C., et al. (1988). Age-specific norms for the Mini-Mental State Exam. *Neurology, 38,* 1565–1568.

Blessed, G., Tomlinson, B. E., & Roth, M. (1968). The association between quantitative measures of dementia and of senile change in the cerebral grey matter of elderly subjects. *The British Journal of Psychiatry, 114,* 797–811.

Borson, S., Scanlan, J. M., Watanabe, J., et al. (2005). Simplifying detection of cognitive impairment: Comparison of the Mini-Cog and Mini-Mental State Examination in a multiethnic sample. *Journal of the American Geriatrics Society, 53,* 871–874.

Brunnstrom, H., Gustafson, L., Passant, U., et al. (2009). Prevalence of dementia subtypes: A 30-year retrospective survey of neuropathological reports. *Archives of Gerontology and Geriatrics, 49,* 146–149.

Canadian Task Force on Preventive Health Care, Pottie, K., Rahal, R., Jaramillo, A., et al. (2016). Recommendations on screening for cognitive impairment in older adults. *Canadian Medical Association Journal, 188*(1), 37–46.

Cannon-Albright, L. A., Foster, N. L., Schliep, K., et al. (2019). Relative risk for Alzheimer disease based on complete family history. *Neurology, 92*(15), e1745–e1753.

Crum, R. M., Anthony, J. C., Bassett, S. S., et al. (1993). Population-based norms for the Mini-Mental State Examination by age and educational level. *The Journal of the American Medical Association, 269*(18), 2386–2391.

Clark, C. M., Pontecorvo, M. J., Beach, T. G., et al. (2012). Cerebral PET with florbetapir compared with neuropathology at autopsy for detection of neuritic amyloid-β plaques: A prospective cohort study. *Lancet Neurology, 11*(8), 669–678.

Damasio, H., Grabowski, T. J., Tranel, D., et al. (1996). A neural basis for lexical retrieval. *Nature, 380,* 499–505.

DiSalvio, N. L., Rosano, C., Aizenstein, H. J., et al. (2020). Gray matter regions associated with functional mobility in community-dwelling older adults. *Journal of the American Geriatrics Society, 68*(5), 1023–1028.

Eastwood, M. R., Lautenschlaeger, E., Corbin, S., et al. (1983). A comparison of clinical methods for assessing dementia. *Journal of the American Geriatrics Society, 31,* 342–347.

Falk, N., Cole, A., & Meredith, T. J. (2018). Evaluation of suspected dementia. *American Family Physician, 97*(6), 398–405.

Faulkner, J. W., & Wilshire, C. E. (2020). Mapping eloquent cortex: A voxel-based lesion-symptom mapping study of core speech production capacities in brain tumour patients. *Brain and Language, 200,* 104710.

Folstein, M. F., Folstein, S. E., McHugh, P. R., et al. (1975). A practical method for grading the cognitive state of patients for the clinician. *Journal of Psychiatric Research, 12,* 189–198.

Galvin, J. E., Roe, C. M., Coats, M. A., et al. (2007). Patient's rating of cognitive ability: Using the AD8, a brief informant interview, as a self-rating tool to detect dementia. *Archives of Neurology, 64,* 725–730.

Galvin, J. E., Roe, C. M., Powlishta, K. K., et al. (2005). The AD8: A brief informant interview to detect dementia. *Neurology, 65,* 559–564.

Hammes, J., Bischof, G. N., Bohn, K. P., et al. (2020). One stop shop: Flortaucipir PET differentiates amyloid positive and negative forms of neurodegenerative diseases [published online ahead of print, 2020 Jul 3]. *The Journal of Nuclear Medicine.* https://doi.org/10.2967/jnumed.120.244061 2020;jnumed.120.244061.

Hampel, H., Burger, K., Teipel, S. J., et al. (2008). Core candidate neurochemical and imaging biomarkers of Alzheimer's disease. *Alzheimer's & Dementia: The Journal of the Alzheimer's Association, 4,* 38–48.

Hanseeuw, B. J., Scott, M. R., Sikkes, S., et al. (2020). Alzheimer's Disease Neuroimaging Initiative. Evolution of anosognosia in Alzheimer's disease and its relationship to amyloid. *Annals of Neurology, 87,* 267–280.

Hansson, O., Zetterberg, H., Buchhave, P., et al. (2006). Association between CSF biomarkers and incipient Alzheimer's disease in patients with mild cognitive impairment: a follow-up study. *Lancet Neurology, 5,* 228–234.

Hu, S. H., Chuang, Y. H., Ting, Y. F., et al. (2018). Prevalence of depressive symptoms in older nursing home residents with intact cognitive function in Taiwan. *Research in Nursing & Health, 41*(3), 292–300. https://doi.org/10.1002/nur.21873. PMID 29574780.

Jorm. A. F. (1994). A short form of the Informant Questionnaire on Cognitive Decline in the Elderly (IQCODE): Development and cross-validation. *Psychological Medicine, 24,* 145–153.

Jorm. A. F. (2004). The Informant Questionnaire on Cognitive Decline in the Elderly (IQCODE): A review. *International Psychogeriatrics, 16,* 275–293.

Jorm, A. F., & Jacomb, P. A. (1989). The Informant Questionnaire on Cognitive Decline in the Elderly (IQCODE): Socio-demographic correlates, reliability, validity and some norms. *Psychological Medicine, 19,* 1015–1022.

Knopman, D. S., & Ryberg, S. (1989). A verbal memory test with high predictive accuracy for dementia of the Alzheimer type. *Archives of Neurology, 46,* 141–145.

Li, Y., Meyer, J. S., Thornby, J., et al. (2001). Depressive symptoms among cognitive normal versus cognitive impaired elderly subjects. *International Journal of Geriatric Psychiatry, 16,* 455–461.

Littlejohns, T. J., Henley, W. E., Lang, I. A., et al. (2014). Vitamin D and the risk of dementia and Alzheimer disease. *Neurology, 83,* 920–928.

Locascio, J. J., Growdon, J. H., & Corkin, S. (1995). Cognitive test performance in detecting, staging, and tracking Alzheimer's disease. *Archives of Neurology, 52*, 1087–1099.

Mesulam, M. M., Thompson, C. K., Weintraub, S., et al. (2015). The Wernicke conundrum and the anatomy of language comprehension in primary progressive aphasia. *Brain, 138*(8), 2423–2437.

Meulen, E. F., Schmand, B., van Campen, J. P., et al. (2004). The seven minute screen: A neurocognitive screening test highly sensitive to various types of dementia. *Journal of Neurology, Neurosurgery, and Psychiatry, 75*, 700–705.

Nasreddine, Z. S., Phillips, N. A., Bedirian, V., et al. (2005). The Montreal Cognitive Assessment, MoCA: A brief screening tool for mild cognitive impairment. *Journal of the American Geriatrics Society 53*(4), 695–699.

Novais, F., & Starkstein, S. (2015). Phenomenology of depression in Alzheimer's disease. *Journal of Alzheimer's Disease, 47*(4), 845–855.

Pfeffer, R. I., Kurosaki, T. T., Harrah, C. H., Jr., et al. (1982). Measurement of functional activities in older adults in the community. *Journal of Gerontology, 37*(3), 323–329.

Price, J. L., & Morris, J. C. (1999). Tangles and plaques in nondemented aging and "preclinical" Alzheimer's disease. *Annals of Neurology, 45*, 358–368.

Rabinovici, G. D., Gatsonis, C., Apgar, C., et al. (2019). Association of amyloid positron emission tomography with subsequent change in clinical management among medicare beneficiaries with mild cognitive impairment or dementia. *The Journal of the American Medical Association, 321*(13), 1286–1294.

Ribot. T. (1881). *Les maladies de la mémoire.* Paris: Félix Alcan.

Rinaldi, P., Mecocci, P., Benedetti, C., et al. (2003). Validation of the five-item geriatric depression scale in elderly subjects in three different settings. *Journal of the American Geriatrics Society, 51*, 694–698.

Saint-Aubert, L., Barbeau, E. J., Péran, P., et al. (2013). Cortical florbetapir-PET amyloid load in prodromal Alzheimer's disease patients. *EJNMMI Research, 3*(1), 43.

Sjöberg, L., Karlsson, B., Atti, A. R., et al. (2017). Prevalence of depression: Comparisons of different depression definitions in population-based samples of older adults. *Journal of Affective Disorders, 221*, 123–131.

Snowdon, D. A., Greiner, L. H., Mortimer, J. A., et al. (1997). Brain infarction and the clinical expression of Alzheimer disease. The Nun Study. *The Journal of the American Medical Association, 277*, 813–817.

Solomon, P. R., Brush, M., Calvo, V., et al. (2000). Identifying dementia in the primary care practice. *International Psychogeriatrics, 12*, 483–493.

Solomon, P. R., Hirschoff, A., Kelly, B., et al. (1998). A 7 minute neurocognitive screening battery highly sensitive to Alzheimer's disease. *Archives of Neurology, 55*, 349–355.

Solomon, P. R., & Murphy, C. A. (2005). Should we screen for Alzheimer's disease? A review of the evidence for and against screening Alzheimer's disease in primary care practice. *Geriatrics, 60*, 26–31.

Solomon, P. R., & Murphy, C. A. (2008). Early diagnosis and treatment of Alzheimer's disease. *Expert Review of Neurotherapeutics, 8*, 769–780.

Solomon, P. R., Ruiz, M. A., Murphy, C. A., et al. (2003). The Alzheimer's Disease Caregiver Questionnaire: Initial validation of a screening instrument. *International Psychogeriatrics, 15*(Suppl. 2), 87.

Sperling, R. A., Aisen, P. S., Beckett, L. A., et al. (2011). Toward defining the preclinical stages of Alzheimer's disease: Recommendations from the National Institute on Aging–Alzheimer's Association workgroups on diagnostic guidelines for Alzheimer's disease. *Alzheimer's Disease, 7*(3), 280–292.

Tonga, J. B., Eilertsen, D. E., Solem, I., et al. (2020). Effect of self-efficacy on quality of life in people with mild cognitive impairment and mild dementia: The mediating roles of depression and anxiety. *American Journal of Alzheimer's Disease and Other Dementias, 35*, 1533317519885264.

Tsolaki, M., Iakovidou, V., Papadopoulou, E., et al. (2002). Greek validation of the seven-minute screening battery for Alzheimer's disease in the elderly. *American Journal of Alzheimer's Disease and Other Dementias, 17*, 139–148.

Turk, K. W., Palumbo, R., Deason, R. G., et al. (2020). False memories: The other side of forgetting. *Journal of the International Neuropsychological Society, 26*(6), 545–556.

3

Subjective Cognitive Decline, Mild Cognitive Impairment, and Dementia

QUICK START: SUBJECTIVE COGNITIVE DECLINE, MILD COGNITIVE IMPAIRMENT, AND DEMENTIA

- A three-step approach to evaluate patients with cognitive decline is suggested:
  - Determining if dementia, mild cognitive impairment, or subjective cognitive decline is present
  - Determining which clinical syndrome is present
  - Determining the disease or diseases that are the cause.
- This three-step approach expands upon the two-step approach proposed in Diagnostic and Statistical Manual of Mental Disorders, 5th Edition (DSM-5) and is consistent with the current National Institutes on Aging–Alzheimer's Association Research Framework.
- The spectrum of changes in memory and cognition in aging includes:
  - Cognitively unimpaired (age-associated memory change, normal aging)
  - Subjective cognitive decline (SCD)
  - Mild cognitive impairment (MCI)/mild neurocognitive disorder
  - Dementia/major neurocognitive disorder.
- Common criteria for dementia include:
  - Significant cognitive decline as
    - reported by the patient, a knowledgeable informant, or observed by the clinician, and
    - documented by formal or informal neuropsychological testing.
  - Cognitive impairment is sufficient to interfere with independence in everyday activities.
- Common criteria for mild cognitive impairment include:
  - Cognitive decline as
    - reported by the patient, a knowledgeable informant, or observed by the clinician, and
    - documented by formal or informal neuropsychological testing.
  - Cognitive impairment does not interfere with independence in everyday activities.
- Common criteria for subjective cognitive decline include:
  - Self-experienced persistent decline in cognitive capacity in comparison with a previously normal status
  - Normal performance on standardized cognitive tests.
- Dementing disorders of aging are now considered on a continuum.
- Most patients have more than one pathology causing their cognitive impairment.

In this chapter we propose a strategy for evaluating patients with concerns about their memory and/or other aspects of cognition that will lead to a diagnosis and treatment plan.

A THREE-STEP APPROACH

In approaching the diagnosis of the diseases that cause dementia, we suggest three steps: (1) determining if subjective cognitive decline, mild cognitive impairment, or dementia is present; (2) determining which clinical syndrome is present; and (3) determining the disease or diseases that are the cause. This strategy expands upon the Diagnostic and Statistical Manual of Mental Disorders, 5th Edition (DSM-5) (American Psychiatric Association, 2013) and is consistent with the current National Institute on Aging and Alzheimer's Association (NIA-AA) Research Framework (Jack et al., 2018). Before delving into each of these steps, it will be useful to have a brief discussion of the spectrum of memory changes, both normal and pathological, that can accompany the aging process.

THE SPECTRUM OF COGNITIVE CHANGES

When we discuss the results of a memory evaluation with a patient and family, we often begin with a discussion of the spectrum of memory and other cognitive changes in aging (Fig. 3.1). We note that thinking and memory change just as other abilities do as people age ("Can you run as fast as you could at age 30?" "Can you still carry heavy boxes of books?"). In general, these age-associated memory changes—those that are part of the typical aging process—are characterized by some reduction in the ability to learn and remember new material (that is, mild changes in recent or short-term memory), as well as difficulty coming up with names of people and places. These changes, although occasionally embarrassing, are generally not considered to be pathological, but rather part of the normal aging process ("senior moments" is one phrase we commonly hear). On the other end of the spectrum are memory deficits that are clearly caused by dementing disorders such as Alzheimer's disease.

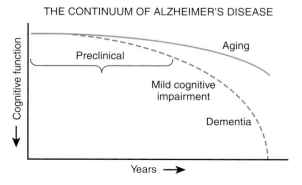

THE CONTINUUM OF ALZHEIMER'S DISEASE

Fig. 3.1 The continuum of cognitive loss in normal aging and disease.

These changes are not part of normal aging, but rather are as a result of a disease process. As a disease process, there is a different continuum that is observed with a different trajectory (see Fig. 3.1). In any disease process leading to dementia there must be a preclinical phase when it is just starting and no changes are noticeable, a frank dementia stage when functional impairment is prominent, and an in-between stage when mild changes in memory are observed and cognitive testing may be abnormal. With this as a backdrop, we begin our evaluation of each patient by determining into which categories they fall: cognitively unimpaired/age-associated memory changes, subjective cognitive decline, mild cognitive impairment, or dementia.

IS DEMENTIA PRESENT?

The first distinction that we endeavor to make is whether the patient meets the criteria for dementia. Dementia is not a disease, but simply a term used to signify the loss of cognitive and functional abilities. Determining that dementia is present requires evaluation of 3 areas: (1) cognition, (2) function, and (3) mood and behavior. These areas are typically evaluated by a combination of interviews with the patient, family (and/or other knowledgeable informant), and neuropsychological testing and questionnaires (see Chapter 2). Below are the criteria for dementia in DSM-5 (where dementia is referred to as a "major neurocognitive disorder"; Box 3.1; see Table 2.2 in Chapter 2 for details on the cognitive domains), and from the National Institute on Aging—Alzheimer's Association workgroup (where dementia from any cause is called "all-cause dementia"; Box 3.2).

As can be seen, the criteria are quite similar, and both include (1) significant cognitive decline as reported by the patient, a knowledgeable informant, or observed by the clinician and (2) documented by formal or informal neuropsychological testing, (3) that the cognitive impairment is sufficient to interfere with independence in everyday activities, and (4) the cognitive impairments are not better explained by delirium or a major psychiatric disorder.

IS MILD COGNITIVE IMPAIRMENT PRESENT?

Even if dementia is not present, it does not mean that the patient's cognition is normal. There is a middle ground between normal, age-appropriate memory changes and

BOX 3.1   Diagnostic and Statistical Manual of Mental Disorders, 5th Edition Criteria for Major Neurocognitive Disorder

A. Evidence of significant cognitive decline from a previous level of performance in one or more cognitive domains (complex attention, executive function, learning and memory, language, perceptual-motor, or social cognition) based on:
   1. Concern of the individual, a knowledgeable informant, or the clinician that there has been a significant decline in cognitive function; and
   2. A substantial impairment in cognitive performance, preferably documented by standardized neuropsychological testing or, in its absence, another quantified clinical assessment.
B. The cognitive deficits interfere with independence in everyday activities (as a result of, at a minimum, requiring assistance with complex instrumental activities of daily living such as paying bills or managing medications).
C. The cognitive deficits do not occur exclusively in the context of a delirium.
D. The cognitive deficits are not better explained by another mental disorder (e.g., major depressive disorder, schizophrenia).

From American Psychiatric Association. (2013). *Diagnostic and statistical manual of mental disorders (DSM-5)* (5th ed.). Arlington, VA: American Psychiatric Association. With permission.

BOX 3.2   National Institute on Aging—Alzheimer's Association All-Cause Dementia Core Clinical Criteria

1. Interfere with the ability to function at work or at usual activities; and
2. Represent a decline from previous levels of functioning and performing; and
3. Are not explained by delirium or major psychiatric disorder;
4. Cognitive impairment is detected and diagnosed through a combination of (1) history-taking from the patient and a knowledgeable informant and (2) an objective cognitive assessment, either a "bedside" mental status examination or neuropsychological testing.
5. The cognitive or behavioral impairment involves a minimum of two of the following domains:
   a. Impaired ability to acquire and remember new information—symptoms include: repetitive questions or conversations, misplacing personal belongings, forgetting events or appointments, getting lost on a familiar route.
   b. Impaired reasoning and handling of complex tasks, poor judgment—symptoms include: poor understanding of safety risks, inability to manage finances, poor decision-making ability, inability to plan complex or sequential activities.
   c. Impaired visuospatial abilities—symptoms include: inability to recognize faces or common objects or to find objects in direct view despite good acuity, inability to operate simple implements, or orient clothing to the body.
   d. Impaired language functions (speaking, reading, writing)—symptoms include: difficulty thinking of common words while speaking, hesitations; speech, spelling, and writing errors.
   e. Changes in personality, behavior, or comportment—symptoms include: uncharacteristic mood fluctuations such as agitation, impaired motivation, initiative, apathy, loss of drive, social withdrawal, decreased interest in previous activities, loss of empathy, compulsive or obsessive behaviors, socially unacceptable behaviors.

Modified from McKhann, G. M., Knopman, D. S., Chertkow, H., et al. (2011). The diagnosis of dementia due to Alzheimer's disease: recommendations from the National Institute on Aging–Alzheimer's Association workgroups on diagnostic guidelines for Alzheimer's disease. *Alzheimer's & Dementia: The Journal of the Alzheimer's Association, 7*, 263–269.

dementia, commonly referred to as mild cognitive impairment (MCI). Just as many diseases can cause dementia, they can also cause mild cognitive impairment. In general, mild cognitive impairment is a less severe version of the particular disease or disorder that is causing dementia (see Fig. 3.1). It is now becoming standard practice when making a diagnosis of mild cognitive impairment to specify the disease or condition that is causing it (e.g., mild cognitive impairment due to Alzheimer's disease). Specifying the disease causing it will lead to an appropriate treatment strategy. Let's again consider criteria from DSM-5 (where it is referred to as a "mild neurocognitive disorder"; Box 3.3; see Table 2.2 in Chapter 2 for details on the cognitive domains), and the National Institute on Aging—Alzheimer's Association workgroup (Box 3.4).

These criteria for mild cognitive impairment are quite similar to each other. Both include (1) cognitive decline as reported by the patient, a knowledgeable informant,

BOX 3.3 Diagnostic and Statistical Manual of Mental Disorders, 5th Edition Criteria for Mild Neurocognitive Disorder

A. Evidence of modest cognitive decline from a previous level of performance in one or more cognitive domains (complex attention, executive function, learning and memory, language, perceptual-motor, or social cognition) based on:
  1. Concern of the individual, a knowledgeable informant, or the clinician that there has been a mild decline in cognitive function; and
  2. A modest impairment in cognitive performance, preferably documented by standardized neuropsychological testing or, in its absence, another quantified clinical assessment.
B. The cognitive deficits do not interfere with independence in everyday activities (as a result of, perseveres in complex instrumental activities of daily living such as paying bills or managing medications, but greater effort, compensatory strategies, or accommodation may be required).
C. The cognitive deficits do not occur exclusively in the context of a delirium.
D. The cognitive deficits are not better explained by another mental disorder (e.g., major depressive disorder, schizophrenia).

From American Psychiatric Association. (2013). *Diagnostic and statistical manual of mental disorders (DSM-5)* (5th ed.). Arlington, VA: American Psychiatric Association. With permission.

BOX 3.4 National Institute on Aging—Alzheimer's Association Summary of Clinical and Cognitive Evaluation for Mild Cognitive Impairment

- Cognitive concern reflecting a change in cognition reported by patient or informant or clinician (as a result of, historical or observed evidence of decline over time)
- Objective evidence of impairment in one or more cognitive domains, typically including memory (as a result of, formal or bedside testing to establish level of cognitive function in multiple domains)
- Preservation of independence in functional abilities
- Not demented.

Modified from Albert, M.S., DeKosky, S.T., Dickson, D., et al., 2011. The diagnosis of mild cognitive impairment due to Alzheimer's disease: recommendations from the National Institute on Aging—Alzheimer's Association workgroups on diagnostic guidelines for Alzheimer's disease. Alzheimers Dement 7, 270–279.

or observed by the clinician and (2) documented by formal or informal neuropsychological testing, and (3) that the cognitive impairment does not interfere with independence in everyday activities. These criteria are also similar to the dementia criteria—with the major difference that independence is preserved in mild cognitive impairment. In general, then, the key distinction is that in dementia the cognitive deficits interfere with day-to-day activities, whereas in mild cognitive impairment they may make these activities more effortful and challenging, but the activities are successfully completed independently.

The National Institute on Aging–Alzheimer's Association Workgroup has recently provided a research framework that provides additional clarification of what it means to be cognitively unimpaired, to have mild cognitive impairment, or to have dementia (Jack et al., 2018) (Box 3.5).

BOX 3.5 National Institute on Aging—Alzheimer's Association Research Framework for Syndromal Staging of Cognitive Continuum

Cognitively Unimpaired
- Cognitive performance within expected range for that individual based on all available information. This may be based on clinical judgment and/or on cognitive test performance (which may or may not be based on comparison to normative data, with or without adjustments for age, education, occupation, sex, etc.).
- Cognitive performance may be in the impaired/abnormal range based on population norms, but performance is within the range expected for that individual.
- A subset of cognitively unimpaired individuals may report subjective cognitive decline and/or demonstrate subtle decline on serial cognitive testing.

Mild Cognitive Impairment
- Cognitive performance below expected range for that individual based on all available information. This may be based on clinical judgment and/or on cognitive test performance (which may or may not be based on comparison to normative data with or without adjustments for age, education, occupation, sex, etc.).
- Cognitive performance is usually in the impaired/abnormal range based on population norms, but this is not required as long as the performance is below the range expected for that individual.

- In addition to evidence of cognitive impairment, evidence of decline in cognitive performance from baseline must also be present. This may be reported by the individual or by an observer (e.g., study partner) or observed by change on longitudinal cognitive testing/behavioral assessments or by a combination of these.
- May be characterized by cognitive presentations that are not primarily amnestic.
- Although cognitive impairment is the core clinical criteria, neurobehavioral disturbance—for example, changes in mood, anxiety, or motivation—may be a prominent feature of the clinical presentation.
- Performs daily life activities independently, but cognitive difficulty may result in detectable but mild functional impact on the more complex activities of daily life, either self-reported or corroborated by a study partner.

Dementia
- Substantial progressive cognitive impairment that affects several domains and/or neurobehavioral symptoms. May be reported by the individual or by an observer (e.g., study partner) or observed by change on longitudinal cognitive testing.
- May be characterized by cognitive presentations that are not primarily amnestic.
- Although cognitive impairment is the core clinical criteria, neurobehavioral disturbance—for example, changes in mood, anxiety, or motivation—may be a prominent feature of the clinical presentation.
- Cognitive impairment and/or neurobehavioral symptoms result in clearly evident functional impact on daily life. No longer fully independent/requires assistance with daily life activities. This is the primary feature differentiating dementia from mild cognitive impairment.
- May be subdivided into mild, moderate, and severe.

Modified from Jack, C. R. Jr., Bennett, D. A., Blennow, K., et al. (Contributors). (2018). NIA-AA Research Framework: Toward a biological definition of Alzheimer's disease. *Alzheimer's & Dementia: The Journal of the Alzheimer's Association, 14*(4), 535–562.

IS SUBJECTIVE COGNITIVE DECLINE PRESENT?

Some patients present to our clinic absolutely certain that their memory has declined over time, yet when we give them detailed neuropsychological testing they perform normally, even when we take into account their age and education. These individuals have subjective cognitive

---

> **BOX 3.6 Criteria for Subjective Cognitive Decline**
>
> - Self-experienced persistent decline in cognitive capacity in comparison with a previously normal status and unrelated to an acute event
> - Normal age-, gender-, and education-adjusted performance on standardized cognitive tests that are used to classify mild cognitive impairment or dementia
> - Does not meet criteria for mild cognitive impairment or dementia
> - Cannot be explained by another psychiatric or neurologic disease, medical disorder, medication, or substance use.

Modified from Jessen, F., Amariglio, R. E., van Boxtel, M., et al. (2014). A conceptual framework for research on subjective cognitive decline in preclinical Alzheimer's disease. *Alzheimer's & Dementia: The Journal of the Alzheimer's Association, 10*, 844–852.

decline (SCD, previously termed *subjective cognitive impairment*) (Jessen et al., 2014) (Box 3.6). There are several reasons why it is relevant to consider this condition. Although the term was introduced and codified mainly for research purposes, it is also useful clinically. One study found that of participants in a memory research center (which may attract individuals with memory concerns), 54% of individuals with subjective cognitive decline developed either mild cognitive impairment or dementia over seven years, compared with only 15% of unimpaired individuals without a cognitive complaint (Reisberg et al., 2010). Another study found that the rate of decline in individuals with subjective cognitive decline was approximately 7% per year (Reisberg et al., 2019). Note that these risks are lower in a community-based sample (Slot et al., 2019). Nevertheless, from a clinical perspective, it makes sense to follow individuals with subjective cognitive decline more closely than unimpaired individuals without a cognitive complaint. After determining whether the patient has dementia, mild cognitive impairment, or subjective cognitive decline, the next step is to determine which clinical syndrome is present.

WHICH CLINICAL SYNDROME IS PRESENT?

Although it has been known since the days that Alois Alzheimer was practicing over 100 years ago that it is difficult to accurately infer the underlying pathology in dementia from the patient's signs and symptoms, this difficulty or disconnect has recently been more explicitly recognized. One reason for this increased recognition is that we now have biomarkers for specific diseases and so we are more aware when we are wrong about an underlying pathology (Rabinovici et al., 2019). We also now have evidence that it is the unusual patient who has a single pathology; most patients have at least two pathologies contributing to their cognitive impairment and many have three or more (Kapasi, DeCarli, & Schneider, 2017).

For example, in the days before using cerebral spinal fluid and positron emission tomography (PET) scans to detect abnormalities of beta amyloid and tau, after evaluating a patient we might make a clinical diagnosis of Alzheimer's disease dementia, knowing that we were likely to be correct when the patient came to autopsy 80% to 90% of the time. We therefore would communicate the diagnosis of "probable Alzheimer's disease" to the patient and family in an honest and confident manner, and then segue into discussions about treatment. Although the clinical diagnosis would be incorrect 10% to 20% of the time, this misdiagnosis would only come to light at autopsy—which few patients would receive.

Today, although our clinical accuracy is still 80% to 90%, because our patients frequently undergo lumbar punctures and PET scans to have their beta amyloid and tau examined, we are now faced with telling one or two out of every ten patients that our clinical diagnosis was wrong and they don't have Alzheimer's disease. Quite understandably, some patients and families become upset that they were told they had "probable Alzheimer's disease" and now they are told they don't have Alzheimer's disease. This is one reason why giving a diagnosis of a clinical syndrome, such as progressive amnestic dysfunction (Mesulam, 2000), may be better than a "probable" disease state.

Once we move from amnestic disorders to disorders affecting other aspects of cognition and behavior, we see that our ability to infer pathology from a clinical evaluation is even more difficult. For example, there was a time that when a patient presented with the signs and symptoms of behavior variant frontotemporal dementia (see Chapter 10) they were given a diagnosis of Pick's disease, thinking that Pick bodies would be found at autopsy. Today, we know that there are at least half a dozen frontotemporal lobar degeneration pathologies

that this patient may have in addition to Pick's disease, and so they are given the syndromic diagnosis of behavioral variant frontotemporal dementia. Other clinical syndromic labels are now also used routinely, such as primary progressive aphasia (see Chapter 9), posterior cortical atrophy (see Chapter 11), and corticobasal syndrome (see Chapter 13). In each case there is the explicit understanding that the exact underlying pathology (or pathologies) cannot be known with complete certainty until autopsy.

Note that, at present, there are not generally accepted syndromes for all presenting clinical disorders. Thus we are currently operating with a hybrid system of some clearly identified clinical syndromes with multiple possible pathologies (behavioral variant frontotemporal dementia and primary progressive aphasia being two examples) and other disorders known by their pathologies (such as dementia with Lewy bodies). This hybrid system is, perhaps, appropriate if some clearly defined clinical syndromes have only one underlying pathology, whereas other syndromes may be caused by a number of different pathologies.

Thus, after it is clear that dementia or mild cognitive impairment is present, the second step is to determine which clinical syndrome is present: whether it is the progressive amnestic dysfunction most commonly seen with Alzheimer's disease, the language disturbance of primary progressive aphasia, or the syndrome seen in dementia with Lewy bodies consisting of parkinsonism, visual hallucinations, and rapid-eye movement (REM) sleep behavior disorder.

A word about treatment. The medications for Alzheimer's disease dementia currently in use—the cholinesterase inhibitors and memantine—treat symptoms, and not underlying pathologies. Moreover, because these medications were developed and evaluated during the time that testing for beta amyloid and tau were not routinely available, the patients who participated in these clinical trials were surely a mixture of individuals with different underlying causes of progressive amnestic dysfunction, including Alzheimer's disease but also limbic-predominant age-related TDP-43 encephalopathy (LATE), vascular dementia, dementia with Lewy bodies, and mixtures of two or more of these pathologies. For this reason, although these medications are U.S. Food and Drug Administration (FDA) approved for "Alzheimer's disease" dementia, we routinely prescribe them for patients with the syndrome of progressive amnestic dysfunction—otherwise known as Alzheimer's clinical syndrome—regardless of their underlying pathology (if known). Future studies will be needed to know if the different pathologies underlying progressive amnestic dysfunction respond differently to the cholinesterase inhibitors and memantine.

WHAT IS THE UNDERLYING PATHOLOGY?

After we have determined that the patient has dementia or mild cognitive impairment (Step 1), and we have characterized their clinical syndrome (Step 2), we can then work on trying to determine the underlying pathology (Step 3). Here knowing the underlying prevalence of the different pathologies is extremely helpful.

When a patient walks into one of our memory clinics, before we even meet them or review their records, we have a good idea of their diagnosis. We can be reasonably confident that they are experiencing memory problems and that in most cases they do have a dementing illness. We know that up to 75% of all dementing illnesses in the elderly (≥65 years) are due in whole or in part to Alzheimer's disease (Fig. 3.2). Because of this prevalence, we start with the working hypothesis for our cognitively impaired patient that Alzheimer's disease is the cause, but we also keep vigilant for the signs of symptoms of other common causes of cognitive impairment. As Fig. 3.2 suggests, by considering

only four other causes of progressive dementias in addition to Alzheimer's disease (dementia with Lewy bodies, vascular dementia, LATE, and the frontotemporal lobar degenerations) we can account for up to 95% of all dementias in the elderly. Fig. 3.3 suggests some overall rules of thumb for considering causes of mild cognitive impairment and dementia other than Alzheimer's disease, and Table 3.1 provides a more exhaustive differential diagnosis. The remainder of the book provides additional information on diagnosing and treating the most common causes of dementing illnesses as well as consideration of less common causes of dementia.

We recognize that the type of patients that we see in our highly specialized setting is certainly not the same in primary care practices or even in general psychiatry or neurology practices. But, in any of these settings, once the age of the patient is known and the diagnosis of dementia or mild cognitive impairment is made, the same strategy that we use would be appropriate.

Lastly, we would note that it is not always possible—or even relevant—to determine the underlying pathology as long as the clinical syndrome is clearly understood. As mentioned earlier, current treatments are based upon clinical syndrome, not pathologic disease. We are hopeful, however, that in the not-too-distant future, disease modifying therapies will be developed for specific disorders. At that time, determining the exact underlying disease will be paramount.

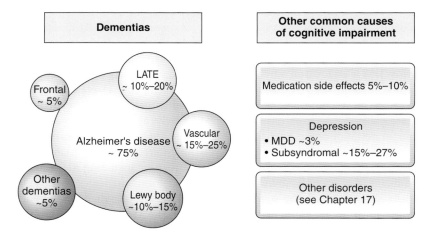

Fig. 3.2 Visual representation of the prevalence and overlap of the common causes of memory loss and other cognitive impairment. *LATE*, Limbic-predominant age-related TDP-43 encephalopathy; *MDD*, major depressive disorder.

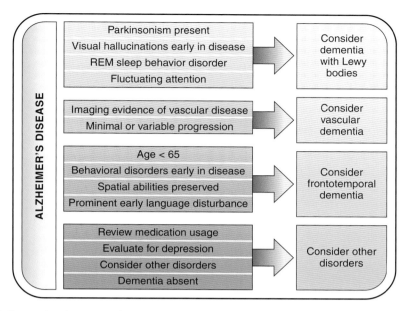

Fig. 3.3 Differential diagnosis of memory loss and other cognitive dysfunction. *REM*, Rapid-eye movement.

TABLE 3.1	Differential Diagnosis by History, Symptom, or Sign	
History, Symptoms, or Signs	**Clinical Syndrome**	**Underlying Etiology**
Memory loss early and prominent	Progressive amnestic dysfunction (also known as Alzheimer's clinical syndrome, dementia of the Alzheimer's type or probable Alzheimer's disease dementia) (see Chapter 4)	Most likely: • Alzheimer's disease (see Chapter 4) Other considerations: • Medication side effects (see Chapter 17) • Limbic-predominant age-related TDP-43 encephalopathy (LATE; see Chapter 6) • Dementia with Lewy bodies (see Chapter 8) • Depression (see Chapter 17) • Vascular dementia (see Chapter 7) • Chronic traumatic encephalopathy (see Chapter 15) • Primary age-related tauopathy (PART; see Chapter 5)
Rigidity, tremor, gait disturbance, and/or parkinsonism present	Parkinsonian syndrome	Most likely • Dementia with Lewy bodies (see Chapter 8) Other considerations • Parkinson's disease (without dementia) • Progressive supranuclear palsy (see Chapter 12) • Corticobasal degeneration (see Chapter 13) • Vascular dementia (see Chapter 7) • Frontotemporal lobar degeneration (see Chapter 10) • Normal pressure hydrocephalus (see Chapter 14) • Chronic traumatic encephalopathy (see Chapter 15) • Creutzfeldt-Jakob disease (see Chapter 16)

(Continued)

TABLE 3.1 **Differential Diagnosis by History, Symptom, or Sign (*Continued*)**		
History, Symptoms, or Signs	**Clinical Syndrome**	**Underlying Etiology**
Fluctuations in attention and alertness early and prominent	None (or "fluctuating syndrome")	Most likely • Dementia with Lewy bodies (see Chapter 8) • Alzheimer's disease (see Chapter 4) • Medication side effects (see Chapter 17) • Systemic illness (see Chapter 17) • Vascular dementia (see Chapter 7) Other considerations • Multiple sclerosis
Visual hallucinations of people and/or animals early and prominent	None (or "visual hallucination syndrome")	Most likely • Dementia with Lewy bodies (see Chapter 8) Other considerations • Alzheimer's disease (see Chapter 4; particularly if "hallucinations" are really memory distortions or misperceptions—thinking husband is father, etc.)
Disturbance of visual function early and prominent	Posterior cortical atrophy (see Chapter 11)	Most likely • Alzheimer's disease (see Chapter 4) • Dementia with Lewy bodies (see Chapter 8) • Corticobasal degeneration (see Chapter 13) Other considerations • Vascular dementia (see Chapter 7) • Creutzfeldt-Jakob disease (see Chapter 16)
Behavioral issues and/or executive dysfunction early and prominent	Behavioral variant frontotemporal dementia (see Chapter 10)	Most likely • Frontotemporal lobar degeneration (see Chapter 10) • Alzheimer's disease (see Chapter 4) Other considerations • Vascular dementia (see Chapter 7) • Dementia with Lewy bodies (see Chapter 8) • Primary age-related tauopathy (PART; see Chapter 5) • Progressive supranuclear palsy (see Chapter 12) • Corticobasal degeneration (see Chapter 13) • Normal pressure hydrocephalus (see Chapter 14) • Chronic traumatic encephalopathy (see Chapter 15) • Primary psychiatric disorders
Language and/or speech dysfunction early and prominent	Primary progressive aphasia or primary progressive apraxia of speech (see Chapter 9)	Most likely • Alzheimer's disease (see Chapter 4) • Frontotemporal lobar degeneration (see Chapter 10) • Progressive supranuclear palsy (see Chapter 12) Other considerations • Corticobasal degeneration (see Chapter 13) • Vascular dementia (see Chapter 7)
History of strokes and/or transient ischemic attacks (TIAs)	Vascular syndrome/vascular cognitive impairment (see Chapter 7)	Most likely • Vascular dementia (see Chapter 7) • Alzheimer's disease (see Chapter 4) Other considerations • Multiple sclerosis

(*Continued*)

TABLE 3.1 Differential Diagnosis by History, Symptom, or Sign (Continued)

History, Symptoms, or Signs	Clinical Syndrome	Underlying Etiology
History of contact sports and/ or multiple concussions	Traumatic encephalopathy syndrome (see Chapter 15)	Most likely • Alzheimer's disease (see Chapter 4) • Chronic traumatic encephalopathy (see Chapter 15)
Progressive limb apraxia, asymmetric motor changes	Corticobasal syndrome (see Chapter 13)	Most likely • Corticobasal degeneration (see Chapter 13) • Alzheimer's disease (see Chapter 4) • Frontotemporal lobar degeneration (see Chapter 10) • Progressive supranuclear palsy (see Chapter 12) • Dementia with Lewy bodies (see Chapter 8) Other considerations • Vascular dementia (see Chapter 7) • Creutzfeldt-Jakob disease (see Chapter 16) • Other (see Chapter 13)
Rapid cognitive deterioration	Rapidly progressing dementia (see Chapter 16)	Most likely • Medication side effects (see Chapter 17) • Acute medical problem (e.g., infection) (see Chapter 17) • Acute neurologic problem (e.g., stroke, subdural hematoma, seizures) (see Chapter 17) Other considerations • Creutzfeldt-Jakob disease (see Chapter 16) • Incorrect history (deterioration actually slow)

REFERENCES

American Psychiatric Association. (2013). *Diagnostic and statistical manual of mental disorders. (DSM-5)* (5th ed.) Arlington, VA: American Psychiatric Association.

Jack, C. R., Jr., Bennett, D. A., Blennow, K., et al. (Contributors). (2018). NIA-AA research framework: Toward a biological definition of Alzheimer's disease. *Alzheimer's & Dementia: The Journal of the Alzheimer's Association, 14*(4), 535–562.

Jessen, F., Amariglio, R. E., van Boxtel, M., et al. (2014). A conceptual framework for research on subjective cognitive decline in preclinical Alzheimer's disease. *Alzheimer's & Dementia: The Journal of the Alzheimer's Association, 10*(6), 844–852.

Kapasi, A., DeCarli, C., & Schneider, J. A. (2017). Impact of multiple pathologies on the threshold for clinically overt dementia. *Acta Neuropathologica, 134*(2), 171–186.

Mesulam. M. M. (2000). *Principles of behavioral and cognitive neurology* (2nd ed.). New York: Oxford University Press.

Rabinovici, G. D., Gatsonis, C., Apgar, C., et al. (2019). Association of amyloid positron emission tomography with subsequent change in clinical management among Medicare beneficiaries with mild cognitive impairment or dementia. *JAMA, 321*(13), 1286–1294.

Reisberg, B., Shulman, M. B., Torossian, C., et al. (2010). Outcome over seven years of healthy adults with and without subjective cognitive impairment. *Alzheimer's & Dementia: The Journal of the Alzheimer's Association, 6*(1), 11–24.

Reisberg, B., Torossian, C., Shulman, M. B., et al. (2019). Two year outcomes, cognitive and behavioral markers of decline in healthy, cognitively normal older persons with global deterioration scale stage 2 (Subjective Cognitive Decline With Impairment). *Journal of Alzheimer's Disease, 67*(2), 685–705.

Slot, R. E. R., Sikkes, S. A. M., Berkhof, J., et al. (2019). Subjective cognitive decline and rates of incident Alzheimer's disease and non-Alzheimer's disease dementia. *Alzheimer's & Dementia: The Journal of the Alzheimer's Association, 15*(3), 465–476.

4

Alzheimer's Disease

QUICK START: ALZHEIMER'S DISEASE

Definition	• Alzheimer's disease is a neurodegenerative disease of the brain characterized by progressive amnestic dysfunction with specific microscopic pathology including senile plaques and neurofibrillary tangles.
Prevalence	• Alzheimer's disease is the most common cause of dementia, affecting approximately 3% of people aged 65 to 74, 17% of people aged 75 to 84, and 32% of people aged 85 and older.
	• Approximately two-thirds of patients with Alzheimer's disease are women, with the overall lifetime risk being 11.6% for men and 21.1% for women.
Genetic risk	• Family history of Alzheimer's disease in a first-degree relative increases the risk between 2-fold and 4-fold, and more distant family relatives with Alzheimer's also increase one's risk.
Cognitive symptoms	• After memory loss, other symptoms develop including word-finding and visuospatial difficulties, and frontal/executive dysfunction including problems with reasoning and judgment.
Diagnostic criteria	• Two widely accepted sets of diagnostic criteria are from the National Institute on Aging–Alzheimer's Association (NIA-AA) workgroup and the Diagnostic and Statistical Manual of Mental Disorders, 5th Edition (DSM-5).
	• For Alzheimer's disease dementia, both criteria require: (1) presence of dementia, (2) deficits in multiple cognitive areas, (3) gradual onset and progression, and (4) ruling out other causes.
	• For mild cognitive impairment due to Alzheimer's disease, both criteria require: (1) presence mild cognitive impairment; (2) deficits in one or more cognitive areas, including memory (for DSM-5) or typically including memory (for NIA-AA); (3) gradual onset and progression; and (4) ruling out other causes.
Behavioral symptoms	• Behavioral and psychiatric symptoms may develop early, including apathy, irritability, agitation, anxiety, and exacerbation of premorbid personality traits.
Treatment	• Cholinesterase inhibitors are U.S. Food and Drug Administration (FDA) approved for the treatment of mild, moderate, and severe Alzheimer's disease dementia.
	• Memantine is FDA approved for the treatment of moderate and severe Alzheimer's disease dementia.
	• The behavioral and psychiatric symptoms of Alzheimer's disease are often more distressing to caregivers than the cognitive ones, and should also be treated.
Top differential diagnoses	• Normal aging, limbic-predominant age-related TDP-43 encephalopathy (LATE), dementia with Lewy bodies, vascular dementia, frontotemporal dementia.

(See Chapters 2 and 3 for additional information.)

An 84-year-old woman was brought in by her daughter for slowly deteriorating thinking and memory over five years. Her phone was disconnected because she forgot to pay the bills, and there was spoiled food in the refrigerator. When interviewed she had pauses in her speech and her daughter often filled in missing words for her. She was not oriented to the day, date, month, or year, nor could she name several common items or recall them a few minutes later. A computed tomography (CT) scan of the head showed an average amount of small vessel ischemic disease for her age (see Chapter 7) and atrophy of hippocampi, temporal lobes, and parietal lobes.

A 78-year-old man and his wife were both concerned that his memory was not as good as it was last year. He used to be able to remember a short grocery list in his head, but now he needed to write it down or he would return with the wrong items. He continued to pay the bills, balance the checkbook, and do household projects, although these tasks now took him longer to complete. Evaluation of memory testing in the office showed that he scored below normal when repeating a brief story containing ten details. His laboratory data were unremarkable, and his magnetic resonance imaging (MRI) scan showed bilateral atrophy in hippocampi, temporal lobes, and parietal lobes.

Both of these patients show a characteristic pattern of symptoms, cognitive testing, and structural brain imaging suggestive of Alzheimer's disease, the first consistent with Alzheimer's disease dementia, the second consistent with mild cognitive impairment (MCI) due to Alzheimer's disease.

PREVALENCE, PROGNOSIS, AND DEFINITION

Alzheimer's disease is a neurodegenerative disease of the brain typically characterized by a prominent memory impairment and having a specific pathology including senile plaques and neurofibrillary tangles (Rabinovici, 2019). Over time, Alzheimer's disease produces neurochemical deficits and prominent brain atrophy. Alzheimer's disease is by far the most common cause of dementia, either by itself or in combination with other disorders. Although the exact prevalence is difficult to ascertain, it is estimated that approximately 5.8 million Americans are living with Alzheimer's disease dementia. The overall prevalence of Alzheimer's disease dementia

in the community is estimated at about 10% in population-based studies. Although there are approximately 200,000 Americans under age 65 living with Alzheimer's, the disease becomes more prevalent with age, with most cases being diagnosed after the age of 65. It is estimated that approximately 3% of people aged 65 to 74 years, 17% of people aged 75 to 84 years, and 32% of people aged 85 years and older have Alzheimer's disease dementia. Worldwide, it is estimated that 50 million people have dementia, comprising 5% of the world's population over age 60 (World Health Organization, 2019). Because the population is aging, the number of individuals with Alzheimer's disease is rapidly rising (Figs. 4.1–4.4). Approximately two-thirds of patients with Alzheimer's disease are women, with the overall lifetime risk being 11.6% for men and 21.1% for women. The incidence of Alzheimer's disease is lower in Asian Americans and higher in American blacks and Hispanics/Latinos compared with non-Hispanic American whites. The average patient with Alzheimer's disease dementia lives approximately 4 to 8 years from diagnosis until death, with the range being approximately 4 to 12 years. On average, the Mini-Mental State Examination (MMSE) and Montreal Cognitive Assessment (MoCA) decline approximately 2 or 3 points per year in these patients. Alzheimer's disease and related dementias are also some of the most expensive health conditions in the USA with a total annual cost for 2019 estimated to be $290 billion for healthcare and long-term care—not including the contribution of unpaid caregivers (Alzheimer's Association, 2019).

ALZHEIMER'S PATHOLOGY

Brain weight is typically reduced in Alzheimer's disease by 100 to 200 grams. Examination of the surface of the brain reveals cortical atrophy of the temporal, parietal, and frontal lobes, as well as the hippocampus (Fig. 4.5). The ventricular system becomes enlarged (Fig. 4.6). The occipital lobes, along with primary sensory and motor cortices, are usually preserved. Microscopically, Alzheimer's pathology consists of two main features, senile plaques and neurofibrillary tangles (Figs. 4.7 and 4.8). Additional microscopic features include selective loss of neurons and synapses, and an increase in the number and activation of astrocytes. Neuropil threads (short, often curly silver-stained fibers) also accumulate in the neocortex. The exact relationship between Aβ,

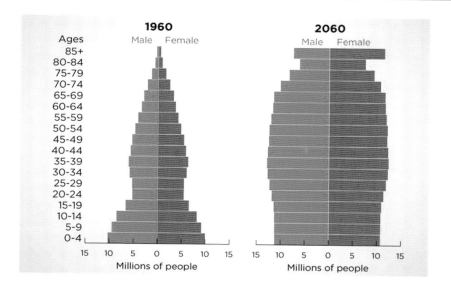

Fig. 4.1 Population of the United States in 1960 and estimated in 2060. (From National Population Projections. (2017). Accessed on January 22, 2020 from www.census.gov/content/dam/Census/library/stories/2018/03/graying-america-pyramid-pillar.jpg.)

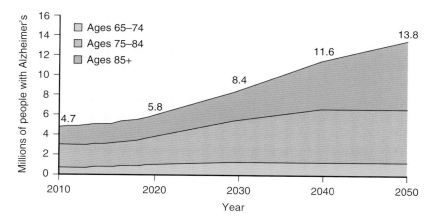

Fig. 4.2 Projected number of people age 65 and older (total and by age group) in the U.S. population with Alzheimer's disease, 2010–2050. (From Alzheimer's Association. (2019). Alzheimer's disease facts and figures. *Alzheimer's & Dementia: The Journal of the Alzheimer's Association. 15*(3), 321–387.)

plaques, tangles, cognitive impairment, and disease progression is an active area of research.

Senile plaques contain a specific type of amyloid, often referred to as β-amyloid or as "Aβ." (Note that the amyloid in Alzheimer's disease is not related to the amyloid in systemic amyloidoses.) Aβ is a 40- or 42-amino acid peptide that is a fragment of a larger, membrane-spanning glycoprotein known as the amyloid precursor protein or APP. The normal function of Aβ is unclear, although it may be part of the brain's immune system (Moir, Lathe, & Tanzi, 2018). Up to 50% of the Aβ found in plaques is Aβ42. Senile plaques are extracellular structures that are composed of Aβ, dystrophic neuritic processes (axons and dendrites), astrocytes

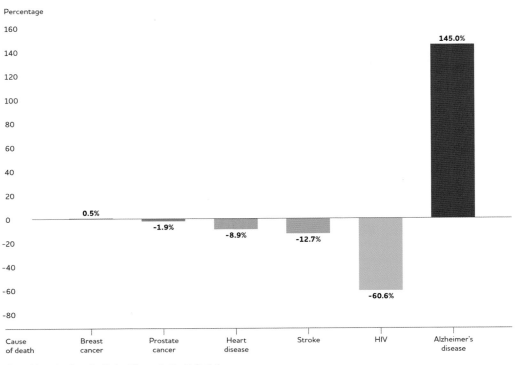

Fig. 4.3 Percentage changes in selected causes of death between 2000 and 2017. (From Alzheimer's Association. (2019). Alzheimer's disease facts and figures. *Alzheimer's & Dementia: The Journal of the Alzheimer's Association, 15*(3), 321–387.)

and their processes, and microglial cells (see Fig. 4.8). When axons and dendrites are disrupted, the communication between neurons becomes impaired. When microglial cells attempt to remove amyloid and remnants of axons and dendrites, an inflammatory reaction can start causing more damage. Under light microscopy senile plaques appear to have a fluffy central core with surrounding thick irregular processes (Fig. 4.9). Various classifications of senile plaques have been proposed, including diffuse and neuritic types. Neuritic plaques are associated with the destruction of axons and dendrites of neurons. Diffuse plaques do not disrupt these neuronal processes, but are thought to be the precursor of neuritic plaques.

Neurofibrillary tangles are intraneuronal cytoplasmic structures that are composed of paired filaments with a regular helical periodicity (see Fig. 4.8). Neurofibrillary tangles appear to be composed primarily of a hyperphosphorylated form of the microtubule-associated protein

tau. Microtubules are one of the three major constituents of the neuronal cytoskeleton, an infrastructural element of neurons that participate in functions such as axonal transport and maintenance of the structural integrity of the cell. Among other roles, tau and other microtubule-associated proteins stabilize the microtubule assembly (think of tau as the support beams or rivets for this system). Although neurofibrillary tangles begin as intracytoplasmic structures, they may remain behind after the neuron dies, forming "ghost" or "tombstone" tangles in the neuropil. Under the microscope neurofibrillary tangles can look like skeins of yarn (see Fig. 4.9).

NEUROCHEMISTRY

A deficit in acetylcholine is the most consistently found alteration of brain chemistry in Alzheimer's disease. Early in the disease there is a loss of choline acetyltransferase and reduced high-affinity choline uptake

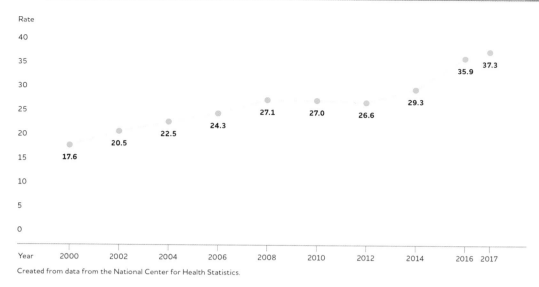

Fig. 4.4 U.S. annual Alzheimer's death rate (per 100,000 people) by year. (From Alzheimer's Association. (2019). Alzheimer's disease facts and figures. *Alzheimer's & Dementia: The Journal of the Alzheimer's Association, 15*(3), 321–387.)

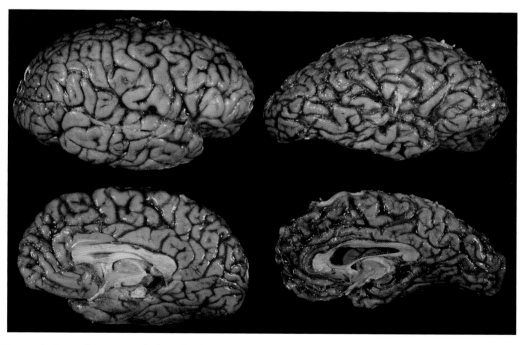

Fig. 4.5 External view of gross pathology in Alzheimer's disease. Comparison of a brain with Alzheimer's disease *(right)* with a healthy brain *(left)*. Note that the meningeal vessels are more prominent in the brain with Alzheimer's disease because the brain gyri have shrunk, revealing the vessels.

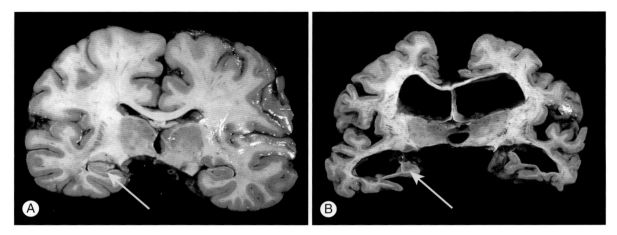

Fig. 4.6 Coronal view of gross pathology in Alzheimer's disease. Coronal view through a brain with Alzheimer's disease **(B)** compared with a healthy brain **(A)**. Note the hippocampus *(arrows)*, intact in the healthy brain and atrophic in the brain with Alzheimer's disease (note also the enlarged ventricles).

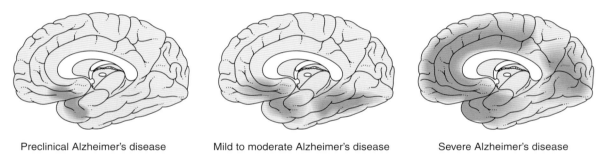

Preclinical Alzheimer's disease   Mild to moderate Alzheimer's disease   Severe Alzheimer's disease

Fig. 4.7 Alzheimer's disease spreads through the brain.

and acetylcholine synthesis (Mesulam et al., 2004). Studies have shown a correlation between the loss of choline acetyltransferase and impairment of cognition (Mesulam, 2004). These data have led to the cholinergic hypothesis of Alzheimer's disease that, in turn, has led to the development of acetylcholinesterase inhibitor therapies to treat this disorder (see Chapter 19). Other studies have shown that, in addition to acetylcholine, many other neurotransmitters also become disrupted as the disease progresses, including norepinephrine, serotonin, glutamate, and dopamine (Fig. 4.10).

DIAGNOSTIC CRITERIA

There are several different clinical diagnostic criteria that are used for Alzheimer's disease. The two most

common are from the Diagnostic and Statistical Manual of Mental Disorders (DSM; current edition 5) and the National Institute on Aging–Alzheimer's Association Criteria (Albert et al., 2011; McKhann et al., 2011) (Boxes 4.1–4.3). Each has provided criteria for Alzheimer's disease dementia (called major neurocognitive disorder due to Alzheimer's disease in DSM-5) and mild cognitive impairment due to Alzheimer's disease (called mild neurocognitive disorder due to Alzheimer's disease in DSM-5).

For Alzheimer's disease dementia, common elements of each are:
- the presence of dementia (see Chapter 3)
- deficits in two or more cognitive areas
- insidious onset and a gradually progressive decline
- no evidence of another etiology that could substantial contribute to the dementia.

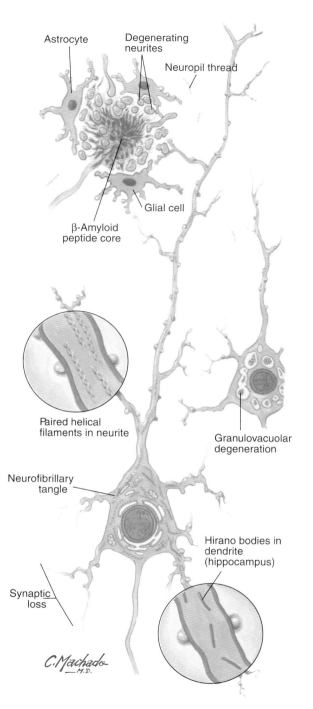

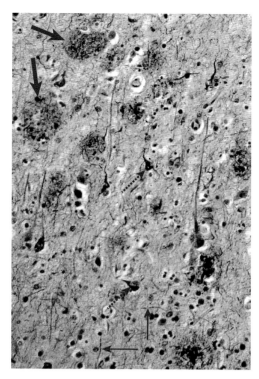

Fig. 4.9 Light microscopic view of Alzheimer's pathology. Plaques *(thick arrows)*, tangles *(dotted arrows)*, and neuropil threads *(thin arrows)* in Alzheimer's disease.

Fig. 4.8 Some of the pathological features in Alzheimer's disease. (Netter illustration from www.netterimages.com. Copyright Elsevier Inc. All rights reserved.)

For mild cognitive impairment due to Alzheimer's disease, the common elements of each are:

- the presence of mild cognitive impairment (see Chapter 3)
- deficits in one or more cognitive areas, including memory (for DSM-5) or typically including memory (for NIA-AA)
- gradual onset and progression
- no evidence of another etiology that could substantially contribute to the mild cognitive impairment.

There is also a more recent National Institute on Aging–Alzheimer's Association research framework (Jack et al., 2018) that offers clarification and simplification of several aspects of the 2011 criteria. First, as described in Chapter 3, they provide new definitions for cognitively unimpaired, mild cognitive impairment, and dementia due to any cause. Second, they separate Alzheimer's disease as a pathologic entity from the Alzheimer's clinical syndrome. Other terms previously used for Alzheimer's

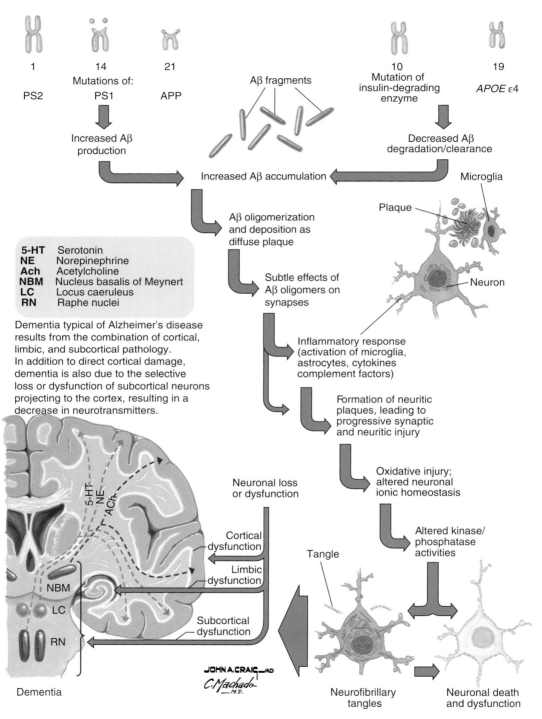

Fig. 4.10 The amyloid cascade hypothesis in Alzheimer's disease. (Netter illustration from www.netterimages.com. Copyright Elsevier Inc. All rights reserved.)

BOX 4.1   **Diagnostic and Statistical Manual of Mental Disorders, 5th Edition Criteria for Major or Mild Neurocognitive Disorder Resulting due to Alzheimer's Disease**

A. The criteria are met for major or mild neurocognitive disorder.

B. There is insidious onset and gradual progression of impairment in one or more cognitive domains (for major neurocognitive disorder, at least two domains must be impaired).

C. Criteria are met for either probable or possible Alzheimer's disease as follows:

For major neurocognitive disorder:
Probable Alzheimer's disease is diagnosed if either of the following is present; otherwise **possible Alzheimer's disease** should be diagnosed.
   1. Evidence of a causative Alzheimer's disease genetic mutation from family history or genetic testing.
   2. All three of the following are present:
      a. Clear evidence of decline in memory and learning and at least one other cognitive domain (based on detailed history or serial neuropsychological testing).
      b. Steadily progressive, gradual decline in cognition, without extended plateaus.
      c. No evidence of mixed etiology (i.e., absence of other neurodegenerative or cerebrovascular disease, or another neurological, mental, or systemic disease or condition likely contributing to cognitive decline).

For mild neurocognitive disorder:
Probable Alzheimer's disease is diagnosed if there is evidence of a causative Alzheimer's disease genetic mutation from either genetic testing or family history.
Possible Alzheimer's disease is diagnosed if there is no evidence of a causative Alzheimer's disease genetic mutation from either genetic testing or family history, and all three of the following are present:
   1. Clear evidence of decline in memory and learning.
   2. Steadily progressive, gradual decline in cognition, without extended plateaus.
   3. No evidence of mixed etiology (i.e., absence of other neurodegenerative or cerebrovascular disease, or another neurological or systemic disease or condition likely contributing to cognitive decline).

D. The disturbance is not better explained by cerebrovascular disease, another neurodegenerative disease, the effects of a substance, or another mental, neurological, or systemic disorder.

From American Psychiatric Association. (2013). *Diagnostic and statistical manual of mental disorders (DSM-5)* (5th ed.). Arlington, VA: American Psychiatric Association.

clinical syndrome include "progressive amnestic dysfunction" (Mesulam, 2000), "probable Alzheimer's dementia," and "dementia of the Alzheimer's type." (We prefer the term *progressive amnestic dysfunction* because it is simple, self-explanatory, and less likely to be confused with the pathologic entity of Alzheimer's disease.) Third, they provide a new definition of biomarkers to help identify when Alzheimer's disease pathology is actually present (which requires evidence of both amyloid and phosphorylated tau deposition in the brain), as well as when neurodegeneration is present (Box 4.4). This framework can be used to simplify the cumbersome nomenclature of the 2011 criteria (McKhann et al., 2011). In this chapter we have provided the 2011 core criteria for probable Alzheimer's disease dementia (see Box 4.2) and mild cognitive impairment due to Alzheimer's disease (see Box 4.3) because of their clinical utility, as well as the 2018 syndromal cognitive stage and biomarker profile table (Table 4.1)—rather than the somewhat confusing 2011 definitions of possible Alzheimer's disease and probable Alzheimer's disease dementia with increased level of certainty.

RISK FACTORS, PATHOLOGY, AND PATHOPHYSIOLOGY

Age is the primary risk factor for Alzheimer's disease. Other risk factors include family history of Alzheimer's disease, female gender, few years of education, medical factors (including strokes, elevated plasma homocysteine levels, obstructive sleep apnea, and other risk factors for cerebrovascular disease), lifestyle choices, and genetic factors, particularly certain allelic forms of the gene coding for apolipoprotein E (APOE). Head injury may also be a risk factor for Alzheimer's disease in addition to dementia with Lewy bodies (see Chapter 8) and chronic traumatic encephalopathy (CTE) (see Chapter 15). Late-onset depression has been associated with increased risk of cognitive decline, although depression may be an early sign of Alzheimer's disease (see Chapter 17). In addition, as many as 90% of individuals with trisomy 21 (Down's syndrome) who die over the age of 30 show Alzheimer's disease pathology in their brains, suggesting that it may be found in all

---

BOX 4.2 **National Institute on Aging–Alzheimer's Association, Probable Alzheimer's Disease Dementia (Also Termed Progressive Amnestic Dysfunction, Alzheimer's Clinical Syndrome, or Dementia of the Alzheimer's Type)**

Probable Alzheimer's disease dementia is diagnosed when the patient:

1. Meets NIA-AA criteria for dementia described in Chapter 3, and in addition, has the following characteristics:
   A. Insidious onset. Symptoms have a gradual onset over months to years, not sudden over hours or days;
   B. Clear-cut history of worsening of cognition by report or observation; and
   C. The initial and most prominent cognitive deficits are evident on history and examination in one of the following categories.
      i. Amnestic presentation: It is the most common syndromic presentation of Alzheimer's disease dementia. The deficits should include impairment in learning and recall of recently learned information. There should also be evidence of cognitive dysfunction in at least one other cognitive domain, as defined in the NIA-AA criteria for dementia described in Chapter 3.
      ii. Nonamnestic presentations:
         • Language presentation: The most prominent deficits are in word-finding, but deficits in other cognitive domains should be present.
         • Visuospatial presentation: The most prominent deficits are in spatial cognition, including object

agnosia, impaired face recognition, simultanagnosia, and alexia. Deficits in other cognitive domains should be present.
         • Executive dysfunction: The most prominent deficits are impaired reasoning, judgment, and problem solving. Deficits in other cognitive domains should be present.
   D. The diagnosis of probable Alzheimer's disease dementia should not be applied when there is evidence of (a) substantial concomitant cerebrovascular disease, defined by a history of a stroke temporally related to the onset or worsening of cognitive impairment; or the presence of multiple or extensive infarcts or severe white matter hyperintensity burden; or (b) core features of dementia with Lewy bodies other than dementia itself; or (c) prominent features of behavioral variant frontotemporal dementia; or (d) prominent features of semantic variant primary progressive aphasia or nonfluent/agrammatic variant primary progressive aphasia; or (e) evidence for another concurrent, active neurological disease, or a non-neurological medical comorbidity or use of medication that could have a substantial effect on cognition.

Modified from McKhann, G. M., Knopman, D. S., Chertkow, H., et al. (2011). The diagnosis of dementia due to Alzheimer's disease: Recommendations from the National Institute on Aging–Alzheimer's Association workgroups on diagnostic guidelines for Alzheimer's disease. *Alzheimer's & Dementia: The Journal of the Alzheimer's Association, 7*, 263–269.

BOX 4.3 **National Institute on Aging–Alzheimer's Association, Clinical and Cognitive Criteria for Mild Cognitive Impairment due to Alzheimer's Disease**

Establish clinical and cognitive criteria for mild cognitive impairment

• Cognitive concern reflecting a change in cognition reported by patient or informant or clinician (i.e., historical or observed evidence of decline over time)
• Objective evidence of impairment in one or more cognitive domains, typically including memory (i.e., formal or bedside testing to establish level of cognitive function in multiple domains)
• Preservation of independence in functional abilities

• Not demented.

Examine etiology of mild cognitive impairment due to Alzheimer's disease pathophysiological process

• Rule out vascular, traumatic, medical causes of cognitive decline, where possible
• Provide evidence of longitudinal decline in cognition, when feasible
• Report history consistent with Alzheimer's disease genetic factors, where relevant.

Modified from Albert, M. S., DeKosky, S. T., Dickson, D., et al. (2011). The diagnosis of mild cognitive impairment due to Alzheimer's disease: Recommendations from the National Institute on Aging–Alzheimer's Association workgroups on diagnostic guidelines for Alzheimer's disease. *Alzheimer's & Dementia: The Journal of the Alzheimer's Association, 7*, 270–279.

BOX 4.4 Amyloid, Tau, Neurodegeneration or AT(N) Biomarker Grouping

A: Aggregated Aβ or associated pathologic state
- Low CSF $A\beta_{42}$ or $A\beta_{42}/A\beta_{40}$ ratio
- Positive amyloid PET

T: Aggregated tau (neurofibrillary tangles) or associated pathologic state
- Elevated CSF phosphorylated tau
- Positive tau PET

(N): Neurodegeneration or neuronal injury
- Atrophy on anatomic MRI
- Decreased metabolism on [18]flurodeoxyglucose (FDG) PET
- Elevated CSF total tau

Note that "(N)" is in parentheses to indicate that, whereas amyloid and phosphorylated tau are specific to Alzheimer's disease, neurodegeneration is nonspecific.

CSF, Cerebrospinal fluid; *MRI*, magnetic resonance imaging; *PET*, positron emission tomography.

Modified from Jack, C. R., Jr., Bennett, D. A., Blennow, K., et al. (Contributors). (2018). NIA-AA research framework: Toward a biological definition of Alzheimer's disease. *Alzheimer's & Dementia: The Journal of the Alzheimer's Association, 14*(4), 535–562.

older individuals with Down's syndrome. Several studies have suggested that having high premorbid intelligence (often correlated with many years of education) may be protective, in addition to healthy lifestyle choices such as physical activity, Mediterranean-style diet, and social engagement (see Chapter 22). Some possible disease-modulating factors have shown mixed results: some studies show a beneficial effect whereas other studies show either no effect or a detrimental effect. The factors with mixed results include estrogen supplementation, certain nonsteroidal antiinflammatory drugs (NSAIDs), certain statin-based lipid-lowering agents, and smoking. Note that intervention trials with NSAIDs and statins have been negative to date (see Chapter 21). One reason that NSAIDs have been suspected as possibly being protective is that inflammation has been postulated as playing an important role in the pathophysiology of Alzheimer's disease (see Fig. 4.10). Lastly, it should also be noted that some of these factors—including but not limited to obesity, diabetes, hypertension, and cardiac disease—may increase the risk of progressive amnestic dysfunction (Alzheimer's clinical syndrome), but not Alzheimer's disease pathology (Vemuri et al., 2012). Nonetheless, we certainly want to encourage our

TABLE 4.1 Alzheimer's Syndromal Cognitive Stage and Biomarker Profile

Biomarker Profile	Syndromal Cognitive Stage		
	Cognitively Unimpaired	**Mild Cognitive Impairment**	**Dementia**
A⁺T⁻(N)⁻	Preclinical Alzheimer's pathologic change	Alzheimer's pathologic change with mild cognitive impairment (MCI)	Alzheimer's pathologic change with dementia
A⁺T⁻(N)⁺	Alzheimer's and concomitant suspected non-Alzheimer's pathologic change, cognitively unimpaired	Alzheimer's and concomitant suspected non-Alzheimer's pathologic change with MCI	Alzheimer's and concomitant suspected non-Alzheimer's pathologic change with dementia
A⁺T⁺(N)⁻ A⁺T⁺(N)⁺	Preclinical Alzheimer's disease	Alzheimer's disease with MCI	Alzheimer's disease with dementia

See Chapter 3 for definition of cognitively unimpaired, mild cognitive impairment, and dementia. See Box 4.3 for definition of biomarkers A, T, and (N). +/− indicates the presence/absence of the biomarker.

Modified from Jack, C. R., Jr., Bennett, D. A., Blennow, K., et al. (Contributors). (2018). NIA-AA research framework: Toward a biological definition of Alzheimer's disease. *Alzheimer's & Dementia: The Journal of the Alzheimer's Association, 14*(4), 535–562.

patients to reduce their risk of dementia, whether from Alzheimer's disease or cerebrovascular pathology. As mentioned in Chapter 3, most clinical dementia results from mixed pathology,

Alzheimer's Disease Is Not Part of Normal Aging

Given that age is the primary risk factor for Alzheimer's disease and that such a high percentage of older adults develop the disease, it is reasonable to wonder whether Alzheimer's disease is simply part of the normal aging process. We do not believe that this idea is correct. Alzheimer's disease is simply more common in aging, as are hypertension, type 2 diabetes, and cancer. At least three lines of evidence support the idea that Alzheimer's is a distinct age-related, but not age-determined, disease. First, many individuals live into their 80s and 90s without evidence of significant cognitive impairment, as do roughly half of centenarians. Second, patients with the accelerated aging disorder progeria do not develop dementia. Third, although autopsies may show some Alzheimer's pathology in the brains of normal older adults without cognitive impairment, the density of these neurofibrillary tangles and senile plaques is markedly lower in these individuals than in those with clinically diagnosed Alzheimer's disease.

Genetic Predisposition

Specific mutations on chromosomes 21, 14, and 1 have been associated with early-onset familial Alzheimer's disease. These patients with autosomal-dominant early-onset disease are relatively rare, and are typically easy to diagnose by family history. Patients with early-onset disease present clinically in their 40s and 50s, and usually family members can detect subtle changes years before clinical onset. The genetics of late-onset Alzheimer's disease has been harder to elucidate. The strongest genetic risk factor for late-onset Alzheimer's disease is the APOE allele. Relative to having an APOE ε3 allele, patients having an APOE ε4 allele are at increased risk of developing Alzheimer's disease (see Fig. 4.10 and 4.11).

Apolipoprotein E

APOE is a major component of lipoproteins and has many normal functions, including lipid transport. The gene coding for APOE is on chromosome 19. The three common isoforms of APOE are APOE-2, APOE-3, and

APOE-4, coded for by alleles ε2, ε3, and ε4, respectively. APOE ε3 is the most common allele in the population, with a frequency of about 78%. Patients with familial and sporadic late-onset Alzheimer's disease (onset after age 55 years) have an approximately 3-fold increased likelihood of having an APOE ε4 allele. Conversely, the likelihood of having an APOE ε2 allele is lower than expected by allelic frequencies alone. Numerous studies have confirmed these findings, which suggest that APOE ε4 is a risk factor for developing Alzheimer's disease, whereas APOE ε2 is a protective factor. In addition to conferring increased risk of developing Alzheimer's disease, having an APOE ε4 allele also lowers the age of onset of the disease compared with those without an ε4 allele who develop it (van der Lee et al., 2018). The majority of studies suggest that the course of Alzheimer's disease is not affected by the presence of an ε4 allele, although a few studies have disagreed with this finding. Neuropathologically, in patients with Alzheimer's disease there is more Aβ deposition in the brains of those with an ε4 allele than in those who have only ε3 alleles.

Should APOE genotyping be ordered routinely? Given the wealth of clinical and basic science data on the relationship between APOE and Alzheimer's disease, the question arises as to whether APOE genotyping should be performed routinely. We would argue that, in general, it is not clinically useful. Although carrying an APOE ε4 allele is a significant risk factor, it is neither necessary nor sufficient to cause Alzheimer's disease. First, approximately half of patients with Alzheimer's disease do not carry an APOE ε4 allele. Second, up to one-quarter of patients with non-Alzheimer's dementias carry an ε4 allele. Third, 10% to 19% of healthy older adults carry one or two ε4 alleles. Fourth, because APOE alleles are present from birth, APOE genotyping cannot be used to distinguish mild Alzheimer's disease from normal aging. Thus using the APOE ε4 allele as a marker of Alzheimer's disease would result in huge numbers of both false positives and false negatives. Although it can be helpful in research, we do not recommend APOE genotyping in clinical practice.

Family History

A family history of Alzheimer's disease in a first-degree relative increases the risk of developing Alzheimer's disease between 2-fold and 4-fold (Lampert et al., 2013), and more distant family relatives with Alzheimer's also increase one's risk (Cannon-Albright et al., 2019). Knowledge of this increase in risk causes many

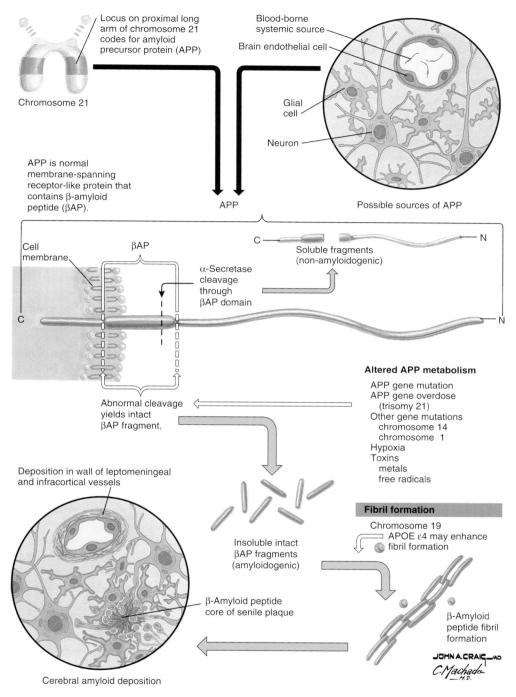

Locus on proximal long arm of chromosome 21 codes for amyloid precursor protein (APP)

Chromosome 21

Blood-borne systemic source

Brain endothelial cell

Glial cell

Neuron

Possible sources of APP

APP is normal membrane-spanning receptor-like protein that contains β-amyloid peptide (βAP).

APP

Cell membrane

βAP

C   N

Soluble fragments (non-amyloidogenic)

α-Secretase cleavage through βAP domain

C   N

Altered APP metabolism

APP gene mutation
APP gene overdose (trisomy 21)
Other gene mutations
  chromosome 14
  chromosome 1
Hypoxia
Toxins
  metals
  free radicals

Abnormal cleavage yields intact βAP fragment.

Deposition in wall of leptomeningeal and infracortical vessels

Insoluble intact βAP fragments (amyloidogenic)

β-Amyloid peptide core of senile plaque

Fibril formation

Chromosome 19
APOE ε4 may enhance fibril formation

β-Amyloid peptide fibril formation

JOHN A. CRAIG—MD
C. Machado—M.D.

Cerebral amyloid deposition

Fig. 4.11 Possible pathways for normal and pathological Aβ processing. (Netter illustration from www.netterimages.com. Copyright Elsevier Inc. All rights reserved.)

middle-aged children of patients with Alzheimer's disease to become apprehensive that they, too, will develop this disorder. We generally point out to these family members that, although the risk of Alzheimer's disease is increased with a family history of the disorder, Alzheimer's disease is unfortunately extremely common as we age, such that everyone is at risk for the disorder, with or without a family history. More importantly, if the overall risk of Alzheimer's disease is about 2.5% between ages 65 and 70, the risk without a family history is probably around 1.5% and the risk with a family history is probably around 3%. Thus, although the relative risk may be doubled, the overall risk is still quite small. See Chapter 30 for more on this important topic.

Gender

As mentioned, approximately two-thirds of patients with Alzheimer's disease are women, with the overall lifetime risk being 11.6% for men and 21.1% for women. This finding cannot solely be explained by the longer life expectancy of women resulting in larger numbers of women living into old age. Factors that have been suggested to explain this phenomenon include hormonal differences between men and women, different lifelong environmental exposures, and differences in years of education. More research is needed on this important topic.

Education

It has been suggested that an increased number of years of education may reduce the risk of Alzheimer's disease, possibly by creating a "cognitive reserve" or a higher mental threshold that delays the onset of clinical symptoms. High educational attainment may also allow patients to compensate for some memory loss (by using memorization strategies, for example), disguising their symptoms and making diagnosis more challenging. Several studies suggest that low educational attainment is a risk factor for Alzheimer's disease: one study found that an uneducated person over the age of 75 years is twice as likely to suffer dementia as is a person who has completed the 8th grade or higher. In another study, low linguistic ability early in life predicted poor cognitive function and Alzheimer's disease in late life (Snowdon et al., 1996; Snowdon, Greiner, & Markesbery, 2000). In the Framingham Heart Disease Study, however, low educational attainment was not found to be a significant risk factor for Alzheimer's disease (although it was for vascular dementia) (Cobb et al., 1995). Overall, we do consider education to be an important factor when considering a patient's risk of Alzheimer's disease.

Trauma

Traumatic head injury associated with loss of consciousness or posttraumatic amnesia has been shown to be a risk factor for Alzheimer's disease, with some studies showing a relative risk greater than two (Fleminger et al., 2003). Several studies have suggested that the risk of Alzheimer's disease related to head injury is mediated through a specific genetic predisposition. One study found a 10-fold increase in Alzheimer's disease in individuals with traumatic head injury and an APOE ε4 allele, whereas no increase in the disease was seen in individuals without an APOE ε4 allele (Mayeux et al., 1995). Chronic traumatic encephalopathy, previously known as dementia pugilistica, may be found in boxers and other individuals with a history of repeated head injury (e.g., football players); its relationship to Alzheimer's disease is still being determined (see Chapter 15). Some speculate that the majority of individuals with a history of multiple concussions who develop progressive amnestic dysfunction have underlying chronic traumatic encephalopathy pathology, and not Alzheimer's disease. However, it is clear from the few studies that included pathology that traumatic brain injury increases the risk of Alzheimer's disease (Mckee & Daneshvar, 2015).

Strokes

Strokes do not cause Alzheimer's pathology, but may contribute to cognitive dysfunction in patients who already have Alzheimer's pathology. Patients who have Alzheimer's pathology as well as small vessel ischemic strokes in the white matter and deep gray structures in the brain (basal ganglia, thalamus) are thus likely to have more cognitive dysfunction and dementia than those without these strokes (Snowdon et al., 1997). Cerebrovascular disease can thereby turn an individual with asymptomatic Alzheimer's pathology into a patient with dementia. It is for this reason that reducing cerebrovascular risk factors can help prevent the development of progressive amnestic dysfunction (Alzheimer's clinical syndrome). Elevated plasma homocysteine levels—a known risk factor for strokes—is also a risk factor for the development of progressive amnestic dysfunction (Seshadri et al., 2002). This effect of homocysteine is likely present because strokes may hasten a clinical diagnosis of dementia in a patient who already has Alzheimer's pathology (Luchsinger et al., 2004; Miller et al., 2002).

COMMON SIGNS, SYMPTOMS, AND STAGES

Alzheimer's disease typically first presents with memory loss for recent information, followed by word-finding difficulties, visuospatial difficulties, and frontal/executive dysfunction. As the disorder progresses, behavioral problems often develop such as irritability, exacerbation of premorbid personality traits, and sometimes aggression. Patients continue to lose function until they require round-the-clock care, usually in a long-term care facility.

As it is currently conceptualized, Alzheimer's disease starts with a preclinical asymptomatic phase, followed by a mild cognitive impairment phase, and then finally a dementia phase which itself is typically divided into different stages. There is also sometimes a subjective cognitive decline phase in-between the asymptomatic and mild cognitive impairment phases (see Chapter 3 for additional information on the different phases). Although there are no universally accepted definitions for the staging of patients with Alzheimer's disease dementia, most clinicians agree that there are at least four stages of the disease—very mild, mild, moderate, and severe—each with its own cognitive, functional, and behavioral issues (Tables 4.2 and 4.3). Note that some patients with mild cognitive impairment due to Alzheimer's disease would also fit with the description below of the 0.5 (very mild) Clinical Dementia Rating.

Mild Cognitive Impairment due to Alzheimer's Disease

Patients with the mild cognitive impairment stage of Alzheimer's disease often begin to show a decline in a single cognitive domain, which is typically memory. Because of this early decline in memory, most of these patients are described as having "amnestic mild cognitive impairment." The decline may, however, be in another cognitive domain, such as language presenting with mild word finding difficulty or executive function presenting with difficulty doing a complicated task (e.g., preparing a multicourse holiday meal). Patients with mild cognitive impairment may also show impairments in more than one cognitive domain, so long as they remain independent in their functional abilities and therefore do not

meet criteria for dementia. One particular difference between patients with mild cognitive impairment due to Alzheimer's disease and those with Alzheimer's disease dementia is that insight is often preserved in patients with mild cognitive impairment. This insight, although often helpful in using compensatory strategies when dealing with memory difficulties, may also lead to depression. This very common secondary depression is certainly one of the reasons that it is easy to confuse mild cognitive impairment due to underlying Alzheimer's pathology with a primary depression causing secondary memory problems. (See the section on Depression and Anxiety in Chapter 17 for more on how to distinguish depression from other etiologies of memory loss.)

Very Mild Alzheimer's Disease Dementia

Patients with very mild Alzheimer's disease dementia show a slight but definite decline in memory, and sometimes in word-finding as well. They tend to be fully oriented, except perhaps for knowing the date. They show slight impairments in judgment and problem-solving, community affairs, and home life and hobbies. For example, balancing the checkbook and keeping track of bills may become more difficult, and they may buy the same grocery items a number of times. They can usually manage their medications with a pill-box or other system of organization. These patients are typically able to prepare simple meals, and can usually be on their own for a few days at a time without getting into trouble. Most patients with very mild Alzheimer's disease dementia are safe to drive, although they may become lost on occasion, particularly when driving at night or to a new location (for more on driving see Chapter 28).

Mild Alzheimer's Disease Dementia

Patients with mild Alzheimer's disease dementia show noticeable declines in memory and often word-finding, and these declines interfere with everyday activities. They usually show some disorientation to time and place. Judgment and problem-solving are moderately impaired. They are unable to function independently in community affairs. They cannot perform complicated hobbies and household tasks, but may still be able to perform simple ones. They are able to perform personal care tasks such as brushing teeth, changing clothes, and bathing, although they may need reminding to do these activities. These patients are usually safe to be on their own for a few hours, but may forget to eat, take medications, bathe,

TABLE 4.2   Clinical Dementia Rating Scale for Alzheimer's Disease Dementia

Clinical Dementia Rating	0 (Normal)	0.5 (Very Mild)	1 (Mild)	2 (Moderate)
MMSE mean (range)	29 (27–30)	25.7 (24–27)	20.0 (16–26)	13.6 (6–17)
MoCA mean (range)	26 (22–30)	21 (19–22)	15 (11–21)	9 (5–12)
Memory (major category)	No memory loss or slight inconsistent forgetfulness	Consistent slight forgetfulness, partial recollection of events, "benign" forgetfulness	Moderate memory loss; more marked for recent events; defect interferes with everyday activities	Severe memory loss; only highly learned material retained; new material rapidly lost
Secondary Categories				
Orientation	Fully oriented	Fully oriented except for slight difficulty with time relationships	Moderate difficulty with time relationships; oriented for place at examination; may have geographic disorientation elsewhere	Severe difficulty with time relationships; usually disoriented to time, often to place
Judgment and problem-solving	Solves everyday problems and handles business and financial affairs well; judgment good in relation to past performance	Slight impairment in solving problems, and understanding similarities and differences	Moderate difficulties in handling problems, understanding similarities and differences; social judgment usually maintained	Severely impaired in handling problems, understanding similarities and differences; social judgment usually impaired
Community affairs	Independent function at usual level in job, shopping, and volunteer and social groups	Slight impairment in these activities	Unable to function independently at these activities although may still be engaged in some; appears normal to casual inspection	No pretense of independent function outside home. Appears well enough to be taken to function outside a family home
Home and hobbies	Life at home, hobbies, and intellectual interests are well maintained	Life at home, hobbies, and intellectual interests slightly impaired	Mild but definite impairment of function at home, more difficult chores abandoned, more complicated hobbies and interests abandoned	Only simple chores preserved; very restricted interests, poorly maintained
Personal care	Fully capable of self-care	Fully capable of self-care	Needs prompting	Requires assistance in dressing, hygiene, keeping of personal effects

MMSE, Mini-Mental State Examination; *MoCA*, Montreal Cognitive Assessment.
Modified from Morris, J. C. (1993). The Clinical Dementia Rating (CDR): current version and scoring rules. *Neurology, 43,* 2412–2414.

TABLE 4.3 Alzheimer's Disease Staging and Clinical Signs

Preclinical, Mild Cognitive Impairment	Mild Alzheimer's Disease	Moderate Alzheimer's Disease	Severe/Late-Stage Alzheimer's Disease
Very mild cognitive decline	Memory loss	Increasing memory loss	Inability to recognize family or to communicate
Memory lapses	Confusion about location or familiar places	Confusion	Lost sense of self
Mild word-finding difficulties	Taking longer to accomplish normal daily tasks	Problems recognizing friends and family	Weight loss
Decline in ability to plan and organize; activities take longer	Trouble handling money and paying bills	Poor judgment leading to bad decisions	Groaning, moaning, grunting
	Poor judgment leading to bad decisions	Difficulty organizing thoughts and thinking logically	Increased sleeping
	Loss of spontaneity and sense of initiative	Inability to learn new things or to cope with new or unexpected situations	Lack of bladder and bowel control
	Mood and personality changes, increased anxiety	Restlessness, agitation, anxiety, tearfulness, wandering	Seizures, skin infections, difficulty swallowing
		Repetitive statements or movement	Aspiration pneumonia
		Delusions, suspiciousness, paranoia	Death

and change their clothes if left alone for a few days. Most patients with mild Alzheimer's disease dementia should not drive, as their judgment, processing speed, and executive and visuospatial function all begin to be impaired.

Moderate Alzheimer's Disease Dementia

In moderate Alzheimer's disease dementia, memory loss is severe; only remote and/or very prominent memories are retained, and almost all new material is rapidly lost. Disorientation to time and place are common. Judgment and problem-solving show severe impairment. Although the patient appears well enough to be taken to activities outside the home, there is no pretense of independent function. Only simple hobbies and household tasks can be maintained. Assistance is needed in personal care activities such as dressing and hygiene, and urinary incontinence often develops. Patients with moderate Alzheimer's disease dementia should not be left alone because of potential issues of wandering, incontinence, and safety.

Severe Alzheimer's Disease Dementia

In the severe stage of Alzheimer's disease, memory is severely impaired and only fragments of memory remain. The patient is typically only oriented to self. Judgment and problem-solving are not possible. The patient appears too ill to be taken to activities outside the home, and the patient is not capable of pursuing hobbies or performing household tasks. The patient requires help with all aspects of personal care and is frequently incontinent of both urine and feces. Patients with severe Alzheimer's disease dementia are usually managed in a long-term care facility.

THINGS TO LOOK FOR IN THE HISTORY

Alzheimer's disease typically starts insidiously with either memory loss or word-finding difficulties. Different family members often date the onset of symptoms to different months or years; such disagreement is common and suggests an insidious onset. Usually symptoms are noticeable for 6 months to several years before coming to the attention of a healthcare professional.

In addition to memory loss and word-finding difficulties, other common signs and symptoms to look for in the history include geographical disorientation (getting lost) and impairments in reasoning, problem-solving, and judgments. Apathy, depression, and anxiety are common in mild cognitive impairment due to Alzheimer's disease and become more noticeable in very mild and mild Alzheimer's disease dementia. Impairment in controlling one's behavior increases as the disease progresses. See Chapter 2 for an in-depth discussion of these and other elements of the history in Alzheimer's disease.

THINGS TO LOOK FOR ON THE PHYSICAL AND NEUROLOGICAL EXAMINATION

In mild cognitive impairment due to Alzheimer's disease and very mild Alzheimer's disease dementia, the physical and neurological examination is typically normal, except for trouble with praxis (see Chapter 13). As the disease progresses into the mild, moderate, and severe dementia stages, a number of neurological signs often develop, including brisk deep tendon reflexes and frontal release signs such as the snout, grasp, and palmomental reflexes. See Chapter 2 for a discussion of these frontal release signs. Although none of these signs are sensitive or specific for Alzheimer's disease, they do suggest that something is wrong in the central nervous system, and thus support the diagnosis of a brain disease of some type (as opposed to, for example, depression or normal aging).

PATTERN OF IMPAIRMENT ON COGNITIVE TESTS

Memory, language, reasoning and judgment, visuospatial function, and attention may all be impaired in Alzheimer's disease. However, in the mild cognitive impairment, very mild, and mild stages there are common patterns that may be observed on cognitive tests that may aid in diagnosis. In addition to the discussions below, please also see Chapters 2 and 3 for additional information on the pattern of cognitive impairment in Alzheimer's disease.

Memory

Although Alzheimer's disease may affect episodic memory in several different ways, one hallmark of the disease is that memory is impaired even when the learning or encoding of information is maximized by multiple rehearsals, and after retrieval demands have been minimized with the use of a multiple-choice recognition test. In other words, even when patients appear to have successfully learned new information by repeating it back over several learning trials, they are typically unable to recall the information and often even to recognize this information on a multiple-choice test (see Appendix C for more information). This type of memory loss is often referred to as a "rapid rate of forgetting," although whether the information has been truly learned or not in the first place has been a matter of debate (e.g., Budson et al., 2007).

From a practical standpoint, this means that in the mild cognitive impairment, very mild, and mild stages of Alzheimer's disease the registration or learning of the items is usually intact, but recall is usually impaired and patients are also unable to choose the registered words from a list (such as on the MoCA). Similarly, on more comprehensive tests that include both recall and recognition components (such as the CERAD word list memory test [Welsh et al., 1992]), there will be a number of words successfully learned in the encoding trials that are not recognized on the recognition test.

Language

In mild cognitive impairment due to Alzheimer's disease language is often normal. In very mild or mild Alzheimer's disease dementia the problems with language are usually due to the combination of an anomia plus an impairment of semantic memory. From a cognitive testing standpoint, two aspects of this impairment are typically found. First, there is an anomia, or impairment in naming uncommon objects. In very mild and mild Alzheimer's disease dementia this impairment may be observed in tests such as the Boston Naming Test (Balthazar et al., 2008). In this test, line drawings of items are presented, with very common items shown at the beginning of the test (e.g., comb) and less common items shown toward the end of the test (e.g., trellis). Although the official Boston Naming Test consists of 60 items, 30- and 15-item versions have been successfully used. Note that only when patients reach the moderate stage of Alzheimer's disease dementia do they typically show difficulty in naming the two items on the MMSE and the three animals on the MoCA.

The second aspect of language that is typically impaired in Alzheimer's disease is the ability to generate an adequate number of words in 1 minute in certain semantic categories, such as "animals," "fruits," and "vegetables." In fact, many patients with very mild and mild disease show impairment on these tests of word generation to categories, but perform normally on tests of word generation to letters. See Chapter 2 and Appendix A for additional discussion of these tests.

Reasoning and Judgment

Patients with Alzheimer's at almost all stages of disease beyond mild cognitive impairment are impaired in their reasoning, judgment, problem-solving, abstraction, and insight. Although an idea of impairment in these abilities is typically best obtained from the history, they may be evaluated in several other ways as well. First, there are a number of standard neuropsychological tests to evaluate this aspect of cognition. Second, impairment in these abilities may also be observed in the clinic by asking patients:

- what they would do in certain situations (e.g., "What would you do if you found an envelope on the street with an address and a stamp on it?"),
- to interpret proverbs (e.g., "What does it mean to say: a rolling stone gathers no moss?"), or
- to make abstractions (e.g., "How are a table and chair alike?").

Visuospatial Function

Visuospatial function is impaired in Alzheimer's disease beyond the mild cognitive impairment stage, and it becomes progressively worse as the disease worsens. In the very mild or mild dementia stage of disease, difficulty with somewhat complex tasks such as clock drawing and copying cubes and intersecting pentagons may be impaired. In later stages even fewer demanding tasks such as copying familiar shapes (such as a triangle) become difficult.

Attention

It is important to differentiate simple versus complex attention. Simple attention, such as counting from 1 to 20, reciting the months of the year forwards, spelling a common word, or performing simple addition (e.g., 2 plus 5) is typically intact in the mild cognitive impairment, very mild, and mild stages of Alzheimer's disease. More complex attention requiring the use of working memory (the ability to maintain information in memory while at the same time manipulating this information), however, is often impaired at the mild stage of the disease. Complex attention includes tasks such as counting from 20 back down to one, reciting the months of the year backwards, spelling a common word backwards,

and performing more complex arithmetic (e.g., subtracting 7s serially from 100).

Examples

On the MMSE, the patient with mild cognitive impairment due to Alzheimer's disease will typically range from 25 to 30, with points lost recalling one to three of the recall items, and perhaps the date. In addition to these items, the patient with very mild Alzheimer's disease dementia may show difficulty with serial 7s/WORLD backwards and intersecting pentagons. Patients in the mild stage of Alzheimer's disease dementia may also show difficulty with the year, month, day, county, city, name of place, floor, the three-step command, and writing a sentence. In the moderate and severe stages of Alzheimer's disease, as language becomes more impaired, patients may show difficulty with the remaining items as well.

On the MoCA patients with mild cognitive impairment due to Alzheimer's disease typically score between 19 and 26, often missing points for delayed recall and perhaps the date. In the very mild and mild stage of Alzheimer's disease dementia patients often have increasing trouble with the alternating number-letter connect-the-dots, 3-dimensional figure copy, and clock hands, serial 7s, and abstraction. Trouble with additional items occurs as the patient progresses into the moderate stage.

LABORATORY STUDIES

There are no routine laboratory studies that support the diagnosis of Alzheimer's disease. It is, of course, important to obtain a number of screening laboratory studies to search for readily treatable causes of cognitive dysfunction, as described in Chapter 2. Tests of cerebrospinal fluid measuring Aβ42, total tau, and phosphorylated tau should be considered in certain circumstances, such as when the patient appears to have a straightforward case of Alzheimer's disease dementia or mild cognitive impairment due to Alzheimer's disease—but is younger than 66 years old—to confirm that this disorder is, in fact, present so that the work-up can be stopped. Please see Chapter 2 for these and additional tests that may be important to consider in the evaluation.

STRUCTURAL IMAGING STUDIES

It should first be clearly stated that Alzheimer's disease cannot be either ruled in or ruled out by the pattern of atrophy observable on a structural imaging scan, or the lack of such atrophy. The primary purpose in obtaining a structural imaging study is to identify or rule out other etiologies that may cause dementia. Thus a structural imaging study is ordered to evaluate for the presence of large strokes, tumors, hemorrhages, hydrocephalus, the extent of small vessel ischemic disease, and other such pathology.

Having stated that structural imaging studies cannot be used to diagnose Alzheimer's disease or to refute it, as mentioned in Chapter 2, it is worthwhile looking to determine whether there is atrophy bilaterally in hippocampi, anterior temporal lobes, and parietal lobes (Fig. 4.12). If this pattern of atrophy is present in combination with the appropriate clinical context it may suggest that Alzheimer's disease pathology is present. Brain atrophy is also one of the signs of neurodegeneration—the (N) in the 2018 AT(N) research framework (see Box 4.4). Structural imaging studies are also invaluable for showing the extent of small vessel ischemic disease that a patient has. Because almost every patient aged 70 years or older has some small vessel ischemic disease, the question for the clinician is whether the extent of the small vessel ischemic disease is a minor, a major, or (rarely) the sole factor in the patient's memory loss. See Fig. 2.3 for an example of an MRI scan of a patient with mild Alzheimer's disease showing atrophy and an average amount of small vessel ischemic cerebrovascular disease. See Fig. 2.4 for a CT scan of a patient with mild Alzheimer's disease showing hippocampal atrophy.

MOLECULAR AND FUNCTIONAL IMAGING STUDIES

Given that all current treatments for dementia are symptomatic and none are specific for a particular pathology (see Section III), neither a functional imaging study (fluorodeoxyglucose positron emission tomography [FDG PET] or ^{99}Tc single photon emission computed tomography [SPECT]), nor a molecular imaging study (amyloid or tau PET) is necessary in the evaluation of the vast majority of patients in whom Alzheimer's disease is suspected. If the history and cognitive examination suggest a case of straightforward Alzheimer's disease in a patient older than age 65 years, the history, physical and neurological examination, cognitive testing, and laboratory and structural imaging studies are sufficient

to make an accurate diagnosis given the high prevalence of Alzheimer's disease in older adults.

Functional and molecular imaging studies are helpful, however, in two circumstances when considering a diagnosis of Alzheimer's disease, as discussed in Chapter 2. First, when the patient is 65 years old or less, we recommend supporting the diagnosis with an amyloid or tau PET scan (or cerebrospinal fluid study) even if the rest of the work-up strongly suggests a case of Alzheimer's disease. The prevalence of Alzheimer's is much lower in someone so young; for this reason, the differential diagnosis is broad, and it becomes as important to "rule in" Alzheimer's disease as it is to "rule out" all other causes of memory loss and dementia. Second, in addition to Alzheimer's disease, when other forms of dementia are being strongly considered, such as frontotemporal dementia, the ^{99}Tc SPECT or FDG-PET metabolic scans can help distinguish between Alzheimer's disease and these other forms of dementia. For additional information see Chapter 2 and Figs. 2.5–2.7. Lastly, tau PET scans are now FDA approved. Following the AT(N) framework described above in Box 4.4 and Table 4.1, some difficult-to-diagnose patients can now undergo both amyloid and tau PET imaging, in addition to MRI, providing the full AT(N) characterization to aid in diagnosis (Fig. 4.13).

DIFFERENTIAL DIAGNOSIS

In our experience, the most common disorders to be confused with Alzheimer's disease are other degenerative dementias. The most common disorder that looks like Alzheimer's is limbic-predominant age-related TDP-43 encephalopathy (LATE, see Chapter 6). If the patient showed behavioral problems and/or personality changes first and foremost, or has prominent problems with reasoning and judgment, then a behavioral variant frontotemporal dementia (see Chapter 10) should be considered. A primary progressive aphasia (see Chapter 9) should be considered if problems with language predominate.

If there are visual hallucinations or visual misperceptions, perhaps around the time of sleep, dementia with Lewy bodies should be considered (see Chapter 8). Dementia with Lewy bodies should also be considered if there is rapid eye movement (REM) sleep behavior disorder or parkinsonism. Note that many patients have the mixed dementia of Alzheimer's disease plus dementia with Lewy bodies. Parkinsonism should also

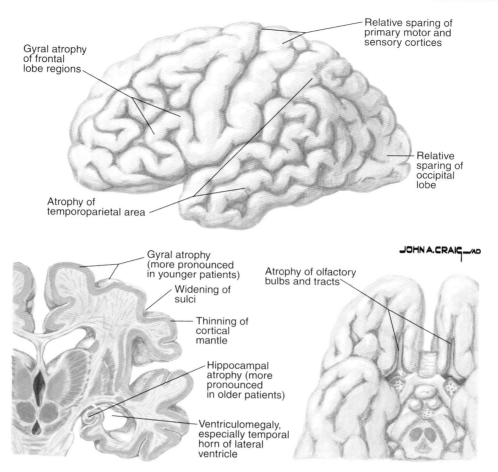

Relative sparing of primary motor and sensory cortices

Gyral atrophy of frontal lobe regions

Relative sparing of occipital lobe

Atrophy of temporoparietal area

Gyral atrophy (more pronounced in younger patients)

Widening of sulci

Thinning of cortical mantle

Hippocampal atrophy (more pronounced in older patients)

Ventriculomegaly, especially temporal horn of lateral ventricle

Atrophy of olfactory bulbs and tracts

JOHN A.CRAIG—AD

Fig. 4.12 Patterns of focal atrophy in Alzheimer's disease. (Netter illustration from www.netterimages.com. Copyright Elsevier Inc. All rights reserved.)

of course lead one to consider Parkinson's disease, and parkinsonian syndromes which affect cognition such as progressive supranuclear palsy (see Chapter 12) and corticobasal degeneration (see Chapter 13).

Vascular dementia should be considered if there are many large or small ischemic strokes on the structural imaging scan (CT or MRI) (see Chapter 7). However, if the history and cognitive examination suggest Alzheimer's disease, then we would argue that the patient most likely has Alzheimer's disease, the symptoms of which may be exacerbated to some extent by the amount of small vessel or other ischemic disease. Whether the patient can be said to have a mixed dementia of Alzheimer's disease plus vascular disease depends upon the amount of vascular disease present on the structural imaging study, and

whether a number of the symptoms are consistent with vascular dementia (see Chapter 7).

TREATMENTS

As discussed in detail in Section III: *Treatment of Memory Loss, Alzheimer's Disease, and Dementia*, current pharmacological therapies to treat Alzheimer's disease include medications approved by the FDA to enhance cognition in Alzheimer's disease (cholinesterase inhibitors and memantine), as well as medications to treat mood, anxiety, agitation, and other behavioral problems (Table 4.4).

For patients with Alzheimer's disease (including those with mild cognitive impairment due to Alzheimer's

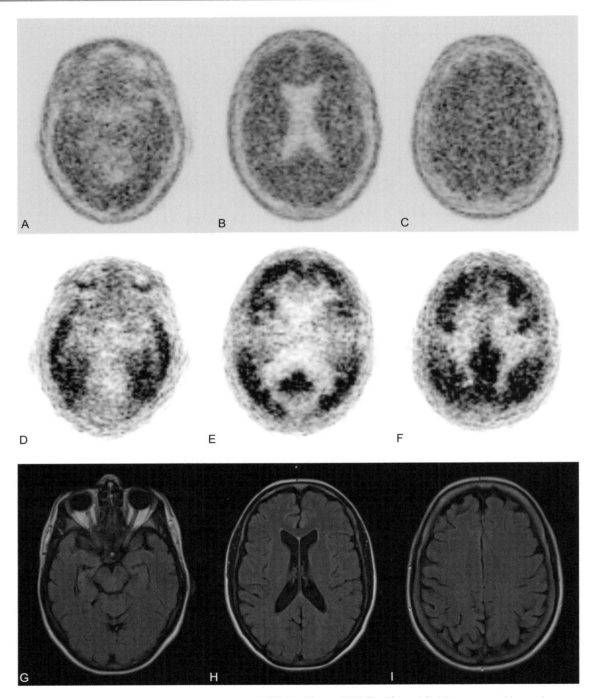

Fig. 4.13 Amyloid positron emission tomography (PET) **(A–C)**, tau PET **(D–F)**, and fluid attenuated inversion recovery (FLAIR) magnetic resonance imaging (MRI) **(G–I)** scans of a patient who has Alzheimer's disease with mild cognitive impairment. According to the National Institute on Aging–Alzheimer's Association research framework she is $A^+T^+(N)^+$ (see Box 4.4 and Table 4.1 for details).

TABLE 4.4 **Medication for Alzheimer's Disease**

Medication Class	U.S. Food and Drug Administration Approved?	Summary of Benefits	Common Side Effects
Cholinesterase inhibitors (see Chapter 19 for comparison of cholinesterase inhibitors)	Yes	Multiple studies demonstrating cognitive, behavioral, and functional benefit	Gastrointestinal (nausea, loose stools), vivid dreams
Memantine (Namenda) (see Chapter 20)	Yes	Multiple studies demonstrating cognitive, behavioral, and functional benefit	Drowsiness and confusion, worse in milder patients
Selective serotonin reuptake inhibitors—particularly those that treat both anxiety and depression (sertraline, escitalopram) (see Chapter 27)	No—off-label use	Treatment if there is depression that often accompanies mild cognitive impairment (MCI) (clinical experience, but no published studies)	Gastrointestinal upset; sexual dysfunction

disease [Petersen, Lopez, & Armstrong, 2018]), we would recommend treatment with a cholinesterase inhibitor: donepezil (Aricept, available as generic), sustained release galantamine (generic), or the rivastigmine (Exelon) patch (oral rivastigmine is not well tolerated). Donepezil (Aricept) has been approved by the FDA for use in mild (including very mild), moderate, and severe Alzheimer's disease dementia, whereas galantamine and rivastigmine (Exelon) have been approved for use in patients with mild and moderate disease. (We would note, however, that we have used galantamine and rivastigmine [Exelon] in patients with severe Alzheimer's disease dementia to good effect as well.) Cholinesterase inhibitors improve memory and other aspects of cognition, improve function, and reduce behavioral and neuropsychiatric symptoms. Cholinesterase inhibitors should be initiated as soon as the diagnosis is established, and continued until the goal of treatment is only hospice, that is, until the goal of treatment is to help the patient die with care, comfort, and dignity. See Chapter 19 for more on this class of medications.

In addition to treatment with cholinesterase inhibitors, in patients with moderate and severe Alzheimer's disease dementia we also recommend a trial of treatment with memantine (generic and Namenda). As discussed in Chapter 20, memantine tends to improve functional and neuropsychiatric symptoms in patients with Alzheimer's disease dementia rather than memory.

Patients with Alzheimer's disease in the mild cognitive impairment, very mild, and mild stages often have preserved insight and are understandably quite depressed and anxious about their memory loss and the fact that they have Alzheimer's disease. Sometimes patients articulate this concern, and sometimes they feel anxious because they know at some level things are wrong even if they cannot say just what it is. In some patients with Alzheimer's disease in the moderate stage, anxiety can manifest itself as agitation. It is therefore not surprising that approximately one-half to two-thirds of patients with Alzheimer's disease benefit from selective serotonin reuptake inhibitor medication (see Chapter 27). In our experience, sertraline (generic and Zoloft) and escitalopram (generic and Lexapro) work best because they treat both depression and anxiety. They are also well tolerated with few side effects in the patient with memory loss and/or dementia.

As patients with Alzheimer's disease progress to moderate and severe dementia stages, additional medications to control behavior may be necessary. Please see Section IV: *Behavioral and Psychological Symptoms of Dementia* for additional information on pharmacological and non-pharmacological treatment of these symptoms.

REFERENCES

Albert, M. S., DeKosky, S. T., Dickson, D., et al. (2011). The diagnosis of mild cognitive impairment due to Alzheimer's disease: Recommendations from the National Institute on Aging–Alzheimer's Association workgroups on diagnostic guidelines for Alzheimer's disease. *Alzheimer's & Dementia: The Journal of the Alzheimer's Association, 7,* 270–279.

Alzheimer's Association. (2019). Alzheimer's disease facts and figures. *Alzheimer's & Dementia: The Journal of the Alzheimer's Association, 15*(3), 321–387.

Balthazar, M. L., Cendes, F., Damasceno, B. P., et al. (2008). Semantic error patterns on the Boston Naming Test in normal aging, amnesic mild cognitive impairment, and mild Alzheimer's disease: Is there semantic disruption? *Neuropsychology, 22,* 703–709.

Budson, A. E., Simons, J. S., Waring, J. D., et al. (2007). Memory for the September 11, 2001, terrorist attacks one year later in patients with Alzheimer's disease, patients with mild cognitive impairment, and healthy older adults. *Cortex; A Journal Devoted to the Study of the Nervous System and Behavior, 43,* 875–888.

Cannon-Albright, L. A., Foster, N. L., Schliep, K., et al. (2019). Relative risk for Alzheimer disease based on complete family history. *Neurology, 92*(15), e1745–e1753.

Cobb, J. L., Wolf, P. A., Au, R., et al. (1995). The effect of education on the incidence of dementia and Alzheimer's disease in the Framingham Study. *Neurology, 45,* 1707–1712.

Fleminger, S., Oliver, D. L., Lovestone, S., et al. (2003). Head injury as a risk factor for Alzheimer's disease: The evidence 10 years on; a partial replication. *Journal of Neurology, Neurosurgery, and Psychiatry, 74,* 857–862.

Jack, C.R., Jr., Bennett, D.A., Blennow, K., et al. (Contributors). (2018). NIA-AA research framework: Toward a biological definition of Alzheimer's disease. *Alzheimer's & Dementia: The Journal of the Alzheimer's Association, 14*(4), 535–562.

Lampert, E. J., Roy Choudhury, K., Hostage, C. A., et al. (2013). Prevalence of Alzheimer's pathologic endophenotypes in asymptomatic and mildly impaired first-degree relatives. *PLoS One, 8,* e60747.

Luchsinger, J. A., Tang, M. X., Shea, S., et al. (2004). Plasma homocysteine levels and risk of Alzheimer disease. *Neurology, 62,* 1972–1976.

Mayeux, R., Ottman, R., Maestre, G., et al. (1995). Synergistic effects of traumatic head injury and apolipoprotein-epsilon 4 in patients with Alzheimer's disease. *Neurology, 45,* 555–557.

Mckee, A. C., & Daneshvar, D. H. (2015). The neuropathology of traumatic brain injury. *Handbook of Clinical Neurology, 127,* 45–66.

McKhann, G. M., Knopman, D. S., Chertkow, H., et al. (2011). The diagnosis of dementia due to Alzheimer's disease: Recommendations from the National Institute on Aging and the Alzheimer's Association Workgroup. *Alzheimer's & Dementia: The Journal of the Alzheimer's Association, 7,* 263–269.

Mesulam, M.-M. (2000). *Principles of behavioral and cognitive neurology* (2nd ed.). New York: Oxford University Press.

Mesulam, M. (2004). The cholinergic lesion of Alzheimer's disease: Pivotal factor or side show? *Learning & Memory, 11,* 43–49.

Mesulam, M., Shaw, P., Mash, D., et al. (2004). Cholinergic nucleus basalis tauopathy emerges early in the aging-MCI-Alzheimer's disease continuum. *Annals of Neurology, 55,* 815–828.

Miller, J. W., Green, R., Mungas, D. M., et al. (2002). Homocysteine, vitamin B6, and vascular disease in Alzheimer's disease patients. *Neurology, 58,* 1471–1475.

Moir, R. D., Lathe, R., & Tanzi, R. E. (2018). The antimicrobial protection hypothesis of Alzheimer's disease. *Alzheimer's & Dementia: The Journal of the Alzheimer's Association, 14*(12), 1602–1614.

Petersen, R. C., Lopez, O., Armstrong, M. J., et al. (2018). Practice guideline update summary: Mild cognitive impairment: Report of the Guideline Development, Dissemination, and Implementation Subcommittee of the American Academy of Neurology. *Neurology, 90*(3), 126–135.

Rabinovici, G. D. (2019). Late-onset Alzheimer disease. *Continuum (Minneap Minn), 25*(1), 14–33.

Seshadri, S., Beiser, A., Selhub, J., et al. (2002). Plasma homocysteine as a risk factor for dementia and Alzheimer's disease. *The New England Journal of Medicine, 346,* 476–483.

Snowdon, D. A., Greiner, L. H., & Markesbery, W. R. (2000). Linguistic ability in early life and the neuropathology of Alzheimer's disease and cerebrovascular disease. Findings from the Nun Study. *Annals of the New York Academy of Sciences, 903,* 34–38.

Snowdon, D. A., Greiner, L. H., Mortimer, J. A., et al. (1997). Brain infarction and the clinical expression of Alzheimer disease. The Nun Study. *The Journal of the American Medical Association, 277,* 813–817.

Snowdon, D. A., Kemper, S. J., Mortimer, J. A., et al. (1996). Linguistic ability in early life and cognitive function and Alzheimer's disease in late life. Findings from the Nun Study. *The Journal of the American Medical Association, 275,* 528–532.

van der Lee, S. J., Wolters, F. J., Ikram, M. K., et al. (2018). The effect of APOE and other common genetic variants on the onset of Alzheimer's disease and dementia: A community-based cohort study. *The Lancet. Neurology, 17*(5), 434–444.

Vemuri, P., Lesnick, T. G., Przybelski, S. A., et al. (2012). Effect of lifestyle activities on Alzheimer disease biomarkers and cognition. *Annals of Neurology, 72,* 730–738.

Welsh, K. A., Butters, N., Hughes, J. P., et al. (1992). Detection and staging of dementia in Alzheimer's disease. Use of the neuropsychological measures developed for the Consortium to Establish a Registry for Alzheimer's Disease. *Archives of Neurology, 49,* 448–452.

World Health Organization, 2019. Risk reduction of cognitive decline and dementia: WHO guidelines. Geneva. Licence: CC BY-NC-SA 3.0 IGO.

Primary Age-Related Tauopathy

An 88-year-old woman came into the clinic with her family because over the last six months she had begun having difficulty balancing her checkbook and taking her medications correctly. Although she had stopped driving some years ago, she was able to independently do her grocery shopping with a list, prepare her meals, pay her bills, do her laundry, and keep her house clean and tidy. Her Mini-Mental State Examination (MMSE) score was 25/30, which was below the mean of 27 and in the lower quartile for her age and eighteen years of education (Master's degree) (Crum et al., 1993). Although her family reported that she had "memory problems," detailed

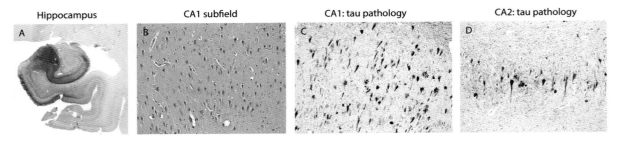

Fig. 5.1 Primary age-related tauopathy (PART). A patient with PART showing severe tau pathology within the hippocampus without beta-amyloid plaque deposition. A low-power view demonstrates tau pathology within the parahippocampal gyrus, subiculum, and hippocampus **(A)**. There is moderate loss of neurons within the CA1 subfield (**B**, Luxol fast blue/hematoxylin and eosin stain). Tau pathology immunostaining shows numerous neurofibrillary pretangles and tangles in CA1 **(C)** and CA2 **(D)** with relative sparing of CA3 and CA4. Magnification: **A**, ~8×; **B–C, B–D**, (Figure courtesy of Dr. Thor Stein.)

neuropsychological testing showed impairment only in the Trailmaking Test Part B. Other neuropsychological tests, including memory for words and stories, naming pictures, word fluency to letters and categories, and the Trailmaking Test Part A were all within one standard deviation of the mean. Her magnetic resonance imaging (MRI) scan showed mild atrophy of hippocampi and frontal lobes bilaterally, not clearly abnormal for age. Despite having some mild functional deficits with her instrumental activities of daily living (checkbook and pills), we felt a diagnosis of mild cognitive impairment (MCI) was most appropriate given that she had no other functional problems and her testing showed impairment in only one cognitive domain. Given that she did not show memory deficits, we did not offer her cholinesterase inhibitors but instead made practical suggestions (such as using a pillbox) to help her maintain her independence. She showed little decline over the next four years before dying in her home at age 92. Her autopsy showed Braak stage IV primary age-related tauopathy (PART).

PREVALENCE, PATHOLOGY, GENETICS, AND DEFINITION

Primary age-related tauopathy (PART) is a new name for the tangles which frequently occur in the hippocampus—particularly the anterior hippocampus—without the amyloid plaques that define Alzheimer's disease (Fig. 5.1). Older names for PART include "tangle-predominant senile dementia," "tangle-only dementia,"

"preferential development of NFT [neurofibrillary tangles] without senile plaques," and "senile dementia of the neurofibrillary tangle type." Although some contend that PART is simply part of Alzheimer's disease (Duyckaerts et al., 2015), the consensus in the field is that it is a different disorder (Crary et al., 2014).

The tangles in PART are similar to those seen in Alzheimer's disease, containing both 3-repeat and 4-repeat tau isoforms. They display a typical paired helical filament morphology. The grading system of PART is from the Braak tangle staging system, although PART-type pathology is generally only seen in Braak stages I through IV (entorhinal to limbic regions) and not stages V and VI (neocortical regions) (Crary et al., 2014).

The majority of individuals with PART are older. In one study, whereas individuals without PART or other neuropathologies died at approximately age 81, those with stage I died age about age 82, those with stages II or III died at about age 88, and those with stage IV died about age 92 (Crary et al., 2014). Another study found the average age at death in individuals with PART to be 88 years (Josephs et al., 2017). Studies of centenarians whose brains come to autopsy show that virtually 100% of those without Alzheimer's amyloid plaques still have neurofibrillary tangles (i.e., PART) in their hippocampus (Jicha & Nelson, 2019). Because PART appears to be inevitable with aging, some speculated that it may be one of the causes of the so-called normal "age-associated memory impairment." It may also be a common cause of MCI in individuals in their 80s, as well as subjective cognitive decline and mild dementia.

One reason that the consensus is that PART is separate from Alzheimer's disease, is that their genetics are different. There has been no observed association between PART and common genetic risk factors for Alzheimer's disease, such as apolipoprotein E status. One study found an association between PART and the microtubule-associated protein tau (MAPT) H_1 haplotype, which has also been associated with another tauopathy, progressive supranuclear palsy (see Chapter 12) (Jicha & Nelson, 2019).

CLINICAL FEATURES, HISTORY, AND PATTERN OF IMPAIRMENT ON COGNITIVE TESTS

There are no published clinical diagnostic criteria for PART. One study showed that before their death, about one-third of individuals with PART were given an MCI diagnosis (67% amnestic MCI, 33% nonamnestic) and two-thirds were given a dementia diagnosis, with Alzheimer's being the most common suspected etiology, 57% for those with MCI and 52% for those with dementia. The authors noted that these rates of a clinical diagnosis of Alzheimer's were considerably lower than those individuals with MCI and dementia and Alzheimer's pathology age autopsy (69% and 86%, respectively), suggesting that clinicians were aware that many of patients with PART didn't look quite like Alzheimer's disease (Teylan et al., 2019).

Another study using subjects from the Mayo Clinic Alzheimer's Disease Research Center and the Mayo Clinic Study of Aging found that their 52 subjects with PART showed very few cognitive deficits (Josephs et al., 2017). These individuals, who were an average of 87 years old when evaluated, had an average MMSE score of 28 (normal), and only showed deficits on the Trailmaking Test Part B and Wechsler Adult Intelligence Scale (WAIS) block design. Other neuropsychological tests and scales were within normal limits including Wechsler Memory Scale-Revised (WMS-R) logical memory delayed recall, Boston Naming Test, controlled oral word association test, auditory verbal learning test (AVLT) delayed recall, and the Unified Parkinson's Disease Rating Scale (UPDRS) (Trailmaking Test Part A results were borderline). These researchers also found a correlation between the Braak stage of these patients and focal atrophy in the left anterior—but not posterior—hippocampus. They

suggested that this lack of involvement of the posterior hippocampus was important as it is this latter region that has been associated with episodic memory dysfunction (Josephs et al., 2017).

Another study correlated MMSE score with PART Braak stage. They found that for Braak stages 0 (no pathology), I, II, III, and IV, average MMSE scores were 28.0, 28.4, 26.5, 25.1, and 24.3, respectively (Crary et al., 2014).

Without biomarkers to identify individuals with PART before death, we can only extrapolate from cross-sectional autopsy data like these to infer the course and prognosis of this disease. Nonetheless, when we combine the results of these three studies, the fact that virtually 100% of centenarians develop PART, and the fact that part of the definition of PART is that it only affects Braak stages I through IV (entorhinal to limbic regions) and not stages V and VI (neocortical regions), we can draw some conclusions.

These data suggest that PART is a mild neurodegenerative disease. It is likely a common cause of the cognitive deficits seen "normal aging," as well as subjective cognitive decline, mild cognitive impairment, and mild dementia. One would not expect individuals who only have PART pathology to reach the moderate to severe stages of dementia. The cognitive deficits are expected to be difficulty with executive function, particularly on timed test involving set shifting and visuospatial function. Although patients and families may complain of "memory" problems, the expectation is that those with pure PART pathology would either perform normally on tests of episodic memory, or they would show a so-called "frontal pattern of memory deficits," with impairment of encoding and delayed recall but intact recognition for those items encoded.

THINGS TO LOOK FOR ON THE PHYSICAL AND NEUROLOGICAL EXAMINATION

There are no elements on the physical or neurological examination that would suggest a diagnosis of PART. Positive findings on the neurological examination (such as tremor, parkinsonism, or focal signs) would make the diagnosis of PART less likely.

LABORATORY STUDIES

There are no laboratory studies to support a diagnosis of PART.

STRUCTURAL IMAGING STUDIES

The pattern of MRI brain atrophy in PART has been examined in a single study which found an association between Braak stage in PART and the grey matter volume in the left anterior hippocampus as well as scattered regions of the cerebellum (Josephs et al., 2017). Thus more extensive brain atrophy would suggest that other or additional pathologies are present.

FUNCTIONAL AND MOLECULAR IMAGING STUDIES

Fluorodeoxyglucose (FDG) positron emission tomography (PET) studies could be used to search for pathologies other than PART, as prominent parietal hypometabolism would suggest Alzheimer's disease (see Chapter 4), occipital hypometabolism would suggest Lewy body dementia (see Chapter 8) or posterior cortical atrophy (see Chapter 11), and frontal hypometabolism would suggest behavioral variant frontotemporal dementia (see Chapter 10). Similarly, negative amyloid PET studies and dopamine transporter single photon emission computed tomography scans would be helpful only in ruling out Alzheimer's and Lewy body diseases, respectively.

DIFFERENTIAL DIAGNOSIS

Individuals with PART would typically present to the clinic with subjective cognitive decline, mild cognitive impairment, or mild dementia in their 80s or 90s. Although complaints of memory problems would be common, testing would reveal primarily a frontal/executive pattern of cognitive impairment. For these reasons, the main differential diagnoses would be vascular cognitive impairment/vascular dementia (see Chapter 7) and early stages of other neurodegenerative diseases including (but not limited to) limbic-predominant age-related TDP-43 encephalopathy (LATE) (see Chapter 6), Alzheimer's (see Chapter 4), and Lewy body diseases (see Chapter 8).

TREATMENTS

There are no known pharmacologic treatments for PART. We recommend the use of memory strategies and memory aids in these patients (see Chapter 22).

REFERENCES

Crary, J. F., Trojanowski, J. Q., Schneider, J. A., et al. (2014). Primary age-related tauopathy (PART): A common pathology associated with human aging. *Acta Neuropathologica, 128*, 755–766.

Crum, R. M., Anthony, J. C., Bassett, S. S., et al. (1993). Population-based norms for the Mini-Mental State Examination by age and educational level. *The Journal of the American Medical Association, 269*(18), 2386–2391.

Duyckaerts, C., Braak, H., Brion, J. P., et al. (2015). PART is part of Alzheimer disease. *Acta Neuropathologica, 129*(5), 749–756.

Jicha, G. A., & Nelson, P. T. (2019). Hippocampal sclerosis, argyrophilic grain disease, and primary age-related tauopathy. *Continuum (Minneapolis, Minn.), 25*(1), 208–233.

Josephs, K. A., Murray, M. E., Tosakulwong, N., et al. (2017). Tau aggregation influences cognition and hippocampal atrophy in the absence of beta-amyloid: A clinico-imaging-pathological study of primary age-related tauopathy (PART). *Acta Neuropathologica, 133*(5), 705–715.

Teylan, M., Besser, L. M., Crary, J. F., et al. (2019). Clinical diagnoses among individuals with primary age-related tauopathy versus Alzheimer's neuropathology. *Laboratory Investigation, 99*(7), 1049–1055.

Limbic-predominant Age-related TDP-43 Encephalopathy

QUICK START: LIMBIC-PREDOMINANT AGE-RELATED TDP-43 ENCEPHALOPATHY

Definition	• In limbic-predominant age-related TDP-43 encephalopathy (LATE), phosphorylated transactive response DNA binding protein of 43 kDa (TDP-43) is found in neuronal cytoplasmic inclusions in the setting of neuronal loss and gliosis in the amygdala, hippocampal CA1 subfield, subiculum, and sometimes inferior temporal and frontal neocortex. Some cases of LATE are associated with hippocampal sclerosis.
Prevalence	• LATE is a common cause of dementia in individuals over the age of 80 years, and becomes more common with each decade of life. In one analysis of individuals whose mean age was about 90, LATE was the third most common cause of dementia (17%) after Alzheimer's (39%) and cerebrovascular disease (25%).
Genetic risk	• LATE has been associated with five genes: ATP-binding cassette sub-family member 9 (ABCC9) on chromosome 12p, apolipoprotein E (APOE) on chromosome 19q, granulin (GRN) on chromosome 17q, potassium channel subfamily M regulatory beta subunit 2 (KCNMB2) on chromosome 3q, and transmembrane protein 106B (TMEM106B) on chromosome 7p.
Cognitive symptoms	• LATE typically begins with isolated mild episodic memory dysfunction and a diagnosis of amnestic mild cognitive impairment. When either hippocampal sclerosis or neocortical involvement is present, additional cognitive domains may be impaired leading to a dementia diagnosis.
Clinical features	• LATE will typically be diagnosed in individuals over the age of 80 with slowly progressing memory problems and structural imaging studies showing relatively isolated (and perhaps severe) hippocampal atrophy. The diagnosis of LATE is supported by negative biomarkers for other neurodegenerative diseases.
Treatment	• Although there are no U.S. Food and Drug Administration (FDA) approved treatments for LATE, it is reasonable to try cholinesterase inhibitors for the treatment of mild cognitive impairment and mild, moderate, and severe dementia. • Memantine can be tried for the treatment of moderate and severe dementia.
Top differential diagnoses	• Normal aging, primary age-related tauopathy (PART), Alzheimer's disease, chronic traumatic encephalopathy.

An 85-year-old man came to see us for slowly progressing memory loss over the last few years. When asked the last time he was remembering normally, his family was unsure, with some family members thinking it might have been five years ago or more. He had mild difficulty with some instrumental activities of daily living, such as needing some assistance with bill paying and filling his pillbox. His testing showed mainly problems with memory, including encoding, recall, and recognition of items, as well as some difficulty with executive function in the timed generation of words to specific letters and the Trailmaking Test Part B alternating number-letter sequencing task. In addition to some nonspecific age-related atrophy, his magnetic resonance imaging (MRI) scan was notable for severe hippocampal atrophy. We made a diagnosis of probable Alzheimer's disease dementia, mild stage, and started him on a cholinesterase inhibitor. He and his family were interested in clinical trials. During a follow-up visit we began the screening process for the trial including, per protocol, scheduling an amyloid positron emission tomography (PET) scan. The PET scan was negative, indicating sparse to no amyloid plaques, inconsistent with a pathologic diagnosis of Alzheimer's disease.

In the age of amyloid and tau imaging, about 10% to 20% of patients that we and other memory centers diagnose with the syndrome of progressive amnestic dysfunction (also called probable Alzheimer's disease, dementia of the Alzheimer's type, and Alzheimer's clinical syndrome) will end up having a pathology other than Alzheimer's disease. Although some of these patients will end up with Lewy body or vascular pathology, we now know of another pathology that causes progressive amnestic dysfunction, mimicking Alzheimer's disease.

PREVALENCE, PROGNOSIS, AND DEFINITION

Limbic-predominant age-related TDP-43 encephalopathy (LATE) is a new name for a disease that frequently mimics Alzheimer's disease and is now recognized to be more prevalent than previously thought. Older names for this disease include "hippocampal sclerosis," "hippocampal sclerosis of aging," "hippocampal sclerosis dementia," "cerebral age-related TDP-43 with sclerosis," and "TDP-43 pathologies in the elderly." LATE is commonly observed in individuals older than age 80 years. In fact, the prevalence of LATE pathology is quite high and increases proportionally with age—unlike Alzheimer's disease pathology, which peaks in the ninth decade and actually decreases over age 100 (Nelson et al., 2019) (Fig. 6.1). Furthermore, using a statistical approach typically used to evaluate the impact of risk factors on disease

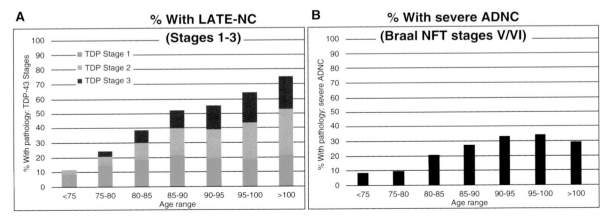

Fig. 6.1 Prevalence of limbic-predominant age-related TDP-43 encephalopathy neuropathologic change (*LATE-NC*) **(A)** compared with severe Alzheimer's disease neuropathologic change (*ADNC*) **(B)** stratified by age in a community-based cohort (Rush University, n = 1376). *NFT, Neurofibrillary tangle; TDP*, TDP-43. (Modified from Nelson, P. T., Dickson, D. W., Trojanowski, J. Q., et al. (2019). Limbic-predominant age-related TDP-43 encephalopathy (LATE): Consensus working group report. *Brain, 142*(6), 1503–1527. Erratum in: *Brain*, 2019 Jul 1; *142*(7), e37.)

prevalence in a population, an analysis of the attributable risk of dementia in individuals with advanced age (mean 89.7 years) found that LATE was the second most common neurodegenerative disease (after Alzheimer's) and the third most common cause of dementia (after Alzheimer's and vascular disease) (Nelson et al., 2019) (Table 6.1). Because our population is aging, we expect that LATE will become an even more important disease in the future (see Fig. 4.1). Women and men appear to be equally likely to have LATE pathology at any given age but, because women live longer than men, there are more women with LATE than men. No racial or ethnic differences for LATE have been reported. Retrospective studies suggest that individuals who have only LATE pathology progress more slowly than those with Alzheimer's pathology, but that progression is swiftest when both pathologies are present (Jicha & Nelson, 2019; Nag et al., 2017; Nelson et al., 2019). Note that multiple pathologies are common in individuals with dementia in their 80s and 90s. Most patients with LATE will therefore also have some Alzheimer's, vascular, or Lewy body pathology as well.

TABLE 6.1 A Statistical Analysis of Attributable Risk From Research Volunteers in Two Clinical-Pathological Studies of Aging from Rush University

Neuropathological Indices	Fraction Attributable % (95% CI)[a]
ADNC	39.4 (31.5–47.4)
Vascular disease pathology[b]	24.8 (17.3–32.1)
LATE-NC	17.3 (13.1–22.0)
α-Synucleinopathy/Lewy body pathology	11.9 (8.4–15.6)

Fractions of dementia of the Alzheimer's type cases that were attributable to individual neuropathological indices in advanced age. In this sample, the mean age of death was 89.7 years with a range of 65–108 years.
[a]95% CIs were derived using bootstrapping.
[b]Vascular pathologies included cerebral amyloid angiopathy, atherosclerosis, arteriolosclerosis, and gross infarcts.
ADNC, Alzheimer's disease neuropathologic change; CI, confidence intervals; LATE-NC, limbic-predominant age-related TDP-43 encephalopathy neuropathologic change.
Modified from Nelson, P. T., Dickson, D. W., Trojanowski, J. Q., et al. (2019). Limbic-predominant age-related TDP-43 encephalopathy (LATE): Consensus working group report. Brain, 142(6), 1503–1527. Erratum in: Brain, 2019 Jul 1; 142(7), e37.

CLINICAL DIAGNOSIS

There are no published clinical diagnostic criteria for LATE. The diagnosis will typically be made in individuals over the age of 80, who are slowly progressing over years, with memory problems predominating (including rapid forgetting of information), and structural imaging studies showing relatively isolated (and perhaps severe) hippocampal atrophy. The diagnosis of LATE is supported by negative biomarkers for other neurodegenerative diseases, such as negative amyloid imaging, negative tau imaging, negative dopamine transporter scan, and normal amyloid and phosphorylated tau in the cerebrospinal fluid (CSF).

PATHOLOGY, PATHOPHYSIOLOGY, AND GENETICS

Nonphosphorylated transactive response DNA binding protein of 43 kDa (TDP-43) is normally found in neuronal cell nuclei (Fig. 6.2). In the pathologic state, phosphorylated TDP-43 is found in neuronal cytoplasmic inclusions in the setting of widespread neuronal loss and frequent gliosis in the hippocampal CA1 subfield, subiculum, and amygdala (Jicha & Nelson, 2019). Although the hippocampal sclerosis that frequently accompanies LATE may be unilateral, TDP-43 pathology is almost always observed bilaterally. TDP-43 inclusions are composed of bundles of 10–20 nm diameter straight filaments frequently accompanied by electron dense granules (Nelson et al., 2019).

In the 2019 LATE neuropathologic change staging system, Stage 1 involves amygdala only, Stage 2 involves amygdala plus hippocampus, and Stage 3 involves amygdala, hippocampus, plus middle frontal gyrus (Nelson et al., 2019). Note that although hippocampal sclerosis is often observed in LATE, it is neither necessary nor sufficient for a diagnosis of LATE neuropathologic change. LATE pathology has also been described in other neocortical regions, as well as olfactory bulb, basal ganglia, and brainstem.

Genetics

Five genes have been reported to confer increased risk for the development of LATE pathology: ATP-binding cassette sub-family member 9 (ABCC9) on chromosome 12p, apolipoprotein E (APOE) on

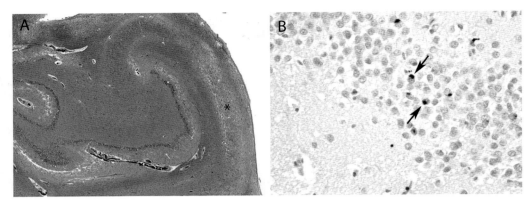

Fig. 6.2 Limbic-predominant age-related TDP-43 encephalopathy (LATE). Hippocampal pathology in LATE typically involves near complete neuronal loss and gliosis within the CA1 subfield without corresponding tau pathology (**A**, *hippocampal sclerosis). Hippocampal sclerosis can be focal and is not always observed. An immunostain for phosphorylated TDP-43 shows abnormal cytoplasmic inclusions within the dentate gyrus of the hippocampus (**B**, *arrows*). Magnification: **A**, 24×; **B**, 400×. (Figure courtesy of Dr. Thor Stein.)

chromosome 19q, granulin (GRN) on chromosome 17q, potassium channel subfamily M regulatory beta subunit 2 (KCNMB2) on chromosome 3q, and transmembrane protein 106B (TMEM106B) on chromosome 7p (Nelson et al., 2019). Of note, granulin and TMEM106B are also associated with increased risk for TDP-43 associated frontotemporal lobar degeneration leading to either behavioral variant frontotemporal dementia (see Chapter 10) or primary progressive aphasia (often semantic variant, see Chapter 9). The apolipoprotein E ε4 allele is also associated with increased risk for the pathology of Alzheimer's disease (see Chapter 4), dementia with Lewy bodies (see Chapter 8), and chronic traumatic encephalopathy (see Chapter 15). There are no other known risk factors for LATE.

COMMON SIGNS, SYMPTOMS, AND STAGES

Retrospective autopsy studies show that when LATE pathology is present without hippocampal sclerosis or neocortical involvement, isolated mild episodic memory dysfunction is the most common cognitive deficit (Fig. 6.3). Most patients at this stage are diagnosed with amnestic mild cognitive impairment (Nag et al., 2017; Wilson et al., 2019). When either hippocampal sclerosis or neocortical involvement of LATE pathology is present, additional cognitive domains are involved and function may be impaired, leading to a dementia diagnosis (Nelson et al., 2019). One study found that in the dementia stage, LATE was misdiagnosed as Alzheimer's disease 91% of the time (Nag et al., 2017).

THINGS TO LOOK FOR IN THE HISTORY

The clinical presentation of LATE is similar to Alzheimer's disease and other causes of progressive amnestic dysfunction. The history will generally be of gradual onset of memory loss over multiple years in an individual over the age of 80 years. In comparison with Alzheimer's disease, the patient is likely to be older, the progression slower, and the course milder (Nag et al., 2017; Nelson et al., 2019; Wilson et al., 2019).

THINGS TO LOOK FOR ON THE PHYSICAL AND NEUROLOGICAL EXAMINATION

There are no elements on the physical or neurological examination that would distinguish LATE from other causes of progressive amnestic dysfunction such as Alzheimer's disease. Positive findings on the neurological examination (such as tremor, parkinsonism, or focal signs) would make the diagnosis of LATE less likely.

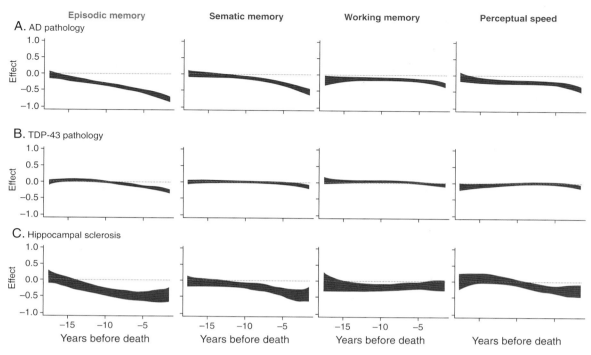

Fig. 6.3 Neurodegenerative disease and change in cognitive domains in **(A)** Alzheimer's disease pathology, **(B)** TDP-43 pathology, and **(C)** hippocampal sclerosis. The *black dotted lines* show the initial association, and the *blue shading* shows 95% confidence intervals of changes in the association as a function of years before death. (Modified from Wilson, R. S., Yang, J., Yu, L., et al. (2019). Postmortem neurodegenerative markers and trajectories of decline in cognitive systems. *Neurology, 92,* e831–e840.)

PATTERN OF IMPAIRMENT ON COGNITIVE TESTS

Episodic memory impairment, including rapid forgetting of information, is expected in all patients with LATE. In pathology Stages 1 (amygdala only) and 2 (amygdala and hippocampus) the cognitive impairment is expected to be mild and limited to memory. Once pathology Stage 3 (amygdala, hippocampus, and neocortex) is reached and/or hippocampal sclerosis is present, episodic memory is expected to be more prominent, and other cognitive domains are often impaired (Nag et al., 2017; Nelson et al., 2019; Wilson et al., 2019).

LABORATORY STUDIES

There are no laboratory studies to support a diagnosis of LATE.

STRUCTURAL IMAGING STUDIES

The pattern of brain atrophy in LATE has been studied and primarily involves amygdala and hippocampus, as well inferior cortical regions of temporal and frontal lobes (Fig. 6.4). Other areas of the cortex are generally spared. In individuals who have LATE and hippocampal sclerosis, the atrophy of the medial temporal lobes may be severe. When comparing the pattern of atrophy observed in LATE to that of Alzheimer's disease, it is notable that the parietal lobe, which is frequently involved in Alzheimer's, is relatively spared in LATE.

FUNCTIONAL AND MOLECULAR IMAGING STUDIES

Although fluorodeoxyglucose (FDG) PET is beginning to be studied in cases suspected to be LATE, no

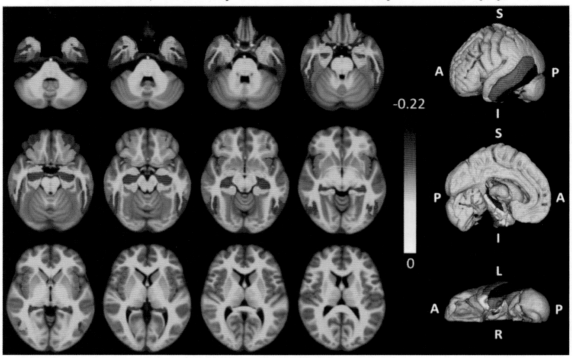

Fig. 6.4 Brain regions affected in limbic-predominant age-related TDP-43 encephalopathy. Darker colors indicate greater brain atrophy in that region. (Modified from Nelson, P. T., Dickson, D. W., Trojanowski, J. Q., et al. (2019). Limbic-predominant age-related TDP-43 encephalopathy (LATE): Consensus working group report. *Brain, 142*(6), 1503–1527. Erratum in: *Brain*, 2019 Jul 1, *142*(7), e37.)

clear pattern of hypometabolism has been identified. Nonetheless, it would be reasonable to assume that patients with isolated LATE pathology would show medial and inferior temporal lobe hypometabolism (Botha et al., 2018), without the prominent parietal hypometabolism seen in Alzheimer's disease (see Chapter 4), occipital hypometabolism seen in Lewy body dementia (see Chapter 8), or frontal hypometabolism seen in behavioral variant frontotemporal dementia (see Chapter 10).

LATE is more likely to be the sole cause of dementia when amyloid and tau PET studies and dopamine transporter SPECT scans are negative, ruling out Alzheimer's and Lewy body diseases, respectively. However, it is also common to have LATE pathology along with Alzheimer's and Lewy body pathology, so a positive amyloid PET, tau PET, or dopamine transporter SPECT does not rule out LATE.

DIFFERENTIAL DIAGNOSIS

Because LATE is a progressive amnestic disorder of late life, beginning with mild cognitive impairment and progressing to dementia, Alzheimer's disease is the main differential diagnosis that should be considered. When hippocampal sclerosis is present, the differential should include other causes of hippocampal sclerosis including epilepsy, hypoxia, and hypoglycemia as well as other neurodegenerative diseases such as Alzheimer's and frontotemporal lobar degeneration.

TREATMENTS

As discussed in Chapter 3, the medications for Alzheimer's disease dementia currently in use—the cholinesterase inhibitors (see Chapter 19) and memantine (see Chapter 20)—treat symptoms, and not underlying pathologies. Because these medications were developed and evaluated during the time that testing for biomarkers (such as beta amyloid and tau) was not routinely available, the patients who participated in these clinical trials were surely a mixture of individuals with different underlying causes of progressive amnestic dysfunction, including LATE, as well as Alzheimer's disease. For this reason, although these medications are Food and Drug Administration (FDA) approved for "Alzheimer's disease" dementia, we recommend trying them for patients with suspected LATE. As described in Chapters 19 and 20, cholinesterase inhibitors should be tried in individuals with mild cognitive impairment or mild, moderate, or severe dementia, and memantine should be tried in individuals with moderate or severe dementia. Future studies will be needed to know if patients with isolated LATE pathology respond better or worse to these medications than do those with isolated Alzheimer's pathology.

REFERENCES

Botha, H., Mantyh, W. G., Murray, M. E., et al. (2018). FDG-PET in tau-negative amnestic dementia resembles that of autopsy-proven hippocampal sclerosis. *Brain, 141,* 1201–1217.

Jicha, G. A., & Nelson, P. T. (2019). Hippocampal sclerosis, argyrophilic grain disease, and primary age-related tauopathy. *Continuum (Minneapolis, Minn.), 25*(1), 208–233.

Nag, S., Yu, L., Wilson, R. S., et al. (2017). TDP-43 pathology and memory impairment in elders without pathologic diagnoses of AD or FTLD. *Neurology, 88,* 653–660.

Nelson, P. T., Dickson, D. W., Trojanowski, J. Q., et al. (2019). Limbic-predominant age-related TDP-43 encephalopathy (LATE): Consensus working group report. *Brain, 142*(6), 1503–1527. Erratum in: *Brain.* 2019 Jul 1, *142*(7), e37.

Wilson, R. S., Yang, J., Yu, L., et al. (2019). Postmortem neurodegenerative markers and trajectories of decline in cognitive systems. *Neurology, 92,* e831–e840.

7

Vascular Cognitive Impairment and Vascular Dementia

QUICK START: VASCULAR COGNITIVE IMPAIRMENT AND VASCULAR DEMENTIA	
Definition	• Vascular cognitive impairment is the overarching term used when cognitive dysfunction is due to cerebrovascular disease (i.e., strokes).
	• Vascular dementia (VaD) occurs when cerebrovascular disease causes cognitive dysfunction that significantly impairs daily functioning.
	• Vascular mild cognitive impairment (VaMCI) occurs when cerebrovascular disease causes cognitive dysfunction that does not significantly impair daily functioning.
	• The exact cerebrovascular disease that can cause cognitive and functional impairment may be varied, and can include:
	Small vessel ischemic disease
	Multiple cortical strokes
	Strategic infarcts
	Cerebral amyloid angiopathy.
Prevalence	• Approximately 5% to 10% of patients with dementia have a pure vascular dementia, that is, dementia entirely due to cerebrovascular disease.
	• Another 10% to 15% of patients with dementia suffer from a mixed dementia of cerebrovascular disease plus a neurodegenerative disease.
	• Almost all patients with cognitive impairment due to a neurodegenerative disease have some cerebrovascular disease that makes at least a small contribution to their cognitive difficulties.
Genetic risk	• The genetic risk is related to the varied underlying cerebrovascular pathology.
	• One disorder, CADASIL (cerebral autosomal dominant arteriopathy with subcortical infarcts and leukoencephalopathy), is due to mutation of the Notch3 gene at the chromosome locus 19p13.
Cognitive symptoms	• Neuropsychological testing typically shows impairment in multiple domains, including attention, frontal/executive function, and speed of processing. Memory impairments are typically secondary to attention and frontal/executive dysfunction.

(Continued)

QUICK START: VASCULAR COGNITIVE IMPAIRMENT AND VASCULAR DEMENTIA (*Continued*)

Diagnostic criteria	• **Mild vascular cognitive impairment (VaMCI):** Impairment in *at least* one cognitive domain and mild to no impairment in instrumental activities of daily living (IADLs)/activities of daily living (ADLs), respectively (independent of the motor/sensory sequelae of the vascular event).
	• **Major vascular cognitive impairment (VaD):** Clinically significant deficits of sufficient severity in *at least* one cognitive domain (deficits may be present in multiple domains) and moderate to severe disruption to IADLs/ADLs (independent of the motor/sensory sequelae of the vascular event).
	• Magnetic resonance imaging (MRI) is the gold standard for a diagnosis of vascular cognitive impairment. If only computed tomography (CT) is available, the diagnostic certainty is lowered to "probable." If neither MRI nor CT are available, the diagnostic certainty is lowered to "possible."
	• Full diagnostic criteria are available from the Vascular Impairment of Cognition Classification Consensus Study (VICCCS) (see Box 7.1) and the Diagnostic and Statistical Manual of Mental Disorders, 5th Edition (DSM-5) (see Box 7.2).
Behavioral symptoms	• Depression is often present.
Treatment	• There are no U.S. Food and Drug Administration (FDA)-approved medications to treat vascular cognitive impairment. However, clinical trials have found both cholinesterase inhibitors and memantine to be helpful. For memory problems we recommend a trial of cholinesterase inhibitors, and for apathy we recommend a trial of memantine.
	• Dextromethorphan/quinidine (Nuedexta) can be used for pseudobulbar affect.
	• Aerobic exercise and Mediterranean-style diets may be beneficial.
	• The underlying cause of the cerebrovascular disease must also be evaluated and treated.
Top differential diagnoses	• Mixed dementia (vascular cognitive impairment plus another neurodegenerative disease such as Alzheimer's disease or Lewy body disease), Alzheimer's disease, depression.

A 74-year-old man presented to the clinic with a 6-year history of cognitive and functional decline. His family reported that his problems began with "small TIAs." When we asked them what they meant, they explained that he appeared to be suffering from transient ischemic attacks, such that in a single day he might show a sudden decline in his speech, handwriting, and gait, which would subsequently improve, although not back to his baseline. Despite earning a degree in engineering, he had difficulty at that time with simple calculations, such as calculating the tip in a restaurant. He also had difficulty remembering a short list of items, and finding his way around a familiar street. His family also reported that he would often cry or laugh either inappropriately or with the least provocation.

His medical history included diabetes mellitus type 2 and hypertension. His review of systems was notable for frequent urinary and occasional fecal incontinence. His neurological examination was notable for brisk reflexes throughout. He had bilateral Babinski responses. On the Montreal Cognitive Assessment (MoCA) he scored 23 out of a possible 30, missing points on the alternating number-letter connect-the-dots, clock hands, serial 7s, and delayed recall (although with category cues and multiple choice he recalled the items he missed on delayed recall).

PREVALENCE, PROGNOSIS, AND DEFINITION

Vascular cognitive impairment (VCI) is now the preferred, overarching term for cognitive impairment due to cerebrovascular disease (i.e., strokes) (Fig. 7.1). When cerebrovascular disease causes cognitive dysfunction but not severe enough to lead to functional impairment, the terms *mild vascular cognitive impairment (mild VCI)* and *vascular mild cognitive impairment (VaMCI)* are used. When cerebrovascular disease causes cognitive dysfunction severe enough to cause impairment of instrumental or basic activities of daily living (see Box 2.2), the terms

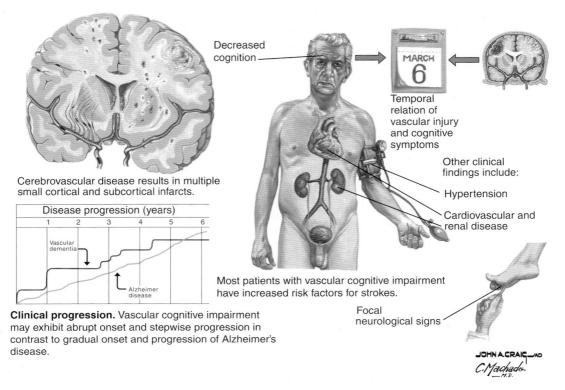

Decreased cognition

Temporal relation of vascular injury and cognitive symptoms

Other clinical findings include:

Hypertension

Cardiovascular and renal disease

Cerebrovascular disease results in multiple small cortical and subcortical infarcts.

Disease progression (years)

Vascular dementia

Alzheimer disease

Most patients with vascular cognitive impairment have increased risk factors for strokes.

Focal neurological signs

Clinical progression. Vascular cognitive impairment may exhibit abrupt onset and stepwise progression in contrast to gradual onset and progression of Alzheimer's disease.

JOHN A. CRAIG—AD
C. Machado—M.D.

Fig. 7.1 Vascular cognitive impairment. (From Netter illustration from www.netterimages.com. Copyright Elsevier Inc. All rights reserved.)

major vascular cognitive impairment (major VCI) and *vascular dementia (VaD)* are used (Table 7.1).

The prevalence of vascular dementia and vascular mild cognitive impairment depends on how they are defined. If vascular dementia is defined such that patients with Alzheimer's disease and other neurodegenerative diseases are excluded, then vascular dementia is a relatively small cause of memory loss and dementia, of the order of 5% to 10% of all dementias, depending upon the particular population (closer to 10% in U.S. veterans, for example). We would describe such patients as having a "pure vascular dementia." Like most older adults, the majority of patients with Alzheimer's disease and other degenerative diseases (such as dementia with Lewy bodies) have some cerebrovascular disease, usually in the form of small vessel ischemic disease. If these patients were also included in the definition of vascular dementia, then the majority of patients with dementia would have vascular dementia or vascular

mild cognitive impairment—along with another type of dementia (Graff-Radford, 2019). It is the unusual patient who has a single pathology; most patients have at least two pathologies contributing to their cognitive impairment and many have three or more (Kapasi, DeCarli, & Schneider, 2017). One study found that vascular disease pathology contributed approximately 25% to late-life dementia due to clinical Alzheimer's disease (Boyle et al., 2019).

We typically classify the cognitively impaired patient with cerebrovascular disease in one of the following ways. If the patient shows no signs of any other etiology of his or her cognitive impairment we would describe him or her as having a "pure vascular dementia" (or "pure vascular mild cognitive impairment," if not demented). If the patient has a neurodegenerative disease (such as Alzheimer's) and they have the average amount of cerebrovascular disease that a nondemented, noncognitively impaired older adult has, we would describe them as

TABLE 7.1 Comparison Between Vascular Dementia, Vascular Mild Cognitive Impairment, Alzheimer's Disease Dementia, and Mild Cognitive Impairment due to Alzheimer's Disease

	Vascular Dementia	Vascular Mild Cognitive Impairment	Alzheimer's Disease Dementia	Mild Cognitive Impairment due to Alzheimer's Disease
Cognitive complaints by patient or family	Present	Present	Present	Present
Cognitive deficits	Present	Present, very mild	Present	Present, very mild
Functional impairment	Present	Absent	Present	Absent
Dementia	Present	Absent	Present	Absent
Likely underlying pathology	Cerebrovascular disease	Cerebrovascular disease	Alzheimer's disease	Alzheimer's disease
Deterioration over time	May occur, but may also remain stable	May occur, but may also remain stable	Always occurs	Occurs if diagnosis correct
U.S. Food and Drug Administration–approved treatment	None	None	Cholinesterase inhibitors, memantine	None
Recommended treatment	Cholinesterase inhibitors	Cholinesterase inhibitors	Cholinesterase inhibitors	Cholinesterase inhibitors
	Memantine if apathy	Memantine if apathy	Memantine if apathy	
	Selective serotonin reuptake inhibitor (SSRI) if depression or anxiety	SSRI if depression or anxiety	SSRI if depression or anxiety	SSRI if depression or anxiety

simply having that neurodegenerative disease (such as Alzheimer's). If the patient has a neurodegenerative disease (such as Alzheimer's) and they have a greater than average amount of cerebrovascular disease—such that it is highly likely that the cerebrovascular disease is making a significant contribution to the patient's dementia—then we would describe them as having a "mixed dementia," and would then further specify, for example, "a mixed dementia of Alzheimer's disease plus vascular dementia" or "a mixed dementia of vascular dementia plus Alzheimer's disease," depending upon which was more prominent (Fig. 7.2), consistent with the current diagnostic criteria (Skrobot et al., 2018) (Box 7.1). Patients classified in this way with a mixed dementia of cerebrovascular disease plus a neurodegenerative disease probably make up 10% to 15% of all dementias.

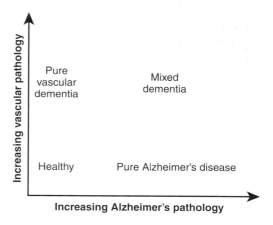

Fig. 7.2 The relationship between vascular and Alzheimer's pathology and clinical diagnosis.

BOX 7.1   Vascular Impairment of Cognition Classification Consensus Study Diagnosis Guidelines

Definitions and Diagnosis of Vascular Cognitive Impairment (VCI)

- Clinical evaluation and neuropsychological protocols should include assessment of executive function, attention, and memory, as well as language and visuospatial function.[a]
- **Mild VCI (vascular mild cognitive impairment; VaMCI):** Impairment in at least one cognitive domain and mild to no impairment in instrumental activities of daily living (IADLs)/activities of daily living (ADLs), respectively (independent of the motor/sensory sequelae of the vascular event).
- **Major VCI (vascular dementia; VaD):** Clinically significant deficits of sufficient severity in at least one cognitive domain (deficits may be present in multiple domains) and moderate to severe disruption to instrumental activities of daily living (IADLs)/activities of daily living (ADLs) (independent of the motor/sensory sequelae of the vascular event).
- Patients given a diagnosis of major VCI (VaD) are subcategorized according to the underlying vascular pathology as appropriate. A clear temporal relationship (within 6 months) between a vascular event and onset of cognitive deficits is only required for a diagnosis of poststroke dementia (PSD).

Subtypes of Major VCI (VaD)

- **Poststroke dementia (PSD):** A patient described as having poststroke dementia may or may not have presented evidence of mild cognitive impairment before stroke. The patient will exhibit immediate and/or delayed cognitive decline that begins within 6 months after a stroke and that does not reverse. Poststroke dementia can result from several different vascular causes and changes in the brain. It encompasses dementia that develops within 6 months of stroke in patients with multiple cortical-subcortical infarcts and strategic infarcts; patients with subcortical ischemic vascular dementia; and those with various forms of neurodegenerative pathology, including Alzheimer's disease. The temporal relationship between the cognitive decline and the stroke differentiates poststroke dementia from other forms of major VCI (VaD).
- **Mixed dementias:** A standalone umbrella subgroup termed "mixed dementias" includes phenotypes representing each combination between vascular and neurodegenerative disease, that is, VCI-Alzheimer's disease, VCI–dementia with Lewy bodies, and so forth.

It is recommended that a patient is referred to as having "VCI-Alzheimer's disease," for example, according to the clinically probable phenotypes, rather than the less-specific "mixed dementia." Where discrimination is possible, the order of terms should reflect the probable relative contribution of the underlying pathology, that is, Alzheimer's disease-VCI or VCI-Alzheimer's disease.

- **Subcortical ischemic vascular dementia:** Small vessel disease is the main vascular cause of subcortical ischemic vascular dementia. Lacunar infarcts and ischemic white matter lesions are the main type of brain lesions, which are located predominantly subcortically. This diagnosis incorporates the overlapping clinical entities of Binswanger's disease and the lacunar state.
- **Multi-infarct dementia:** Multi-infarct dementia is used to indicate the presence of multiple large cortical infarcts and their likely contribution to the dementia.

"Probable" and "Possible" — Terms for the Availability of Evidence

- Magnetic resonance imaging is a "gold-standard" requirement for a **clinical diagnosis of VCI**.[a]
- **Probable mild VCI (VaMCI)** or **probable major VCI (VaD)** is the appropriate diagnostic category if computed tomography imaging is the only means of imaging available.[a]
- **Possible mild VCI (VaMCI)** or **possible major VCI (VaD)** would be appropriate diagnoses if neither MRI nor computed tomography imaging were available.
- In diagnosis of VCI when full clinical assessment of the cognitive impairment due to the clinical event is impaired by aphasia, patients with documented evidence of normal cognitive function (e.g., annual cognitive evaluations) before the clinical event that caused aphasia could be classified as having probable mild VCI (VaMCI) or major VCI (VaD) if imaging is available, and the assessment of activities of daily living should be made where possible. If imaging is not available, the classification should be possible mild VCI (VaMCI) or major VCI (VaD).

Those at Risk of VCI

- It is recommended that greater consideration for diagnosis be given to people who are at risk of VCI if they present with at least 6 months of sustained impairment (even if very mild), rather than transient

(Continued)

BOX 7.1 Vascular Impairment of Cognition Classification Consensus Study Diagnosis Guidelines (*Continued*)

impairment, as identified through caregiver reporting and clinical observation. All other potential causes of sustained impairment (e.g., depression or vitamin D deficiency) should have been excluded.

Exclusions From Diagnosis
- Drug/alcohol abuse/dependence within the last 3 months of first recognition of impairment or delirium.

[a]National Institute of Neurological Disorders–Canadian Stroke Network guidelines are recommended.

Modified from Skrobot, O. A., Black, S. E., Chen, C., et al. (2018). Progress toward standardized diagnosis of vascular cognitive impairment: Guidelines from the Vascular Impairment of Cognition Classification Consensus Study. *Alzheimer's & Dementia: The Journal of the Alzheimer's Association, 14*(3), 280–292.

CRITERIA

There are many published criteria for vascular dementia. Two that we find helpful are those from the Vascular Impairment of Cognition Classification Consensus Study (VICCCS; Skrobot et al., 2018) and the DSM-5; they can be found below in Boxes 7.1 and 7.2. (See Boxes 3.1 and 3.3 for DSM-5 criteria for major and mild neurocognitive disorder.) Both criteria include that:
- the cognitive disorder can be major or mild
- history, exam, and/or neuroimaging evidence of cerebrovascular events is required
- cognitive deficits in attention, processing speed, and frontal-executive function are common
- a temporal relationship between cognitive deficits and cerebrovascular events is supportive.

RISK FACTORS, PATHOLOGY, AND PATHOPHYSIOLOGY

The major risk factors for vascular dementia and vascular mild cognitive impairment are, of course, the risk factors for cerebrovascular disease in general, with the major ones being hypertension, heart disease, smoking, and diabetes. See Box 7.3 for additional common risk factors.

Terminology can be confusing. Cerebrovascular disease can cause cognitive impairment and dementia in a variety of ways. Below we discuss three different pathologies—small vessel ischemic vascular disease, multiple cortical strokes, and strategic infarcts—each using different words to describe the same underlying process. Although the etiology of these pathologies may be very different (as described in detail below), they all come under the rubric of cerebrovascular disease, which is also known as vascular disease, or strokes, or infarcts. In each of these disorders there is a lack of blood flow to a

BOX 7.2 Diagnostic and Statistical Manual of Mental Disorders, 5th Edition Criteria for Major or Mild Vascular Neurocognitive Disorder

A. The criteria are met for major or mild neurocognitive disorder.
B. The clinical features are consistent with a vascular etiology, as suggested by either of the following:
   1. Onset of the cognitive deficits is temporally related to one or more cerebrovascular events.
   2. Evidence for decline is prominent in complex attention (including processing speed) and frontal-executive function.
C. There is evidence of the presence of cerebrovascular disease from history, physical examination, and/or neuroimaging considered sufficient to account for the neurocognitive deficits.
D. The symptoms are not better explained by brain disease or systemic disorder.

Probable vascular neurocognitive disorder is diagnosed if one of the following is present; otherwise **possible vascular neurocognitive disorder** should be diagnosed:
1. Clinical criteria are supported by neuroimaging evidence of significant parenchymal injury due to cerebrovascular disease (neuroimaging-supported).
2. The neurocognitive syndrome is temporally related to one or more documented cerebrovascular events.
3. Both clinical and genetic (e.g., cerebral autosomal dominant arteriopathy with subcortical infarcts and leukoencephalopathy) evidence of cerebrovascular disease is present.

Possible vascular neurocognitive disorder is diagnosed if the clinical criteria are met but neuroimaging is not available and the temporal relationship of the neurocognitive syndrome with one or more cerebrovascular events is not established.

From American Psychiatric Association. (2013). *Diagnostic and Statistical Manual of Mental Disorders (DSM-5)* (5th ed.). Arlington, VA: American Psychiatric Publishing, Inc.

part of the brain, which dies, causing the injury. Because there is a lack of blood flow, they could also each be called "ischemic": ischemic vascular disease, ischemic stroke, an ischemic infarct. The fourth pathology discussed below, cerebral amyloid angiopathy, can cause a part of the brain to die as a result of bleeding rather than lack of blood flow. But when bleeding occurs, damaging the brain tissue, the terms cerebrovascular disease, vascular disease, stroke, and infarct all apply to the resulting injury. Moreover, these four different types of cerebrovascular disease can cause a variety of different types of signs and symptoms depending on where the damage occurs (Fig. 7.3 and Table 7.2).

Small Vessel Ischemic Disease

Small vessel ischemic disease (also known as microinfarcts and subcortical ischemic vascular disease) is thought to be due to two processes, lipohyalinosis and microemboli. Lipohyalinosis is a process in which an eosinophilic material deposits in the connective tissue of the wall of deep penetrating arteries, leading to infarctions. Lipohyalinosis is thought to be secondary to damaged cerebrovascular autoregulation occurring with hypertension and aging. Microemboli can block small penetrating arteries of the brain, leading to infarctions. Microemboli may be due to atheroma, normal or abnormal clotting, and heart disease. Most individuals aged 70 years or older have some small vessel ischemic disease. Studies show that cortical

microinfarcts are often associated with cerebral amyloid angiopathy pathology, whereas deep microinfarcts are associated with arteriosclerosis (Arvanitakis et al., 2017). By itself, a small amount of small vessel ischemic disease does not typically cause noticeable cognitive impairment or dementia. Moderate or large amounts of small vessel ischemic disease, however, can cause cognitive impairment and dementia.

Multi-Infarct Dementia

Multi-infarct dementia is typically the result of multiple cortical strokes. Cortical strokes are most commonly caused by large emboli, which usually originate from the heart (often related to disrupted flow due to atrial fibrillation or ischemic myocardium), the carotid arteries, or the aorta. Multi-infarct dementia occurs when the patient suffers a number of cortical strokes.

Strategic Infarct Dementia

Strategic infarct dementia occurs when a focal lesion (or lesions), often quite small, damages a brain region that is critical for cognitive brain function. The lesions are typically lacunar infarcts or embolic strokes, although hypertensive hemorrhages can also damage these regions. There are many critical brain regions where even a small stroke could disrupt cognitive function in this manner, including the medial temporal lobes (hippocampal formation, entorhinal cortex, parahippocampal cortex), angular gyrus, cingulate gyrus, thalamus, fornix, basal forebrain, caudate, and globus pallidus (see Table 7.2).

Cerebral Amyloid Angiopathy

Cerebral amyloid angiopathy is caused by deposits of β-amyloid, predominantly $A\beta_{40}$, in the media of small- to medium-sized arteries in the leptomeninges and superficial cortex, particularly in the parieto-occipital, temporoparietal, and sometimes frontal regions. It is more common in patients with Alzheimer's disease. Thickening and hyalinization of the involved vessel walls may lead to hemorrhage. Hemorrhages typically occur in the superficial cortex and may be multicentric. Research now shows that cerebral amyloid angiopathy contributes to ischemic strokes as well as bleeding strokes (Graff-Radford, 2019).

Other

Other types of cerebrovascular disease may also lead to cognitive impairment. Hypoperfusion of the brain may occur regionally if there is a focal stenosis of a major

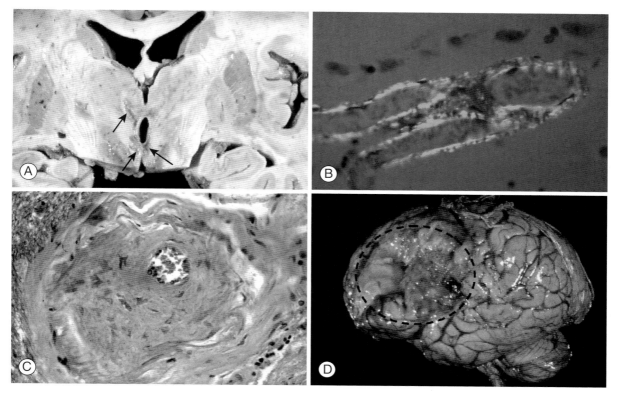

Fig. 7.3 Pathology of vascular dementia. Bilateral thalamic lesions are strategic infarcts (**A**, from a "top of the basilar" stroke, *arrows*), birefringent cerebral amyloid angiopathy in a small blood vessel (**B**), large cortical infarct easily visible on the surface of the brain (**D**, *dotted circle*), and lipohyalinosis of a small vessel (**C**).

artery or globally if there is cardiovascular insufficiency. Hemorrhages caused by hypertension may occur in strategic areas such as the thalamus. There are several relatively rare genetic disorders that can cause vascular cognitive impairment, including CADASIL (cerebral autosomal dominant arteriopathy with subcortical infarcts and leukoencephalopathy), which is caused by mutation of the Notch3 gene at the chromosome locus 19p13 (Federico et al., 2005). CADASIL, which may be as common as five in 100,000, typically presents first with migraine and then with multiple subcortical strokes, leading eventually to dementia, motor and sensory deficits, and death (Pantoni et al., 2010).

COMMON SIGNS, SYMPTOMS, AND STAGES

The signs and symptoms that will be present with cognitive impairment due to cerebrovascular disease

depend upon both the type of cerebrovascular disease and the particular brain structures affected.

Small Vessel Ischemic Disease

Small vessel ischemic disease most commonly occurs in the subcortical white matter. Because most of the brain's white matter is involved in transferring information to or from the frontal lobes, patients with large amounts of small vessel ischemic disease often show signs and symptoms of frontal subcortical dysfunction. Dysfunction of frontal subcortical regions often leads to difficulty focusing and maintaining attention. Also disrupted is working memory, the ability to keep a number of items in mind and mentally manipulate them (see Appendix C). Gait is often affected leading to a "frontal" or "magnetic gait" (called by the French the "*marche à petits pas*," walk of little steps), in which patients describe their feet feeling like they are stuck on the floor. Incontinence is common, even with mild

TABLE 7.2   Stroke Lesion Location and Possible Signs and Symptoms

Lesion Location	Possible Signs and Symptoms
Frontal cortex: left	Word-finding difficulties, Broca's aphasia, poor attention, disinhibition, right hemiparesis
Frontal cortex: right	Poor attention, left neglect, disinhibition, left hemiparesis; can be silent
Basal ganglia: left	Aphasia, right hemiparesis
Basal ganglia: right	Left neglect, left hemiparesis
Temporal cortex: left	Aphasia
Temporal cortex: right	Left neglect
Medial temporal lobe: left or right	Memory loss (left more likely to produce deficits for verbal information, right deficits for nonverbal information)
Parietal cortex: left	Wernicke's aphasia, calculation difficulties
Parietal cortex: right	Confusion, left neglect; can be silent
Thalamus: left	Aphasia, memory loss, disinhibition, right sensory disturbances
Thalamus: right	Left neglect, memory loss, disinhibition, left sensory disturbances
Occipital cortex: left	Visual defects, reading difficulty, confusion, agitation
Occipital cortex: right	Visual defects, confusion; can be silent
Multiple subcortical small vessel strokes	Slowing of cognition, frontal/executive dysfunction, disinhibition, incontinence, weakness, frontal gait

BOX 7.4   Pseudobulbar Affect

The term "pseudobulbar affect" is often used to indicate the loss of cortical control of emotions, such as when patients show inappropriate laughing and crying. Usually these signs of emotion come out with minimal provocation, although they sometimes occur without any discernible trigger. A common example is that patients may cry when they hear about items on a news broadcast that are sad, but not the sort of thing that would have caused them to come to tears in the past. Pseudobulbar affect is usually caused by disruption of frontal subcortical white matter tracts, which is commonly caused by cerebrovascular disease but may also be caused by normal pressure hydrocephalus, multiple sclerosis, cerebral palsy, and traumatic brain injury, along with less common disorders. Pseudobulbar affect can also be seen in Alzheimer's disease and the majority of dementias. Pseudobulbar affect can be treated with the combination pill dextromethorphan/quinidine (Nuedexta) (see Chapter 27).

impairment of cognition. Pseudobulbar affect is also often seen (Box 7.4). Note that small vessel ischemic disease is the only form of cerebrovascular disease that does not typically cause a stepwise progression (Sachdev et al., 2014). Also note that, as described below, cerebral amyloid angiopathy—which can be part of Alzheimer's disease—can cause small vessel ischemic disease and that not all T2 hyperintensities on MRI scans represent ischemic strokes.

Multi-Infarct Dementia

Multi-infarct dementia, being as a result of multiple cortical strokes, usually presents with clinical signs and symptoms referable to the particular region of the cortex affected. These cortical strokes are usually detected clinically, but strokes in the right frontal and right parietal cortices may first be detected during a work-up for dementia. Common signs and symptoms include poor attention, aphasia, disinhibition, hemiparesis, impairment of vision, and other sensory modalities (see Table 7.2).

Strategic Infarct Dementia

Strategic infarct dementia also typically presents with signs and symptoms referable to the particular region of the brain affected by the infarct. Many cases of poststroke dementia are because of strategic infarcts

(Skrobot et al., 2018). Common signs and symptoms include poor attention, slurred speech (dysarthria), aphasia, incontinence, hemiparesis, and impaired coordination (see Table 7.2).

Cerebral Amyloid Angiopathy

Cerebral amyloid angiopathy is usually present along with concomitant Alzheimer's disease. Thus patients with cerebral amyloid angiopathy often first present with symptoms of Alzheimer's disease, and then the more focal symptoms related to the ensuing hemorrhages may become manifest. However, the most common manifestation of cerebral amyloid angiopathy is developing between one and a dozen microhemorrhages, which are generally asymptomatic and detected incidentally on an MRI scan. When symptomatic, several features of cerebral amyloid angiopathy separate it from other cerebrovascular causes of cognitive impairment. First, it has a predilection for affecting the cortex of the temporoparietal–occipital junction. The symptoms resulting from damage to this region can be varied, and may include visual disturbances (which may be bizarre, such as multiple fragmented images), Wernicke's aphasia, word-finding difficulties, and visuospatial impairment. Second, despite the fact that the pathology is related to the rupture of blood vessels and hemorrhage, the symptoms can often present over a number of minutes, rather than all at once as often occurs in a hypertensive hemorrhage or embolic stroke. The last thing that should be mentioned about cerebral amyloid angiopathy is that it can contribute to ischemic strokes as well as hemorrhages. Thus one aspect of the pathology of Alzheimer's disease can cause both hemorrhagic and ischemic strokes.

THINGS TO LOOK FOR IN THE HISTORY

Signs and symptoms of strokes and/or TIAs are the most important events to look for in the history. Sudden symptoms are the key: abrupt weakness or numbness of a limb or part of the face, precipitous loss of vision, sudden loss of speech, and so on. Most patients with more than average cerebrovascular disease will have a history of one or more of such events. A history of risk factors should also be compiled (see Box 7.3).

THINGS TO LOOK FOR ON THE PHYSICAL AND NEUROLOGICAL EXAMINATION

Focal signs suggesting strokes should be sought on the neurological examination, such as a subtle hemiparesis, facial droop, ptosis, neglect, visual field cut, etc. Although nonspecific, signs of corticospinal tract dysfunction such as brisk reflexes and extensor plantars (Babinski's sign) are almost invariably present, and usually floridly abnormal. Frontal release signs, including a grasp, snout, and palmomental reflexes, are also commonly present.

PATTERN OF IMPAIRMENT ON COGNITIVE TESTS

Although the specific impairment that will be observed on cognitive tests in a patient with vascular cognitive impairment depends upon the specific location and type of the cerebrovascular disease, there are some general principles that are useful. The two aspects of neuropsychological function that are impaired in most patients with cerebrovascular disease are frontal/executive function and the speed of cognition, because of the fact that small vessel ischemic disease typically affects the frontal subcortical white matter tracts.

Attention

Attention is generally impaired in vascular dementia. Difficult tasks for these patients include tasks that require information to be kept "in mind" in working memory, such as counting backwards by 7s or 3s, spelling words backwards, or reciting the months of the year backwards.

Language

Word-finding difficulties are extremely common in all types of vascular dementia. True aphasia is uncommon in vascular dementia due solely to small vessel ischemic disease, but is often seen in multi-infarct and strategic infarct dementia.

Memory

Episodic memory shows a "frontal pattern": encoding is often impaired, as is free recall, whereas relative preservation is typically seen when tasks that assist in retrieval are used, such as cued recall, multiple choice, and yes/no recognition.

Reasoning and Judgment

Reasoning and judgment are typically impaired, both because working memory is reduced, impairing the patient's ability to keep various alternatives and details in mind, and because the frontal lobe's ability to inhibit impulsive responses is impaired.

Visuospatial Function

Visuospatial function is typically intact with small vessel ischemic disease, but can be quite impaired with multi-infarct and strategic infarct dementia.

LABORATORY STUDIES

There are no laboratory studies that are useful in either confirming or ruling out vascular cognitive impairment. If vascular cognitive impairment is diagnosed, however, a cerebrovascular work-up should be undertaken that will require a number of laboratory studies.

STRUCTURAL IMAGING STUDIES

The key to making a diagnosis of a vascular cognitive impairment is the structural imaging study. To make the diagnosis of pure vascular dementia or vascular mild cognitive impairment there needs to be sufficient cerebrovascular disease present on the CT or MRI scan to explain the degree of cognitive impairment. To make a diagnosis of a mixed dementia, with vascular cognitive impairment as a contributing factor, there needs to be more cerebrovascular disease present on the CT or MRI scan than is commonly present in an older adult without cognitive impairment. It is, of course, difficult to succinctly articulate exactly how much cerebrovascular disease may be present without significant cognitive impairment.

To complicate matters, we now know that in patients with Alzheimer's disease pathologically, some parietal white matter disease and enlarged perivascular spaces—two causes of white matter hyperintensities on T2 MRI scans—are due to Wallerian degeneration from the Alzheimer's disease rather than small vessel ischemic disease (Banerjee et al., 2017; McAleese et al., 2017). Thus it is essential to distinguish between white matter lesions on MRI and actual subcortical ischemic strokes. Figs. 7.4, 7.5, and 7.6 show imaging studies of patients with pure vascular dementia. Figs. 7.7 and 7.8 show cerebral amyloid angiopathy and superficial siderosis, respectively.

FUNCTIONAL AND MOLECULAR IMAGING STUDIES

Functional and molecular imaging studies are useful in excluding neurodegenerative diseases such as Alzheimer's disease or frontotemporal dementia.

DIFFERENTIAL DIAGNOSIS

There are several aspects to consider in the differential diagnosis. First, are the lesions observed in the imaging study because of cerebrovascular disease? Or some other pathology such as multiple sclerosis, progressive multifocal leukoencephalopathy, or Wallerian degeneration from Alzheimer's disease (Banerjee et al., 2017; McAleese et al., 2017)? Second, is the patient's cerebrovascular disease because of the ordinary causes of stroke such as hypertension, diabetes, and smoking, or to another disorder such as a vasculitis or vasculopathy? Third, as discussed, does the patient have pure vascular cognitive impairment, or is it a mixed disorder, vascular plus Alzheimer's disease or plus dementia with Lewy bodies? The answers to these questions are important as they will invariably lead to different treatments.

TREATMENTS (SEE ALSO TABLE 7.1)

If the patient has the common scenario of a mixed dementia of vascular cognitive impairment plus either Alzheimer's disease or dementia with Lewy bodies, treatment should proceed with medications appropriate to those disorders, such as cholinesterase inhibitors and memantine. If the patient has a pure vascular dementia, although there are no FDA-approved treatments, there are a number of studies which have investigated the treatment of vascular dementia. A meta-analysis (Kavirajan & Schneider, 2007) found that all randomized controlled trials for vascular dementia showed improvement on cognitive subscales, although only a few showed improvement on clinical, behavioral, or functional scales. The studies examined included three donepezil (Aricept) (Black et al., 2003; Roman et al., 2005; Wilkinson et al., 2003), two galantamine (Razadyne) (Auchus et al., 2007;

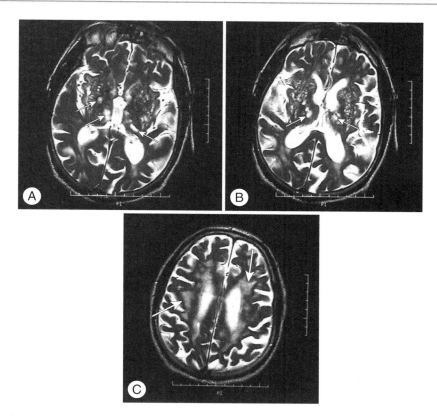

Fig. 7.4 T2-weighted magnetic resonance imaging scan of a patient with pure vascular dementia due to strategic infarcts and small vessel ischemic disease. Note the multiple bright areas in the deep gray structures of the brain including basal ganglia and thalamus **(A** and **B)** and the periventricular subcortical white matter **(C)** indicating strategic infarcts (*thin arrows*, not all infarcts indicated) and small vessel ischemic disease (*thick arrows*, not all disease indicated).

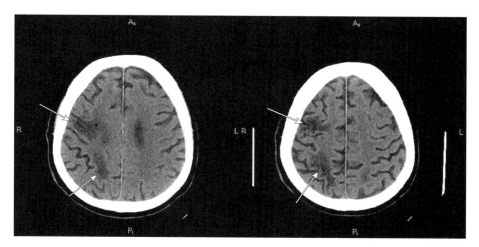

Fig. 7.5 Computed tomography scan of a patient with pure vascular dementia due to multi-infarct dementia. Note the two large right-hemisphere hypodensities (*arrows*) caused by embolic strokes which extend from subcortical to cortical regions.

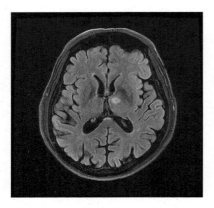

Fig. 7.6 T2-fluid attenuated inversion recovery (FLAIR) magnetic resonance imaging scan of a patient with post-stroke vascular dementia due to a single strategic infarct in the left anterior nucleus of the thalamus. Perhaps because memory loss is typically noticed more when verbal information cannot be remembered and the thalamus is more likely to experience strokes compared with the hippocampus and other components of Papez's circuit (see Appendix C), a stroke in the left anterior thalamic nucleus is the most common strategic infarct dementia we see.

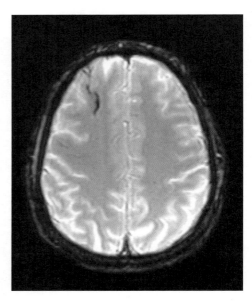

Fig. 7.8 Susceptibility-weighted magnetic resonance imaging scan of a patient with superficial siderosis. One cause of superficial siderosis is cerebral amyloid angiopathy bleeding in the subarachnoid space, which was the case in this patient with Alzheimer's disease.

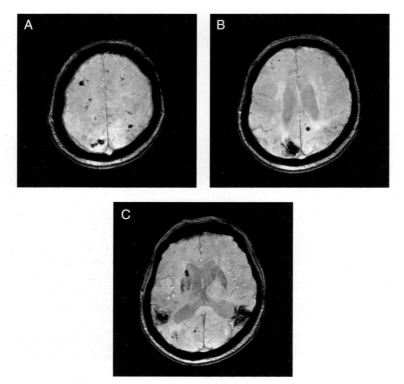

Fig. 7.7 Susceptibility-weighted magnetic resonance imaging scan of a patient Alzheimer's disease and cerebral amyloid angiopathy **(A, B,** and **C)**. The multiple *black dots* and *patches* throughout the brain parenchyma show hemosiderin deposition from small, medium, and large cerebral amyloid angiopathy bleeds.

Erkinjuntti et al., 2002), one rivastigmine (Exelon) (Moretti et al., 2003), and two memantine (Namenda) (Orgogozo et al., 2002; Wilcock, Mobius, & Stoffler, 2002) trials (see also Ballard et al., 2008; Erkinjuntti et al., 2008).

It is our experience that the majority of patients with a pure vascular cognitive impairment and resultant memory problems show improvement in their memory with cholinesterase inhibitors (see Chapter 19). Memantine (see Chapter 20) is also often helpful when problems such as apathy occur. We would therefore recommend a trial of these medications in patients with a pure vascular cognitive impairment when those symptoms are present. Pseudobulbar affect (see Box 7.4) can be treated with the combination pill dextromethorphan/quinidine (Nuedexta) (see Chapter 27).

All patients with cerebrovascular disease will benefit from regular aerobic exercise (Liu-Ambrose et al., 2016) and a Mediterranean-style diet (Valls-Pedret et al., 2015). Lastly, the underlying cause of the cerebrovascular disease must also be evaluated and treated.

REFERENCES

Arvanitakis, Z., Capuano, A. W., Leurgans, S. E., et al. (2017). The relationship of cerebral vessel pathology to brain microinfarcts. *Brain Pathology, 27*(1), 77–85.

Auchus, A. P., Brashear, H. R., Salloway, S., et al. (2007). Galantamine treatment of vascular dementia: A randomized trial. *Neurology, 69*, 448–458.

Ballard, C., Sauter, M., Scheltens, P., et al. (2008). Efficacy, safety and tolerability of rivastigmine capsules in patients with probable vascular dementia: The VantagE study. *Current Medical Research and Opinion, 24*, 2561–2574.

Banerjee, G., Kim, H. J., Fox, Z., et al. (2017). MRI-visible perivascular space location is associated with Alzheimer's disease independently of amyloid burden. *Brain, 140*(4), 1107–1116.

Black, S., Roman, G. C., Geldmacher, D. S., et al. (2003). Efficacy and tolerability of donepezil in vascular dementia: Positive results of a 24-week, multicenter, international, randomized, placebo-controlled clinical trial. *Stroke, 34*, 2323–2330.

Boyle, P. A., Yu, L., Leurgans, S. E., et al. (2019). Attributable risk of Alzheimer's dementia due to age-related neuropathologies. *Annals of Neurology, 85*, 114–124.

Erkinjuntti, T., Gauthier, S., Bullock, R., et al. (2008). Galantamine treatment in Alzheimer's disease with cerebrovascular disease: Responder analyses from a randomized, controlled trial (GAL-INT-6). *Journal of Psychopharmacology, 22*, 761–768.

Erkinjuntti, T., Kurz, A., Gauthier, S., et al. (2002). Efficacy of galantamine in probable vascular dementia and Alzheimer's disease combined with cerebrovascular disease: A randomised trial. *Lancet, 359*, 1283–1290.

Federico, A., Bianchi, S., Dotti, M. T., et al. (2005). The spectrum of mutations for CADASIL diagnosis. *Neurological Science, 26*, 117–124.

Graff-Radford. J. (2019). Vascular cognitive impairment. *Continuum (Minneapolis, Minn.), 25*(1), 147–164.

Kapasi, A., DeCarli, C., & Schneider, J. A. (2017). Impact of multiple pathologies on the threshold for clinically overt dementia. *Acta Neuropathologica, 134*(2), 171–186.

Kavirajan, H., & Schneider, L. S. (2007). Efficacy and adverse effects of cholinesterase inhibitors and memantine in vascular dementia: A meta-analysis of randomised controlled trials. *Lancet Neurology, 6*, 782–792.

Liu-Ambrose, T., Best, J. R., Davis, J. C., et al. (2016). Aerobic exercise and vascular cognitive impairment: A randomized controlled trial. *Neurology, 87*(20), 2082–2090.

McAleese, K. E., Walker, L., Graham, S., et al. (2017). Parietal white matter lesions in Alzheimer's disease are associated with cortical neurodegenerative pathology, but not with small vessel disease. *Acta Neuropathologica, 134*(3), 459–473.

Moretti, R., Torre, P., Antonello, R. M., et al. (2003). Rivastigmine in subcortical vascular dementia: A randomized, controlled, open 12-month study in 208 patients. *American Journal of Alzheimer's Disease and Other Dementias, 18*, 265–272.

Orgogozo, J. M., Rigaud, A. S., Stoffler, A., et al. (2002). Efficacy and safety of memantine in patients with mild to moderate vascular dementia: A randomized, placebo-controlled trial (MMM 300). *Stroke, 33*, 1834–1839.

Pantoni, L., Pescini, F., Nannucci, S., et al. (2010). Comparison of clinical, familial, and MRI features of CADASIL and NOTCH3-negative patients. *Neurology, 74*, 57–63.

Roman, G. C., Wilkinson, D. G., Doody, R. S., et al. (2005). Donepezil in vascular dementia: Combined analysis of two large-scale clinical trials. *Dementia and Geriatric Cognitive Disorders, 20*, 338–344.

Sachdev, P., Kalaria, R., O'Brien, J., et al. (2014). Diagnostic criteria for vascular cognitive disorders: A VASCOG statement. *Alzheimer Disease and Associated Disorders, 28*, 206–218.

Skrobot, O. A., Black, S. E., Chen, C., et al. (2018). Progress toward standardized diagnosis of vascular cognitive impairment: Guidelines from the Vascular Impairment of Cognition Classification Consensus Study. *Alzheimer's & Dementia: The Journal of the Alzheimer's Association, 14*(3), 280–292.

Valls-Pedret, C., Sala-Vila, A., Serra-Mir, M., et al. (2015). Mediterranean diet and age-related cognitive decline: A randomized clinical trial. *JAMA Internal Medicine, 175*(7), 1094–1103.

Wilcock, G., Mobius, H. J., & Stoffler, A. (2002). A double-blind, placebo-controlled multicentre study of memantine in mild to moderate vascular dementia (MMM500). *International Clinical Psychopharmacology, 17*, 297–305.

Wilkinson, D., Doody, R., Helme, R., et al. (2003). Donepezil in vascular dementia: A randomized, placebo-controlled study. *Neurology, 61*, 479–486.

8

Dementia With Lewy Bodies

QUICK START: DEMENTIA WITH LEWY BODIES

Definition	• Dementia with Lewy bodies (DLB) is a neurodegenerative disease of the brain characterized:
	  • clinically by dementia, fluctuating attention and alertness, visual hallucinations, rapid-eye movement (REM) sleep behavior disorder, and parkinsonism, and
	  • pathologically by Lewy body formation and abnormal alpha-synuclein metabolism.
	• Mild cognitive impairment with Lewy bodies is similar to DLB but with preserved or minimally affected function.

Prevalence	• DLB is one of the most common neurodegenerative diseases of the brain, accounting for approximately 7.5% of all dementias in secondary care. It frequently co-occurs with Alzheimer's and/or vascular pathology.
Genetic risk	• There are familial cases of DLB related to mutations or repeats of the alpha-synuclein gene located on chromosome 4. Most patients, however, do not show abnormalities of this gene.
Cognitive and other symptoms	• Impairment in attention, executive function, and visuospatial ability are often prominent. Memory impairment may or may not be prominent initially. • Sleep disturbances are common in DLB, and often leads to disrupted circadian rhythm, fluctuating levels of attention and alertness, and REM sleep behavior disorder.
Summary of diagnostic criteria	Essential for a diagnosis: • Dementia. Core clinical features: • Fluctuating cognition with pronounced variations in attention and alertness. • Recurrent visual hallucinations, typically well-formed and detailed. • REM sleep behavior disorder, which may precede cognitive decline. • One or more spontaneous features of parkinsonism: bradykinesia, rest tremor, or rigidity.

(Continued)

QUICK START: DEMENTIA WITH LEWY BODIES (*Continued*)

Indicative biomarkers:
- Reduced dopamine transporter uptake in basal ganglia demonstrated by SPECT or PET imaging.
- Abnormal (low uptake) [123]iodine-MIBG myocardial scintigraphy.
- Polysomnographic confirmation of REM sleep without atonia.

Probable DLB can be diagnosed if:
  a. Two or more core clinical features of DLB are present, with or without the presence of indicative biomarkers, or
  b. Only one core clinical feature is present, but with one or more indicative biomarkers.

Possible DLB can be diagnosed if:
  a. Only one core clinical feature of DLB is present, with no indicative biomarker evidence, or
  b. One or more indicative biomarkers is present but there are no core clinical features.

Treatment	• Cholinesterase inhibitors are beneficial; rivastigmine (Exelon) has been approved by the U.S. Food and Drug Administration (FDA). • Other medications, including levodopa/carbidopa (Sinemet), memantine, selective serotonin reuptake inhibitors, pimavanserin, and atypical antipsychotics, may be used with caution.
Top differential diagnoses	• Alzheimer's disease, mixed dementia (DLB plus Alzheimer's disease), vascular dementia, progressive supranuclear palsy, corticobasal degeneration, and chronic traumatic encephalopathy.

A 65-year-old man came to the clinic complaining of cognitive difficulties. He had been forgetful for about a year, often confused, and was unable to use the television remote. Although he was generally oriented to the day, date, month, and year, he would get lost—even on familiar routes. He could no longer balance his checkbook or learn a new computer program. He had less volume in his voice, less expression in his face, and his walking had slowed down. On review of systems he admitted to having visual hallucinations of people and animals—which he did not mention for fear of being considered crazy. When asked about sleep, his wife noted that for more than five years he had been kicking and sometimes punching or wrestling her while asleep, such that she often ended up sleeping in a different bed. On examination he had masked facies, increased tone, cogwheeling, and a shuffling gait.

PREVALENCE, PROGNOSIS, AND DEFINITION

Dementia with Lewy bodies (DLB) is a neurodegenerative disease of the brain characterized clinically by dementia, fluctuating attention and alertness, visual hallucinations, rapid-eye movement (REM) sleep behavior disorder, and/or parkinsonism, and pathologically by Lewy body formation and abnormal alpha-synuclein metabolism. Parkinson's disease dementia (PDD) is a clinical diagnosis of dementia occurring in someone who already has Parkinson's disease diagnosed at least one year before the onset of dementia. Pathologically, the cognitive deficits in Parkinson's disease dementia are usually due to Lewy bodies, although they may be due to other pathologies, such as Alzheimer's disease. Lewy body dementia is the "umbrella" term for a clinical diagnosis of either DLB or PDD. Mild cognitive impairment with Lewy bodies is prodromal dementia with Lewy bodies, that is, similar to dementia with Lewy bodies but with preserved or minimally affected function. Parkinson's disease mild cognitive impairment (PD-MCI) is a clinical diagnosis of mild cognitive impairment in someone who already has Parkinson's disease. It may be a prodromal stage of either dementia with Lewy bodies or Parkinson's disease dementia, depending upon how quickly the cognitive symptoms start after the diagnosis of Parkinson's disease. Lastly, Lewy body disease refers to the pathologic state of Lewy bodies in the brain seen in both Lewy body dementia and Parkinson's disease (Armstrong, 2019). (See Table 8.1.)

TABLE 8.1 Comparison Between Alzheimer's and Lewy Body Diseases

| | Lewy Body Diseases | | | | | Alzheimer's Diseases | |
| | | | | Lewy Body Dementia | | | |
	Parkinson's Disease	Parkinson's Disease Mild Cognitive Impairment	Mild Cognitive Impairment With Lewy Bodies	Parkinson's Disease Dementia	Dementia With Lewy Bodies	Mild Cognitive Impairment Due to Alzheimer's Disease	Alzheimer's Disease Dementia
Motor symptoms	Parkinsonism present	Parkinsonism present	Parkinsonism may or may not be present. Tremor less likely	Parkinsonism present	Parkinsonism may or may not be present. Tremor less likely	None	None (until the late stages)
Cognitive deficits	Essentially none	Mild visuospatial, attentional, and executive function deficits	Mild visuospatial, attentional, and executive function deficits	Visuospatial, attentional, and executive function prominent	Visuospatial, attentional, and executive function prominent	Mild memory, word finding, visuospatial, and executive function	Memory, word finding, visuospatial, and executive function prominent
Behavioral and psychological symptoms	Anxiety, depression, and apathy common. Rapid-eye movement (REM) sleep behavior disorder may be present.	Anxiety, depression, and apathy common. Hallucinations and REM sleep behavior disorder may be present.	Anxiety, depression, and apathy common. Hallucinations and REM sleep behavior disorder may be present.	Anxiety, depression, apathy common, plus others as disease progresses. Hallucinations and REM sleep behavior disorder may be present.	Anxiety, depression, apathy common, plus others as disease progresses. Hallucinations and REM sleep behavior disorder often present.	Anxiety and depression common	Anxiety, depression, apathy common, plus others as disease progresses
Bodily function	Anosmia and constipation common	Anosmia and constipation common	Anosmia and constipation common	Anosmia and constipation common	Anosmia and constipation common	Anosmia common	Anosmia common
Activities of daily living	No impairment from cognition	No impairment from cognition	No impairment from cognition	Impaired from cognition	Impaired from cognition	No impairment from cognition	Impaired from cognition

(Continued)

TABLE 8.1 Comparison Between Alzheimer's and Lewy Body Diseases (Continued)

	Lewy Body Diseases				Alzheimer's Diseases	
			Lewy Body Dementia			
	Parkinson's Disease	Parkinson's Disease Mild Cognitive Impairment	Mild Cognitive Impairment With Lewy Bodies	Parkinson's Disease Dementia	Dementia With Lewy Bodies	Mild Cognitive Impairment Due to Alzheimer's Disease	Alzheimer's Disease Dementia
Underlying pathology	Lewy bodies in brainstem	Lewy bodies in brainstem plus Lewy bodies in cortex and/or Alzheimer's pathology	Lewy bodies in cortex±brainstem. May also have Alzheimer's pathology	Lewy bodies in brainstem plus Lewy bodies in cortex (high likelihood) and/ or Alzheimer's pathology (low likelihood)	Lewy bodies in cortex± brainstem. High likelihood of concomitant Alzheimer's pathology	Alzheimer's pathology	Alzheimer's pathology

Does all this terminology seem a bit confusing? In practice, Parkinson's disease mild cognitive impairment and Parkinson's disease dementia are not difficult to diagnose because they are essentially the development of mild cognitive impairment and dementia, respectively, in a patient with established Parkinson's disease. In this chapter, we will focus on understanding dementia with Lewy bodies and its prodromal state, mild cognitive impairment with Lewy bodies, so that these disorders can be distinguished from others that they are commonly confused with, including Alzheimer's disease (see Chapter 4), progressive supranuclear palsy (see Chapter 12), corticobasal degeneration (see Chapter 13), and chronic traumatic encephalopathy (see Chapter 15).

Dementia with Lewy bodies is either the second or third most common neurodegenerative cause of dementia in the older adult after Alzheimer's disease (see Chapter 4) or Alzheimer's and limbic-predominant age-related TDP-43 encephalopathy (LATE) (see Chapter 6), depending upon the age range of those studied (Boyle et al., 2019). One meta-analysis found the incidence of new cases of dementia with Lewy bodies to be 3.8%, with a prevalence of about 4.2% in the community and 7.5% of all dementias in secondary care (Vann Jones & O'Brien, 2014). Another study found the incidence in a county in Minnesota was estimated at 5.9 per 100,000 (Savica et al., 2013).

Although some studies have suggested that the prognosis of patients with dementia with Lewy bodies is similar to those with Alzheimer's disease, other studies suggest that patients with dementia with Lewy bodies show a more rapid decline in function, leading to earlier nursing home placement and death. Our clinical experience is that most patients with dementia with Lewy bodies do progress more rapidly than those with Alzheimer's disease. The combination of parkinsonism, dementia, and visual hallucinations typically leads to nursing home placement in 2 to 6 years, and death in 3 to 8 years. One study found median survival of patients with dementia with Lewy bodies to be 3.7 years (Price et al., 2017), and another found survival of patients with Parkinson's disease dementia to be 4.5 years (Hely et al., 2008). There are, however, exceptions of patients who show a much slower disease progression.

Note that many patients with dementia with Lewy bodies also meet clinical and pathological criteria for Alzheimer's disease, with some studies suggesting an overlap of greater than 90% (Merdes et al., 2003). Thus many patients have a mixed dementia of Alzheimer's disease and dementia with Lewy bodies.

CRITERIA AND DIAGNOSIS

The most important features of dementia with Lewy bodies are dementia (which must of course always be present), rapid-eye movement (REM) sleep behavior disorder, fluctuating cognition, visual hallucinations, and parkinsonism (Fig. 8.1). Criteria for mild cognitive impairment with Lewy bodies have been published (McKeith et al., 2020). Although technically for research, they are immediately useful, as patients with mild cognitive impairment, preserved independent function, and features of dementia with Lewy bodies commonly present to the clinic. See Boxes 8.1–8.3 for a summary of the current clinical diagnostic criteria (see Chapter 3 for the Diagnostic and Statistical Manual of Mental Disorders, 5th Edition general criteria for major and mild neurocognitive disorder). Regarding the parkinsonism, note that up to 25% of patients with autopsy-proven dementia with Lewy bodies showed no signs of parkinsonism during life, perhaps due to having mainly cortical and little brainstem pathology. Note that biomarkers can now be used in support of a probable dementia with Lewy bodies diagnosis, namely reduced dopamine transporter uptake in basal ganglia demonstrated by single photon emission computed tomography (SPECT) or positron emission tomography (PET) imaging, abnormal (low uptake) ^{123}iodine–meta-iodobenzylguanidine (MIBG) myocardial scintigraphy, and polysomnographic confirmation of REM sleep without atonia.

Regarding the characteristics of the dementia, it may appear identical to Alzheimer's disease, with memory problems being prominent, or memory may be relatively normal with major difficulties present in attention, executive function, and visuospatial ability. If the dementia appears quite similar to that of Alzheimer's disease, it is reasonable to presume that (as is common in patients with dementia with Lewy bodies) Alzheimer's pathology of senile plaques and neurofibrillary tangles is likely present along with Lewy bodies and abnormal alpha-synuclein metabolism. Patients with dementia with Lewy bodies can, however, have prominent memory problems without Alzheimer's pathology (Kang et al., 2019).

Determining whether "fluctuating cognition" is present is quite difficult for most clinicians, for the simple reason that all dementing illnesses produce waxing and

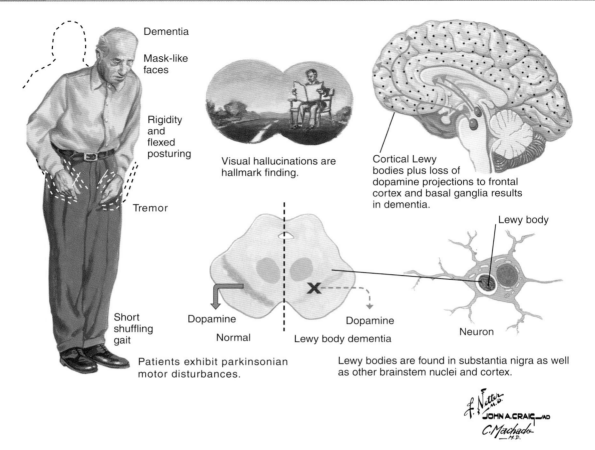

Fig. 8.1 Major clinical and pathological abnormalities in dementia with Lewy bodies. (Netter illustration from www. netterimages.com. Copyright Elsevier Inc. All rights reserved.)

waning, with some days and times of day better than others. In our experience, the key aspect of fluctuating cognition to look for is relative dramatic fluctuations of alertness and/or attention that impact functional abilities (Bradshaw et al., 2004). In one patient we cared for, this manifested rather dramatically: the patient literally fell asleep during dinner and could not be awakened. Quite reasonably, the family was concerned that he had suffered a stroke or other catastrophic medical illness, and he was taken by ambulance to the hospital. By the time he reached the hospital he had awakened, and was back to baseline (the work-up, including magnetic resonance imaging [MRI], electroencephalogram [EEG], and laboratory studies, was unrevealing). Other patients who we have cared for have had similar, although less dramatic, alterations in alertness.

Visual hallucinations are perhaps the most definitive criteria for dementia with Lewy bodies, and are related to the degree of pathology (Jacobson et al., 2014). In our experience actual well-formed hallucinations of people or animals are simply not present in other disorders (see below for discussion). The hallucinations are usually visual, and are almost always of people or animals, although they are sometimes described as large "bugs." These hallucinations are remarkable in several ways. First, patients with mild dementia may be fully or partially aware that they are having hallucinations. We have had many patients who can both describe in detail their hallucinations and also know, at least some of the time, that they are not real (i.e. they do not always have a delusional component). During a consultation, one patient said that he could see a man curled up under

BOX 8.1 Revised Criteria for the Clinical Diagnosis of Probable and Possible Dementia With Lewy Bodies

Essential for a diagnosis:

Dementia defined as progressive cognitive decline sufficient to interfere with normal social or occupational function, or with usual daily activities. Deficits on tests of attention, executive function, and visuospatial ability may be prominent and occur early. Memory impairment is usually evident with progression.

Core clinical features (the first three typically occur early and may persist):
- Fluctuating cognition with pronounced variations in attention and alertness.
- Recurrent visual hallucinations that are typically well formed and detailed.
- Rapid-eye movement (REM) sleep behavior disorder, which may precede cognitive decline.
- One or more spontaneous features of parkinsonism: bradykinesia, rest tremor, or rigidity.

Supportive clinical features:
- Severe sensitivity to antipsychotic agents.
- Postural instability.
- Repeated falls.
- Syncope or other transient episodes of unresponsiveness.
- Severe autonomic dysfunction (e.g., constipation, orthostatic hypotension, urinary incontinence).
- Hypersomnia.
- Hyposmia.
- Hallucinations in other modalities.
- Systematized delusions.
- Apathy, anxiety, and depression.

Indicative biomarkers:
- Reduced dopamine transporter uptake in basal ganglia demonstrated by single photon emission computed tomography (SPECT) or positron emission tomography (PET) imaging.
- Abnormal (low uptake) [123]iodine-meta-iodobenzylguanidine (MIBG) myocardial scintigraphy.
- Polysomnographic confirmation of rapid-eye movement sleep without atonia.

Supportive biomarkers:
- Relative preservation of medial temporal lobe structures on computed tomography/magnetic resonance imaging scan.
- Generalized low uptake on SPECT/PET perfusion/metabolism scan with reduced occipital activity ± the cingulate island sign on fluorodeoxyglucose-PET imaging.
- Prominent posterior slow-wave activity on electroencephalogram with periodic fluctuations in the pre-alpha/theta range.

Probable dementia with Lewy bodies (DLB) can be diagnosed if:
a. Two or more core clinical features of DLB are present, with or without the presence of indicative biomarkers, or
b. Only one core clinical feature is present, but with one or more indicative biomarkers.

Probable DLB should not be diagnosed on the basis of biomarkers alone.

Possible DLB can be diagnosed if:
a. Only one core clinical feature of DLB is present, with no indicative biomarker evidence, or
b. One or more indicative biomarkers is present but there are no core clinical features.

DLB is less likely:
a. In the presence of any other physical illness or brain disorder, including cerebrovascular disease, sufficient to account in part or in total for the clinical picture, although these do not exclude a DLB diagnosis and may serve to indicate mixed or multiple pathologies contributing to the clinical presentation, or
b. If parkinsonian features are the only core clinical feature and appear for the first time at a stage of severe dementia.

Modified from McKeith, I. G., Boeve, B. F., Dickson, D. W., et al. (2017). Diagnosis and management of dementia with Lewy bodies: Fourth consensus report of the DLB Consortium. *Neurology, 89*(1), 88–100.

BOX 8.2 Research Criteria for the Clinical Diagnosis of Probable and Possible Mild Cognitive Impairment With Lewy Bodies

Essential for a diagnosis is mild cognitive impairment defined by:
- Concern by the patient, informant, or clinician regarding cognitive decline.
- Objective evidence of impairment in one or more cognitive domains, more likely to be attention-executive and/or visual processing deficits.
- Preserved or minimally affected performance of previously attained independence in functional abilities, which do not meet the criteria for dementia.

Core clinical features:
- Fluctuating cognition with variations in attention and alertness.
- Recurrent visual hallucinations.
- Rapid-eye movement (REM) sleep behavior disorder.
- One or more spontaneous cardinal features of parkinsonism: bradykinesia, rest tremor, or rigidity.

Proposed biomarkers:
- Reduced dopamine transporter uptake in basal ganglia demonstrated by single photon emission computed tomography or positron emission tomography.
- Polysomnographic confirmation of rapid-eye movement sleep without atonia.
- Reduced meta-iodobenzylguanidine (MIBG) uptake on myocardial scintigraphy.

Probable mild cognitive impairment with Lewy bodies can be diagnosed if:
- Two or more core clinical features are present, with or without the presence of a proposed biomarker, or
- Only one core clinical feature is present, but with one or more proposed biomarkers.

Probable mild cognitive impairment with Lewy bodies should not be diagnosed based on biomarkers alone.

Possible mild cognitive impairment with Lewy bodies can be diagnosed if:
- Only one core clinical feature is present, with no proposed biomarkers, or
- One or more of the proposed biomarkers is present, but there are no core clinical features.

Supportive clinical features:
- Severe sensitivity to antipsychotic agents.
- Postural instability.
- Repeated falls.
- Syncope or other transient episodes of unresponsiveness.
- Prolonged or recurrent delirium.
- Autonomic dysfunction (e.g., constipation, orthostatic hypotension, urinary incontinence).
- Hypersomnia.
- Hyposmia.
- Hallucinations in other modalities including passage and sense of presence phenomena.
- Systematized delusions.
- Apathy, anxiety, and depression.

Potential biomarkers of mild cognitive impairment with Lewy bodies:
- Quantitative electroencephalogram showing slowing and dominant frequency variability.
- Relative preservation of medial temporal lobe structures on structural imaging (computed tomography/magnetic resonance imaging [CT/MRI]).
- Insular thinning and gray matter volume loss on MRI.
- Low occipital uptake on perfusion/metabolism scan.

Mild cognitive impairment plus supportive clinical features or potential biomarkers are insufficient to diagnose mild cognitive impairment with Lewy bodies but may raise suspicion of it and prompt biomarker investigation.

Supportive clinical features or potential biomarkers may add weight to an existing mild cognitive impairment with Lewy bodies diagnosis.

Mild cognitive impairment with Lewy bodies is less likely in the presence of any other physical illness or brain disease, including cerebrovascular disease, sufficient to account in part or in total for the clinical picture, although these do not exclude a mild cognitive impairment with Lewy bodies diagnosis and may serve to indicate mixed or multiple pathologies contributing to the clinical presentation.

Modified from McKeith, I. G., Ferman, T. J., Thomas, A. J., et al. (2020). Research criteria for the diagnosis of prodromal dementia with Lewy bodies. *Neurology, 94*, 743–755.

BOX 8.3   Diagnostic and Statistical Manual of Mental Disorders, 5th Edition Criteria for Major or Mild Neurocognitive Disorder With Lewy Bodies

A. The criteria are met for major or mild neurocognitive disorder.

B. The disturbance has insidious onset and gradual progression.

C. The disorder meets a combination of core diagnostic features and suggestive diagnostic features for either probable or possible neurocognitive disorder with Lewy bodies.

For probable major or mild neurocognitive disorder with Lewy bodies, the individual has two core features, or one suggestive feature with one or more core features. For possible major or mild neurocognitive disorder with Lewy bodies, the individual has only one core feature, or one or more suggestive features.

  1. Core diagnostic features:

    a. Fluctuating cognition with pronounced variations in attention and alertness.

    b. Recurrent visual hallucinations that are well formed and detailed.

    c. Spontaneous features of parkinsonism, with onset subsequent to the development of cognitive decline.

  2. Suggestive diagnostic features:

    a. Meets criteria for rapid-eye movement sleep behavior disorder.

    b. Severe neuroleptic sensitivity.

D. The disturbance is not better explained by cerebrovascular disease, another neurodegenerative disease, the effects of a substance, or another mental, neurological, or systemic disorder.

From American Psychiatric Association (2013). *Diagnostic and statistical manual of mental disorders (DSM-5)* (5th ed.). Arlington, VA: American Psychiatric Publishing, Inc.

---

the desk, but knew that this could not be real. In other cases, the hallucinations can be incredibly realistic, and typically as the dementia progresses there is usually no ability of the patient to separate them from reality. One patient asked his wife why she was not serving dinner to the other people sitting at the table. Another patient thought she was petting an imaginary dog in the waiting room. And another patient used to see little children playing in the corner of the room. This last patient was thought initially to be suffering from a psychotic depression (she had lost a child) until the correct diagnosis was made. Unfortunately, she had already received several courses of electroconvulsive therapy that may have exacerbated her hallucinations and dementia. The cause of visual hallucinations in Lewy body dementia is unknown. One study found an association between the concentration of Lewy bodies in the temporal lobe and well-formed visual hallucinations (Harding, Broe, & Halliday, 2002). However, the hallucinations may also relate to sleep disturbances, as discussed below. Although less common, hallucinations may be in other sensory modalities, including auditory, olfactory, and tactile. Visual hallucinations may also be preceded by prodromal symptoms of seeing things fleetingly "out of the corner of one's eye" and/or a feeling of a presence (without an abnormal visual perception).

True Hallucinations?

Many families of patients who are suffering from dementias other than dementia with Lewy bodies inform us that the patient is having hallucinations. A common example is the patient with Alzheimer's disease who reports that she was talking with her mother last night, even though her mother died many years ago. Another example is the patient who reports that people were up having a party in her house all night long. Typically these symptoms are not true hallucinations but are instead memory distortions (thinking that a real memory from long ago happened recently), confabulations, or delusions. Memory distortions and delusions can usually be easily distinguished from true hallucinations because in the former case the patient is never observed to be actively hallucinating. Interestingly, all of these symptoms—true hallucinations, memory distortions, confabulations, and delusions—will often improve, at least partly, with cholinesterase inhibitors. Thus cholinesterase inhibitors should always be used before atypical antipsychotics to treat these symptoms.

Sleep Disturbances

Although we are all normally paralyzed during REM sleep, those with REM sleep behavior disorder are not, and these individuals act out their dreams while sleeping. These actions can be disturbing and even frightening or life threatening to their sleeping partners. It has been noted for a number of years that REM sleep behavior disorder can be one of the earliest signs of dementia with Lewy bodies (Ferman et al., 2002). One clue as to the reason for this association comes from a patient with dementia with Lewy bodies whose brain at autopsy showed a marked loss of brainstem monoaminergic nuclei (including locus caeruleus and substantia nigra) that inhibit cholinergic neurons in the pedunculopontine nucleus, which usually cause paralysis during REM sleep (Turner et al., 2000). When suspecting that a patient may have dementia with Lewy bodies, it is therefore important to ask whether the patient ever acts out his or her dreams while sleeping, or simply moves around a lot in their sleep. Probably the most common sign of this disorder is that the sleeping partner complains that the patient has begun kicking them at night, and frequently by the time the history is taken the spouse has sought refuge by sleeping in another bed! For patients who sleep alone, a telltale sign is that all the covers and pillows are kicked out and strewn about or the patient may actually fall out of bed.

The association of dementia with Lewy bodies and disturbances in alertness, visual hallucinations, and REM sleep behavior disorder has led researchers to investigate whether many of the symptoms of dementia with Lewy bodies are related to a sleep disorder. Harper et al. (2004) have found that, although both patients with Alzheimer's disease and those with dementia with Lewy bodies have disrupted circadian rhythms, the disruption was greatest in those with dementia with Lewy bodies (Harper et al., 2004). It may be that in dementia with Lewy bodies disruption of circadian rhythm causes loss of alertness owing to drowsiness or actual sleep, and REM phenomena breaking into wakeful consciousness cause the well-formed visual hallucinations.

RISK FACTORS, PATHOLOGY, AND PATHOPHYSIOLOGY

Other than age (mean of approximately 75 years) and male sex there are no known risk factors for dementia with Lewy bodies. Its pathology involves neurodegeneration associated with abnormal alpha-synuclein metabolism and formation of Lewy bodies and Lewy neurites in various brain regions including brainstem, basal

forebrain, limbic regions, and neocortical regions (Fig. 8.2). The pathophysiology is due not only to the direct loss of neurons, but also to neuronal loss in brainstem centers that produce neurotransmitters, including the substantia nigra (producing dopamine) and the nucleus basalis of Meynert (producing acetylcholine) (Grothe et al., 2014). Thus patients with dementia with Lewy bodies have reduced levels of cortical dopamine and acetylcholine, which has important treatment implications (see later).

There are familial cases of dementia with Lewy bodies related to mutations or repeats of the alpha-synuclein gene located on chromosome 4. Most patients with dementia with Lewy bodies, however, do not show abnormalities of this gene.

COMMON SIGNS, SYMPTOMS, AND STAGES

As described in more detail in the section Criteria and Diagnosis, above, the most important features of dementia with Lewy bodies are dementia, fluctuating cognition, visual hallucinations, REM sleep behavior disorder, and parkinsonism.

When considering the stages of dementia with Lewy bodies, there are at least two axes to consider. The first axis is that of distribution of Lewy bodies in the brain. Those patients who initially have more Lewy bodies in their brainstem will present with the motor symptoms of Parkinson's disease. Those patients who present with Lewy bodies more evenly distributed throughout the brainstem, basal forebrain, limbic regions, and neocortical regions usually present with both cognitive impairment and parkinsonism. And those patients who present with mainly cortical Lewy bodies present with cognitive impairment. The second axis to consider is that of disease severity, because each of these patients can demonstrate mild, moderate, or severe magnitude of motor and cognitive symptoms.

THINGS TO LOOK FOR IN THE HISTORY

It is generally not difficult to make the diagnosis of dementia with Lewy bodies in patients who begin with idiopathic Parkinson's disease and develop dementia and prominent visual hallucinations within one year. For those patients who do not have early or prominent

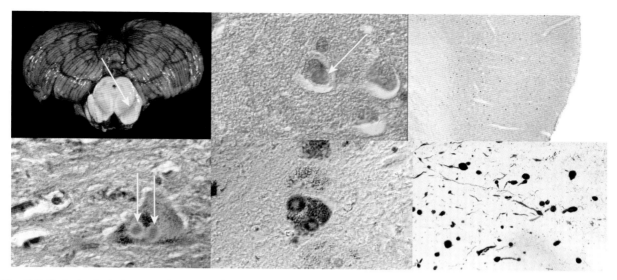

Fig. 8.2 Pathological changes that occur in dementia with Lewy bodies. Clockwise from top left: gross view of the brain through the midbrain to show the pallor of the substantia nigra (should be black, see *arrow*); high-power view showing the eosinophilic (*pink* in color) Lewy body *(arrow)* in a cortical neuron; low-power view of Lewy bodies in the cortex; alpha-synuclein stain technique to visualize only Lewy bodies and Lewy neurites; two Lewy bodies *(rings)* stare up at us via a ubiquitin stain; and high-power view of Lewy bodies in the substantia nigra—note the two Lewy bodies in a single large neuron.

parkinsonism, the diagnosis can be more difficult—and, as mentioned, 20% to 25% of autopsy-proven patients with dementia with Lewy bodies never develop parkinsonism.

A number of signs and symptoms may often be harbingers of the disorder. REM sleep behavior disorder may be present for years preceding the clinical onset of cognitive impairment. Other sleep disturbances, such as nightmares, difficulty distinguishing dreams from being awake, and daytime drowsiness, are common. Brief episodes of poor attention and/or being poorly responsive may also be present early on. In addition to visual hallucinations, visual perceptual difficulties and misperceptions may be prominent early on. Some patients present with the clinical syndrome of posterior cortical atrophy (see Chapter 11). One example is of a patient we cared for who could not see well enough to distinguish different types of paper money; he was referred to us by his ophthalmologist, who found nothing wrong with his eyes. Autonomic dysfunction may also occur early in the course, leading to orthostatic hypotension, cardiovascular instability, urinary incontinence, constipation, impotence, eating and swallowing difficulties, falls, and

syncope. Lastly, anxiety, depression, and apathy may precede the clinical onset of dementia with Lewy bodies, but these symptoms are common in most dementias.

Because dementia with Lewy bodies is a common cause of dementia, and patients and families may not volunteer information about hallucinations, sleep disturbances, and other relevant symptoms, we recommend that clinicians simply incorporate many of the important signs and symptoms of this disorder into their history of present illness and review of systems, probing for:

- fluctuating levels of alertness or periods of being relatively unresponsive
- visual hallucinations of people or animals
- hallucinations in other modalities
- a disturbance of gait
- falls
- a tremor
- rigidity and other signs of parkinsonism
- acting out dreams during sleep or other abnormal movements while sleeping
- difficulty distinguishing dreams from reality when transitioning from sleep.

THINGS TO LOOK FOR ON THE PHYSICAL AND NEUROLOGICAL EXAMINATION

Parkinsonism is the main feature of dementia with Lewy bodies that can be identified in the physical and neurological examination (although signs of autonomic dysfunction can also sometimes be observed). The parkinsonism is generally similar to age-matched, nondemented patients with Parkinson's disease in overall severity, but shows greater symmetry, axial involvement, postural instability, and facial impassivity, and less tremor. It is important to keep in mind that a lack of parkinsonism does not exclude the disorder because up to 25% of autopsy-proven patients with dementia with Lewy bodies showed no clinical signs of parkinsonism. Consistent with this finding is that the diagnostic guidelines do not require that parkinsonism is present.

PATTERN OF IMPAIRMENT ON COGNITIVE TESTS

It had been thought that in patients with pure dementia with Lewy bodies, cognitive impairment is most prominent on measures of attention, visuospatial, and executive function with relative sparing of memory. However, recent studies suggest that patients with pure dementia with Lewy bodies can also have prominent memory problems without Alzheimer's pathology (Kang et al., 2019). Moreover, in the common scenario in which there is an underlying mixed dementia with Alzheimer's pathology as well as cortical Lewy bodies, the cognitive deficits in these patients may be similar to those of Alzheimer's disease. Further research will be needed to determine whether the common belief that cuing improves the memory impairment in patients with pure dementia with Lewy bodies more than in patients with Alzheimer's disease is correct.

LABORATORY, SLEEP, AND ELECTROENCEPHALOGRAPHY STUDIES

There are no laboratory, genetic, or cerebrospinal fluid studies that are helpful in either confirming or ruling out dementia with Lewy bodies. Polysomnography to confirm REM sleep without atonia is helpful when the history is not clear whether the patient has REM sleep behavior disorder or another sleep disorder. Although we do not recommend the routine use of EEG to diagnoses dementia, one may see prominent posterior slow-wave activity with periodic fluctuations in the pre-alpha/theta range.

STRUCTURAL IMAGING STUDIES

There are no features of dementia with Lewy bodies that can be observed on structural imaging. Pure dementia with Lewy bodies is less likely when there is prominent medial temporal atrophy, commonly associated with Alzheimer's disease and LATE. Such atrophy does not, however, lessen the possibility of a mixed dementia of Alzheimer's disease or LATE plus dementia with Lewy bodies.

FUNCTIONAL IMAGING STUDIES

There are two types of functional imaging studies which can be helpful in confirming the diagnosis of dementia with Lewy bodies. Standard SPECT (^{99m}Tc-HMPAO) or PET (fluorodeoxyglucose [FDG]) imaging will often (but not invariably) show occipital hypoperfusion on SPECT imaging (Fig. 8.3) and occipital hypometabolism on PET imaging (Mak et al., 2014), sometimes with sparing of the cingulate, producing the so-called "cingulate island sign." (This is in contrast to classic Alzheimer's disease, in which the cingulate is involved.) Occipital hypometabolism is not specific for dementia with Lewy bodies, however, because it can also be seen in posterior cortical atrophy as a result of underlying Alzheimer's pathology (Whitwell et al., 2017). Functional imaging showing reduction in dopamine transporter activity by either SPECT or PET using specialized tracers is the imaging "gold standard" (Mak et al., 2014) but is not available at all centers (Fig. 8.4).

When the diagnosis of dementia with Lewy bodies is relatively straightforward, there is no reason to obtain a functional imaging study. In the complicated case, however, obtaining such a study can be helpful. Which you choose depends mainly upon your differential diagnosis and which studies are available in your institution.

DIFFERENTIAL DIAGNOSIS

The first issue that we bear in mind when considering a diagnosis of dementia with Lewy bodies is whether the

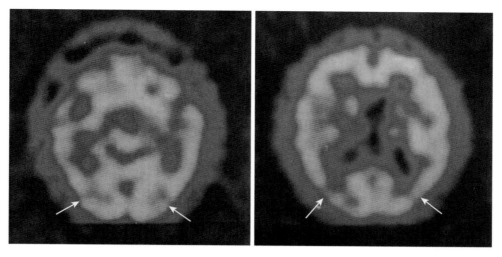

Fig. 8.3 Single photon emission computed tomography scan in a patient with dementia with Lewy bodies. Note decreased occipital function *(arrows)*.

patient's dementia would be best characterized by that diagnosis alone, Alzheimer's disease alone, or both (see Table 8.1). If the patient meets criteria for both dementias, then the patient has a mixed dementia: dementia with Lewy bodies plus Alzheimer's disease. After Alzheimer's disease, the main differential diagnosis of dementia with Lewy bodies includes vascular dementia (see Chapter 7), progressive supranuclear palsy (see Chapter 12), multiple system atrophy, corticobasal degeneration (see Chapter 13), and chronic traumatic encephalopathy (CTE) (see Chapter 15). Creutzfeldt-Jakob disease (see Chapter 16) should also be considered, although the pace of the dementia will usually distinguish between these disorders.

Vascular dementia (see Chapter 7) should be considered if there are many large or small ischemic strokes on the structural imaging scan (computed tomography [CT] or MRI). Strokes in the basal ganglia can produce parkinsonism. However, if the history and cognitive examination strongly suggest dementia with Lewy bodies, then we would argue that the patient most likely has dementia with Lewy bodies, although the dementia may be exacerbated to some extent by small vessel ischemic disease. If the small vessel disease is moderate to severe, yet the patient has clear signs of dementia with Lewy bodies, such as visual hallucinations or REM sleep behavior disorder, then diagnosis of a mixed dementia of dementia with Lewy bodies plus vascular dementia is most appropriate.

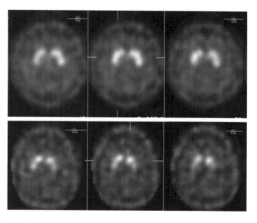

Fig. 8.4 Negative *(top)* and positive *(bottom)* dopamine transporter positron emission tomography scans. Note the asymmetric loss of signal in the striatum in the bottom panel in a patient with dementia with Lewy bodies, showing more of a "period shape" than the normal "comma shape."

Progressive supranuclear palsy (see Chapter 12) should be considered if there is an abnormality of vertical gaze (particularly downgaze), axial rigidity (rigidity of the neck and trunk), difficulty swallowing, and frequent falls. Corticobasal degeneration (see Chapter 13) should be considered if there are strong asymmetric findings, such as focal or asymmetric rigidity or dystonia, inability to control a limb or apraxia of the limb, visual or sensory hemineglect, and focal or asymmetric myoclonus. Chronic traumatic encephalopathy (see Chapter 15) should be considered if there is any history of repetitive head trauma from sports (boxing, football, rugby, etc.), military service, or other cause; a history of such exposures should be routinely elicited.

Lastly, there are several nondementia conditions that could be confused with dementia with Lewy bodies in that they may cause cognitive impairment, fluctuating cognition, repeated falls, and transient unexplained loss of consciousness. These conditions include medication side-effects, complex partial seizures (including temporal lobe epilepsy), multiple sclerosis, and cardiac dysfunction (particularly arrhythmias).

TREATMENTS (TABLE 8.2)

Anticholinergic medications should be avoided because they may impair cognition, cause confusion, aggravate

or cause visual hallucinations, and often exacerbate behavioral disturbances. Benzodiazepines, antipsychotics, and dopamine agonists can also worsen cognition and/or behavior (Armstrong, 2019).

Regarding symptomatic treatment, the FDA has approved the rivastigmine (Exelon) patch to treat Parkinson's disease dementia, which is essentially the same pathological entity as dementia with Lewy bodies. Cholinesterase inhibitors (see Chapter 19) have been shown in a number of studies to improve both cognition and neuropsychiatric/behavioral symptoms in patients with dementia with Lewy bodies (Meng et al., 2019). The most careful of these studies are two rivastigmine (Exelon) studies, one in patients labeled "dementia with Lewy bodies" (McKeith et al., 2000) and the other in patients labeled "Parkinson's disease dementia" (Emre et al., 2004). Smaller and less controlled studies have found similar results with donepezil (Aricept) (Ravina et al., 2005) and galantamine (Razadyne) (Bhasin et al., 2007). Our clinical experience agrees with a recent meta-analysis that

Medication Class	Medication and U.S. Food and Drug Administration (FDA) Approval?	Recommendations
TABLE 8.2 **Medical Treatment for Dementia With Lewy Bodies**		
Cholinesterase inhibitors	Rivastigmine (Exelon patch) is FDA approved to treat Parkinson's disease dementia (dementia with Lewy bodies). Donepezil (Aricept) and galantamine can be used "off-label"	Try in all patients to improve cognition as well as neuropsychiatric and behavioral symptoms, including hallucinations.
Memantine	Memantine (Namenda) "off-label"	Consider when trying to effect improvement in apathy and other symptoms in patients with moderate-to-severe dementia.
Melatonin	Over the counter	Use to reduce rapid-eye movement sleep behavior disorder and fluctuations.
Selective serotonin reuptake inhibitors (SSRIs)	Sertraline (Zoloft) and escitalopram (Lexapro) "off-label"	Consider if depression and/or anxiety is present.
Dopaminergic agents	Levodopa/carbidopa (Sinemet) "off-label"	Use with caution to improve movement when needed for function; can worsen hallucinations.
Selective serotonin 2A receptor inverse agonists	Pimavanserin (Nuplazid) FDA approved for hallucinations and delusions associated with Parkinson's disease	Use with caution after trying cholinesterase inhibitors, SSRIs, and nonpharmacologic approaches.
Atypical antipsychotics	Quetiapine (Seroquel) and risperidone (Risperdal) "off-label"	Use with great caution to improve frightening hallucinations; can worsen cognition and parkinsonism.

found cholinesterase inhibitors can improve cognitive, neuropsychiatric, and behavioral symptoms in patients with dementia with Lewy bodies (Meng et al., 2019). Interestingly, this meta-analysis found that whereas donepezil did not produce more adverse events than placebo, rivastigmine did, suggesting that rivastigmine should be used with additional caution.

The motor symptoms of parkinsonism are generally best treated with levodopa (along with carbidopa, usually referred to as Sinemet) in low dose. Side effects, however, in patients with dementia with Lewy bodies can include confusion and worsening of (or causing) visual hallucinations. Thus, as a general rule of thumb, levodopa is initiated only when the patient has significant functional impairment, such as difficulty getting out of a car or off a toilet.

Memantine (Namenda), as discussed in Chapter 20, enhances dopamine in addition to any effects on glutamate at the N-methyl-D-aspartic (NMDA) acid receptor. Thus, like levodopa, memantine has the potential to be useful but it could also make things worse. This view is supported by the literature: some reports are of patients benefiting and some are of patients worsening; a meta-analysis suggests a slight improvement in global function (Meng et al., 2019). We do not recommend routine use of memantine, but do recommend giving memantine a try when neuropsychiatric symptoms, particularly apathy, are not responsive to cholinesterase inhibitors.

Successfully treating hallucinations is difficult, and pharmacological treatment should be initiated when hallucinations become threatening or otherwise problematic. Moreover, the goal of treatment should not be to eliminate hallucinations, but only to make them no longer frightening and functionally impairing. If the patient is not already on cholinesterase inhibitors, these should always be tried first, as they invariably lessen the frequency and/or intensity of hallucinations. Pimavanserin (Nuplazid) is a selective serotonin 2A receptor inverse agonist FDA approved for hallucinations and delusions associated with Parkinson's disease. A recent study showed that pimavanserin worked as well, if not better, in such patients who also showed cognitive impairment (Mini-Mental State Examination scores from 21 to 24) and were taking cholinesterase inhibitors and/or memantine (Espay et al., 2018). Atypical antipsychotics should be used as third-line treatment for such symptoms. Quetiapine (Seroquel) at bedtime is generally used because it is less likely to worsen parkinsonism, although risperidone (Risperdal) may be more efficacious. Traditional neuroleptics, such as haloperidol (Haldol), should essentially never be used because they are highly likely to worsen parkinsonism. Even atypical antipsychotics may worsen cognition and parkinsonism. (Please carefully review Chapter 27 before treating with an atypical antipsychotic.)

REM sleep behavior disorder is best treated with melatonin. Orthostatic hypotension should be first addressed by reducing relevant medications (such as dopamine agonists and possibly antihypertensive drugs) and nonpharmacologic strategies, such as rising slowly. If these approaches are not successful, the usual medications can be tried. Constipation is best treated with increased water intake and consumption of fiber and dried fruits (such as raisins and prunes); over-the-counter approaches can also be used. Sialorrhea can be treated with botulinum toxin injections, glycopyrrolate, ipratropium bromide spray, and atropine drops (Armstrong, 2019). As in Alzheimer's disease, depression and anxiety are common in patients with dementia with Lewy bodies who have mild disease and preserved insight. If these symptoms are present, we again recommend a selective serotonin reuptake inhibitor such as sertraline (Zoloft) (see Chapter 27).

Lastly, although few studies have looked at the impact of exercise and physical activity for patients with dementia with Lewy bodies specifically, there is increasing evidence regarding the benefits of such activities to body and mind in healthy older adults and patients with Parkinson's disease (Mak et al., 2017). We therefore recommend physical exercise (as tolerated) and a healthy, Mediterranean-style diet to the majority of our dementia with Lewy body patients.

REFERENCES

Armstrong. M. J. (2019). Lewy body dementias. *Continuum (Minneapolis, Minn.)*, 25(1), 128–146. https://doi.org/10.1212/CON.0000000000000685. PMID: 30707190.

Bhasin, M., Rowan, E., Edwards, K., et al. (2007). Cholinesterase inhibitors in dementia with Lewy bodies: A comparative analysis. *International Journal of Geriatric Psychiatry*, 22, 890–895.

Boyle, P. A., Yu, L., Leurgans, S. E., et al. (2019). Attributable risk of Alzheimer's dementia due to age-related neuropathologies. *Annals of Neurology*, 85, 114–124.

Bradshaw, J., Saling, M., Hopwood, M., et al. (2004). Fluctuating cognition in dementia with Lewy bodies and Alzheimer's disease is qualitatively distinct. *Journal of Neurology, Neurosurgery, and Psychiatry, 75*(3), 382–387.

Emre, M., Aarsland, D., Albanese, A., et al. (2004). Rivastigmine for dementia associated with Parkinson's disease. *The New England Journal of Medicine, 351*, 2509–2518.

Espay, A. J., Guskey, M. T., Norton, J. C., et al. (2018). Pimavanserin for Parkinson's disease psychosis: Effects stratified by baseline cognition and use of cognitive-enhancing medications. *Movement Disorders, 33*(11), 1769–1776.

Ferman, T. J., Boeve, B. F., Smith, G. E., et al. (2002). Dementia with Lewy bodies may present as dementia and REM sleep behavior disorder without parkinsonism or hallucinations. *Journal of the International Neuropsychological Society, 8*, 907–914.

Grothe, M. J., Schuster, C., Bauer, F., et al. (2014). Atrophy of the cholinergic basal forebrain in dementia with Lewy bodies and Alzheimer's disease dementia. *Journal of Neurology, 261*, 1939–1948.

Harding, A. J., Broe, G. A., & Halliday, G. M. (2002). Visual hallucinations in Lewy body disease relate to Lewy bodies in the temporal lobe. *Brain, 125*, 391–403.

Harper, D. G., Stopa, E. G., McKee, A. C., et al. (2004). Dementia severity and Lewy bodies affect circadian rhythms in Alzheimer disease. *Neurobiology of Aging, 25*, 771–781.

Hely, M. A., Reid, W. G., Adena, M. A., et al. (2008). The Sydney multicenter study of Parkinson's disease: The inevitability of dementia at 20 years. *Movement Disorders, 23*(6), 837–844.

Jacobson, S. A., Morshed, T., Dugger, B. N., et al. (2014). Plaques and tangles as well as Lewy-type alpha synucleinopathy are associated with formed visual hallucinations. *Parkinsonism & Related Disorders, 20*, 1009–1014.

Kang, S. W., Jeon, S., Yoo, H. S., et al. (2019). Effects of Lewy body disease and Alzheimer disease on brain atrophy and cognitive dysfunction. *Neurology, 92*(17), e2015–e2026.

Mak, E., Su, L., Williams, G. B., et al. (2014). Neuroimaging characteristics of dementia with Lewy bodies. *Alzheimer's Research & Therapy, 6*, 18.

Mak, M. K., Wong-Yu, I. S., Shen, X., et al. (2017). Long-term effects of exercise and physical therapy in people with Parkinson disease. *Nature Reviews Neurology, 13*(11), 689–703.

McKeith, I., Del Ser, T., Spano, P., et al. (2000). Efficacy of rivastigmine in dementia with Lewy bodies: A randomised, double-blind, placebo-controlled international study. *Lancet, 356*, 2031–2036.

McKeith, I. G., Boeve, B. F., Dickson, D. W., et al. (2017). Diagnosis and management of dementia with Lewy bodies: Fourth consensus report of the DLB Consortium. *Neurology, 89*(1), 88–100.

McKeith, I. G., Ferman, T. J., Thomas, A. J., et al. (2020). Research criteria for the diagnosis of prodromal dementia with Lewy bodies. *Neurology, 94*, 743–755.

Meng, Y. H., Wang, P. P., Song, Y. X., et al. (2019). Cholinesterase inhibitors and memantine for Parkinson's disease dementia and Lewy body dementia: A meta-analysis. *Experimental and Therapeutic Medicine, 17*(3), 1611–1624.

Merdes, A. R., Hansen, L. A., Jeste, D. V., et al. (2003). Influence of Alzheimer pathology on clinical diagnostic accuracy in dementia with Lewy bodies. *Neurology, 60*, 1586–1590.

Price, A., Farooq, R., Yuan, J. M., et al. (2017). Mortality in dementia with Lewy bodies compared with Alzheimer's dementia: A retrospective naturalistic cohort study. *BMJ Open, 7*(11), e017504.

Ravina, B., Putt, M., Siderowf, A., et al. (2005). Donepezil for dementia in Parkinson's disease: A randomised, double blind, placebo controlled, crossover study. *Journal of Neurology, Neurosurgery, and Psychiatry, 76*, 934–939.

Savica, R., Grossardt, B. R., Bower, J. H., et al. (2013). Incidence of dementia with Lewy bodies and Parkinson disease dementia. *JAMA Neurology, 70*, 1396–1402.

Turner, R. S., D'Amato, C. J., Chervin, R. D., et al. (2000). The pathology of REM sleep behavior disorder with comorbid Lewy body dementia. *Neurology, 55*, 1730–1732.

Vann Jones, S. A., & O'Brien, J. T. (2014). The prevalence and incidence of dementia with Lewy bodies: A systematic review of population and clinical studies. *Psychological Medicine, 44*(4), 673–683.

Whitwell, J. L., Graff-Radford, J., Singh, T. D., et al. (2017). 18F-FDG PET in posterior cortical atrophy and dementia with Lewy bodies. *Journal of Nuclear Medicine, 58*(4), 632–638.

9

Primary Progressive Aphasia and Apraxia of Speech

QUICK START: PRIMARY PROGRESSIVE APHASIA AND APRAXIA OF SPEECH

Definition and etiology	• Primary progressive aphasia (PPA) is a clinical syndrome characterized by progressive language dysfunction. There are three variants:
	  • Logopenic variant is most often associated with Alzheimer's disease pathology.
	  • Semantic variant (also called semantic dementia or temporal variant frontotemporal dementia) is most often associated with TDP-43 pathology.
	  • Nonfluent/agrammatic variant (also called progressive nonfluent aphasia) is most often associated with tau pathology.
	• Primary progressive apraxia of speech (PPAOS) is an impairment in the production of speech sounds in the absence of language impairment (also called progressive apraxia of speech [PAOS]). It is most often associated with tau pathology.

Prevalence and genetic risk	• Impairments of speech and language are common in neurodegenerative diseases. • The number of patients who meet criteria for primary progressive aphasia or primary progressive apraxia of speech is relatively small. • Genetic risk will depend upon underlying etiology; most individuals with primary progressive aphasia or apraxia of speech have no family history.
Cognitive and behavioral symptoms	• In the logopenic variant of primary progressive aphasia there is hesitant speech, difficulty naming and finding words, and phonologic and/or repetition errors, with no loss of comprehension and preserved grammar. • In the semantic variant of primary progressive aphasia there is a loss of memory for words, starting with anomia, continuing with impaired comprehension of single words, and ultimately leading to impaired comprehension of objects as well. Speech is fluent with normal rate and minimal syntactic errors. • In the nonfluent/agrammatic variant of primary progressive aphasia there is a reduction in the ability to produce speech characterized by slow, effortful, apraxic speech; grammatical errors; short sentences; reduced phrase length; omission of articles (a, an, the); and difficulty pronouncing words, somewhat similar to that of a patient with Broca's aphasia. • Characteristics of primary progressive apraxia of speech include slow rate, articulatory distortions, distorted sound substitutions, and segmentation of syllables.

(Continued)

QUICK START: PRIMARY PROGRESSIVE APHASIA AND APRAXIA OF SPEECH (*Continued*)

Diagnostic criteria	• Primary progressive aphasia core criteria
	• Inclusion: (1) Most prominent clinical feature is difficulty with language; (2) these deficits are the principal cause of impaired function; (3) aphasia is the most prominent deficit at onset and for the initial phases of the disease. (For exclusion criteria see Box 9.1.)
	• For specific criteria for the logopenic, semantic, and nonfluent/agrammatic variants, see Boxes 9.2–9.4.
	• For features of primary progressive apraxia of speech, see Boxes 9.5 and 9.6.
Treatment	• Treatment is supportive. Speech therapy and communication devices are helpful for some patients.
Top differential diagnoses	• Alzheimer's disease, behavioral variant frontotemporal dementia, vascular cognitive impairment, progressive supranuclear palsy, corticobasal degeneration.

A 59-year-old man presents with progressive difficulty talking over several years. Although he knows what he wants to say, he has difficulty saying it and he is frequently frustrated. His family has gotten into the habit of suggesting words and phrases for him. His speech is slow, halting, and nonfluent with grammatical errors. When asked to perform simple commands ("point to the ceiling," "point to the way you would go to get out of this room") his comprehension seems intact, but when tested with syntactically complex sentences ("The lion was eaten by the tiger, which one is dead?" and "Pick up the cup after writing with the pen"), he makes errors.

Communication problems are common in neurodegenerative diseases. Patients with Alzheimer's disease, for example, almost always manifest word-finding difficulties and impaired comprehension of language at some point in the disease course. Patients with corticobasal degeneration and progressive supranuclear palsy often show apraxia of speech. Some patients with progressive speech disorders, however, do not meet criteria for any neurodegenerative disorder—at least at the time of presentation. For this reason, the classification of patients into the different syndromes of primary progressive aphasia (PPA) and primary progressive apraxia of speech (PPAOS) is useful.

PREVALENCE, DEFINITION, AND PATHOLOGY

Primary progressive aphasia and primary progressive apraxia of speech are not diseases. They are clinical syndromes that patients may manifest, with varying underlying neurodegenerative disease etiologies (Table 9.1).

• Primary progressive aphasia is divided into three variants:
  • Logopenic variant (often abbreviated to lvPPA).
  • Semantic variant (also called semantic dementia or temporal variant frontotemporal dementia; often abbreviated to svPPA or SD or tv-FTD). The average age of onset is about age 60 years, although one-quarter of cases present after age 70 years. Prevalence is estimated to range from 2.5 to 7.3 per 100,000, equal in men and women. Median survival is 10 to 13 years after diagnosis (Botha & Josephs, 2019).
  • Nonfluent/agrammatic variant (also called progressive nonfluent aphasia; often abbreviated to naPPA or agPPA or PNFA). The average age of onset is about age 60 years. Prevalence is estimated to range from 0.5 to 3.9 per 100,000, equal in men and women (Botha & Josephs, 2019).
• Primary progressive apraxia of speech is an impairment in the production of speech sounds in the absence of language impairment (also called progressive apraxia of speech; often abbreviated to PPAOS or PAOS). Age of onset ranges from the fifth to the ninth decade of life, with two-thirds of cases presenting over age 65 years. Prevalence is estimated to be approximately 4.4 per 100,000, equal in men and women (Botha & Josephs, 2019).

Although impairments of language are common in neurodegenerative diseases, the number of patients who meet criteria for primary progressive aphasia or apraxia

TABLE 9.1 Pathological and Anatomical Correlates of Primary Progressive Aphasia and Primary Progressive Apraxia of Speech

Feature	Logopenic Variant Primary Progressive Aphasia	Semantic Variant Primary Progressive Aphasia	Nonfluent/ Agrammatic Variant Primary Progressive Aphasia	Primary Progressive Apraxia of Speech
Underlying etiology and pathology	Alzheimer's disease (96%) Frontotemporal lobar degeneration (TDP-43 & tau 4%)	Frontotemporal lobar degeneration (TDP-43 80%, tau 6%) Alzheimer's disease (14%)	Frontotemporal lobar degeneration (tau 67%, TDP-43 19%, other 4%) Alzheimer's disease (10%)	Progressive supranuclear palsy (38%) corticobasal degeneration or other tauopathy (62%)
Cortical atrophy or hypometabolism	Left temporoparietal	Anterior temporal, often left greater than right	Left posterior frontoinsular	Superior premotor, supplementary motor

From Botha and Josephs (2019), Gorno-Tempini et al. (2011), Grossman (2012), Josephs et al. (2014), Jung, Duffy, and Josephs (2013), Santos-Santos et al. (2018), Wicklund et al. (2014).

of speech is quite small. Risk factors, pathology, pathophysiology, prognosis, and age of presentation all depend upon underlying etiology: for example, those patients with underlying frontotemporal lobar degeneration or progressive supranuclear palsy often present in their 50s and 60s, whereas patients with underlying Alzheimer's disease pathology typically present in their 70s and 80s.

CRITERIA

Criteria for primary progressive aphasia consists of core criteria (Box 9.1) plus additional criteria for each variant (Boxes 9.2–9.4). Note that patients who meet the core criteria but have a combination of both agrammatism and semantic impairments at early stages of disease can be described as having "mixed primary progressive aphasia" (Mesulam & Weintraub, 2014). Primary progressive apraxia of speech is diagnosed by a list of common features (Box 9.5) plus criteria for diagnosis (Box 9.6).

COMMON SIGNS, SYMPTOMS, AND STAGES (TABLE 9.2)

Logopenic Variant Primary Progressive Aphasia

The pattern of speech impairment in logopenic variant primary progressive aphasia is common, one that you

BOX 9.1 Primary Progressive Aphasia Core Criteria

Inclusion: Criteria 1–3 must be answered positively.
1. Most prominent clinical feature is difficulty with language
2. These deficits are the principal cause of impaired daily living activities
3. Aphasia should be the most prominent deficit at symptom onset and for the initial phases of the disease

Exclusion: Criteria 1–4 must be answered negatively.
1. Pattern of deficits is better accounted for by other non-degenerative nervous system or medical disorders
2. Cognitive disturbance is better accounted for by a psychiatric diagnosis
3. Prominent initial episodic memory and visuoperceptual impairments are present
4. Prominent, initial behavioral disturbance is present

Modified from Gorno-Tempini, M. L., Hillis, A. E., Weintraub, S., et al. (2011). Classification of primary progressive aphasia and its variants. *Neurology, 76*, 1006–1014.

have likely heard in a patient with Alzheimer's disease dementia. Speech is hesitant, there is difficulty finding words and naming, there are often phonologic errors, and there is difficulty repeating sentences. Grammar is preserved and there is no loss of comprehension. One sign

---

BOX 9.2   Logopenic Variant Primary Progressive Aphasia Criteria

A. Clinical Diagnosis of Logopenic Variant Primary Progressive Aphasia

Both of the following core features must be present:

1. Impaired single-word retrieval in spontaneous speech and naming
2. Absence of definite grammar and comprehension impairment

At least three of the following other features must be present:

1. Speech (phonologic) errors in spontaneous speech and naming
2. Impaired repetition of sentences and phrases
3. Spared single-word comprehension and object knowledge
4. Spared motor speech

B. Imaging-Supported Logopenic Variant Diagnosis

In addition to fulfilling clinical criteria, imaging must show one of the following results:

1. Predominant left posterior perisylvian or parietal atrophy
2. Predominant left posterior perisylvian or parietal hypoperfusion or hypometabolism on SPECT or PET

Modified from Gorno-Tempini, M. L., Hillis, A. E., Weintraub, S., et al. (2011). Classification of primary progressive aphasia and its variants. *Neurology, 76,* 1006–1014 as suggested by Mesulam and Weintraub (2014).

BOX 9.3   Semantic Variant Primary Progressive Aphasia Criteria

A. Clinical Diagnosis of Semantic Variant Primary Progressive Aphasia

Both of the following core features must be present:

1. Impaired confrontation naming
2. Impaired single-word comprehension

A least three of the following other diagnostic features must be present:

1. Impaired object knowledge, particularly for low-frequency or low-familiarity items
2. Surface dyslexia or dysgraphia
3. Spared repetition
4. Spared speech production (grammar and motor speech)

B. Imaging-Supported Semantic Variant Primary Progressive Aphasia Diagnosis

In addition to fulfilling clinical criteria, imaging must show one of the following results:

1. Predominant anterior temporal lobe atrophy
2. Predominant anterior temporal hypoperfusion or hypometabolism on SPECT or PET

Modified from Gorno-Tempini, M. L., Hillis, A. E., Weintraub, S., et al. (2011). Classification of primary progressive aphasia and its variants. *Neurology, 76,* 1006–1014.

---

that a patient is showing word-finding difficulties is when the family has slipped into the habit of filling in the word for the patient when he or she hesitates. By definition, of course, the patient with logopenic variant primary progressive aphasia does not meet criteria for Alzheimer's disease or another neurodegenerative disease when they present. However, because the underlying pathology in these patients is most likely Alzheimer's disease (see Table 9.1), patients with logopenic variant primary progressive aphasia typically show more clinical features of Alzheimer's disease (see Chapter 4) as they progress.

Semantic Variant Primary Progressive Aphasia (Videos 9.1–9.4)

Semantic variant primary progressive aphasia could be described as a loss of memory for words. The disorder often starts as problems with word-finding and naming difficulties (anomia), but progresses to include impaired word comprehension and ultimately impaired

comprehension of objects as well. The naming deficit in semantic variant primary progressive aphasia is often referred to as a two-way naming deficit because patients have difficulty naming an object when shown its picture, and also describing an object when given its name. They have difficulty in word-to-picture matching, identifying the right color for objects (e.g., yellow for banana), and knowing which objects belong together (e.g., dental floss with toothbrush rather than hairbrush). This difficulty occurs because these patients lose the meaning of what things are. It is as if they lived in a culture without bananas or dental floss, and so therefore they would not know the right color for the banana, or what the floss is used for. (For additional explanation, see Appendix C.) Manifestations of the behavioral variant of frontotemporal dementia may occur in patients with semantic variant primary progressive aphasia later in the course of their disease, as most of these patients have underlying frontotemporal dementia pathology (usually TDP-43; see Chapter 10). Note that semantic dementia is sometimes distinguished from semantic variant

---

BOX 9.4 Nonfluent/Agrammatic Variant Primary Progressive Aphasia Criteria

A. Clinical Diagnosis of Nonfluent/Agrammatic Variant Primary Progressive Aphasia

At least one of the following core features must be present:

1. Agrammatism in language production
2. Effortful, halting speech with inconsistent speech sound errors and distortions (apraxia of speech)

A least two of three of the following other features must be present:

1. Impaired comprehension of syntactically complex sentences
2. Spared single-word comprehension
3. Spared object knowledge

B. Imaging-Supported Nonfluent/Agrammatic Variant Primary Progressive Aphasia Diagnosis

In addition to fulfilling clinical criteria, imaging must show one of the following results:

1. Predominant left posterior fronto-insular atrophy
2. Predominant left posterior fronto-insular hypoperfusion or hypometabolism on SPECT or PET

Modified from Gorno-Tempini, M. L., Hillis, A. E., Weintraub, S., et al. (2011). Classification of primary progressive aphasia and its variants. *Neurology, 76*, 1006–1014.

BOX 9.5 Primary Progressive Apraxia of Speech Features

Patients must not meet criteria for primary progressive aphasia or other neurodegenerative disorder. Features ordered from most to least prevalent, with features 1–5 present in all subjects studied:

1. Slow overall speech rate
2. Lengthened intersegment durations (between sounds, syllables, words, or phrases; possibly filled, including intrusive schwa ["ehh" sound])
3. Increased sound distortions or distorted sound substitutions with increased utterance length or increased syllable/word articulatory complexity
4. Syllable segmentation within words >1 syllable
5. Sound distortions
6. Syllable segmentation across words in phrases/sentences
7. Audible or visible articulatory groping; speech initiation difficulty; false starts/restarts
8. Lengthened vowel and/or consonant segments
9. Distorted sound substitutions
10. Deliberate, slowly sequenced, segmented, and/or distorted (including distorted substitutions) speech sequential motion rates in comparison with speech alternating motion rates
11. Increased sound distortions or distorted sound substitutions with increased speech rate
12. Distorted sound additions (not including intrusive schwa ["ehh" sound])
13. Sound or syllable repetitions
14. Sound prolongations (beyond lengthened segments)
15. Inaccurate (off-target in place or manner) speech alternating motion rates (as in rapid repetition of "puh puh")
16. Reduced words per speech breath group relative to maximum vowel duration

Modified from Josephs, K. A., Duffy, J. R., Strand, E. A., et al. (2012). Characterizing a neurodegenerative syndrome: Primary progressive apraxia of speech. *Brain, 135*, 1522–1536.

---

primary progressive aphasia. In the semantic variant, the meaning of the word is lost but the knowledge of the object is retained. In semantic dementia the knowledge of the object is lost as well. For example, a patient with semantic variant primary progressive aphasia may have lost the meaning of the word fork, but still knows what it is used for and how to eat with it. A patient with semantic dementia may not know what such an object is or what it is used for, as if they grew up in a culture without forks.

Nonfluent/Agrammatic Primary Progressive Aphasia

In nonfluent/agrammatic primary progressive aphasia, patients have slow, effortful speech with errors in grammar and/or praxis of speech—the motor planning and sequencing of the lips, tongue, and breath necessary for articulate speech. They often have word-finding difficulties, speak in short sentences, omit the articles (a, an, the), and show difficulty in pronouncing words, similar to that of a patient with Broca's aphasia. Comprehension

is intact, except for syntactically complex sentences, such as "the lion was eaten by the tiger." Repetition is impaired, even for single words. The ability to converse becomes reduced over time, with many patients eventually becoming monosyllabic or mute. Most patients with nonfluent/agrammatic primary progressive aphasia are aware of their language difficulties, which are understandably quite frustrating for them. Manifestations of the behavioral variant of frontotemporal dementia may occur in patients with nonfluent/agrammatic primary progressive

BOX 9.6   Criteria for a Diagnosis of Primary Progressive Apraxia of Speech

Inclusion
- Insidious onset and progressive worsening of speech disturbance
- Apraxia of speech is the only or dominant speech disturbance at the time of testing
- Dysarthria can be present but must be less severe than apraxia of speech
- Any evidence of aphasia is considered equivocal

Exclusion
- Pattern of deficits is better accounted for by other non-degenerative nervous system or medical disorders, or by a psychiatric diagnosis

- Unequivocal evidence for aphasia on detailed language/neuropsychological testing (i.e., the patient may meet root criteria for primary progressive aphasia)
- Dysarthria deemed to be more severe than apraxia of speech
- Prominent initial symptoms that would suggest another neurodegenerative disorder, including typical and atypical Alzheimer's disease, behavioral variant frontotemporal dementia, progressive supranuclear palsy, corticobasal syndrome, and motor neuron disease.

Modified from Botha, H., Josephs, K. A. (2019). Primary progressive aphasias and apraxia of speech. *Continuum (Minneapolis, Minn.)*, *25*(1), 101–127.

TABLE 9.2   Clinical Characteristics of Primary Progressive Aphasia and Primary Progressive Apraxia of Speech

Feature	Logopenic Variant Primary Progressive Aphasia	Semantic Variant Primary Progressive Aphasia	Nonfluent/Agrammatic Variant Primary Progressive Aphasia	Primary Progressive Apraxia of Speech
Impaired grammar	—	—	Typically present	—
Apraxia of speech	—	—	Often present	Present
Impaired comprehension	—	Single words	Only for syntactically complex sentences	—
Impaired naming	Present	Present	—	—
Impaired object knowledge	—	Present	—	—
Paraphasia	Present	Sometimes present	Present	—
Speech rate	Moderately reduced	Normal	Significantly reduced	Significantly reduced
Impaired repetition	Sentences and phrases	—	Single words	Single words
Surface dyslexia or dysgraphia	—	Present		—

From Gorno-Tempini et al. (2011), Jung et al. (2013), Mesulam and Weintraub (2014).

aphasia later in the course of their disease, as most of these patients have underlying frontotemporal dementia pathology (usually tau; see Chapter 10). See Videos 9.5 to 9.7 for examples of spontaneous speech, and Videos 9.8 to 9.13 for performance during cognitive testing.

Primary Progressive Apraxia of Speech (Videos 9.14 and 9.15)

Patients with primary progressive apraxia of speech are impaired in the motor planning and sequencing of the lips, tongue, and breath necessary for articulate speech.

Speech is slow with articulatory groping, distorted articulation, sound substitutions, false starts and restarts, segmentation of syllables, and increased difficulty with utterance length. Similar to nonfluent/agrammatic primary progressive aphasia, the ability to converse becomes reduced over time, with many patients eventually becoming monosyllabic or mute. In primary progressive apraxia of speech, language itself is not disordered; that is, although there is impaired speech output there is no aphasia, making it different from nonfluent/agrammatic primary progressive aphasia. For this reason, writing or typing may be preserved in primary progressive apraxia of speech. Primary progressive apraxia of speech is also different from dysarthria, in that the problem is not solely because of weakness of lips, tongue, and other vocal apparatus. Over time, most patients with primary progressive apraxia of speech develop parkinsonian signs, with bradykinesia and masked facie being most common. Other signs observed included axial rigidity, other apraxias, and eye movement abnormalities. In one study 38% of patients developed a progressive supranuclear palsy-like syndrome that included severe parkinsonism, near mutism, dysphagia with choking, vertical supranuclear gaze palsy or slowing, balance difficulties with falls, and urinary incontinence (Josephs et al., 2014) (see Chapter 12).

THINGS TO LOOK FOR IN THE HISTORY

In general, when disorders of communication such as primary progressive aphasia and primary progressive apraxia of speech are severe enough to cause functional impairments in daily life (which is part of the core criteria for primary progressive aphasia), patients and families notice and complain. The job of the clinician is to first figure out which disorder of speech and/or language is present based on the information presented in this chapter, and then to look for signs and symptoms that could indicate whether the diagnosis of another neurodegenerative disorder is more appropriate. For example, if a patient presents with word-finding difficulties and a diagnosis of logopenic variant primary progressive aphasia is being considered, symptoms of episodic memory deficits should be elicited, as such patients may be better characterized as having Alzheimer's disease with word-finding difficulties, if memory deficits are equally or more prominent than language deficits.

THINGS TO LOOK FOR ON THE PHYSICAL AND NEUROLOGICAL EXAMINATION

Although there are no particular signs on the physical or neurological examination to suggest primary progressive aphasia, it is critical to pay close attention to comprehension and production during conversation, and to have the patient repeat sounds, single words, phrases, and sentences. Because many patients with this disorder have underlying frontotemporal dementia pathology, signs of motor neuron disease should be sought for, including brisk reflexes, extensor plantars, fasciculations, and muscle wasting. (Up to 10% of patients with motor neuron disease also show signs and symptoms of behavioral variant frontotemporal dementia; see Chapter 10.)

In patients for whom a diagnosis of primary progressive apraxia of speech is being considered, the examination should look for nonverbal oral apraxias. These can be tested by asking the patient to blow, cough, click their tongue, and perform similar movements. There may also be signs of parkinsonism including bradykinesia, masked facie, and axial

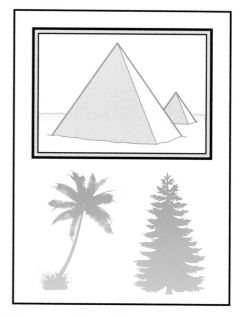

Fig. 9.1 The Pyramids and Palm Trees test. The goal of the test is for the patient to correctly point out which of the two lower pictures is most associated with the upper picture.

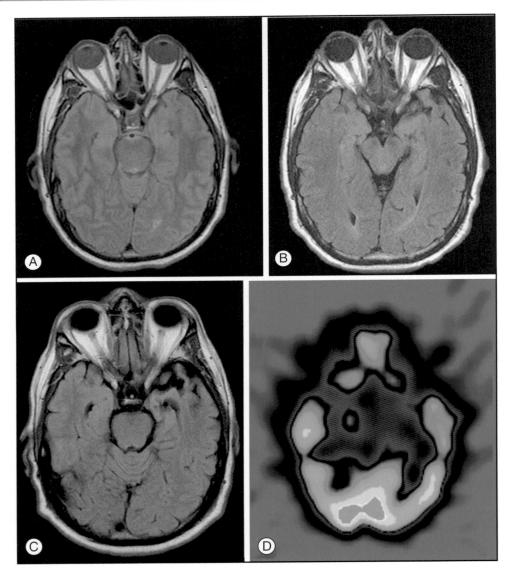

Fig. 9.2 Imaging studies of a patient with semantic variant primary progressive aphasia over time. Magnetic resonance imaging scans showing the temporal lobes at the level of the optic nerve from **(A)** 2005, **(B)** 2007, and **(C)** 2012. Note the progressive atrophy in the left anterior temporal lobe (*upper right side of image*). **(D)** A single photon emission computed tomography scan from 2008 shows hypoperfusion of the left anterior temporal lobe (*right side of image*).

rigidity. Signs of progressive supranuclear palsy (such as eye movement abnormalities) and corticobasal degeneration (such as apraxias) should also be sought, as one of these underlying disorders may be present (see Chapters 12 and 13).

PATTERN OF IMPAIRMENT ON COGNITIVE TESTS

When considering one of these disorders it is essential to evaluate language in addition to other cognitive domains. To characterize the language impairment a number of tests can be used. Some of the common ones include the Controlled Oral Word Fluency (see Video 9.16), Category Fluency (see Video 9.17), Boston Naming Test (see Video 9.12), the Boston Diagnostic Aphasia Battery, the Western Aphasia Battery–revised, part V of DeRenzi and Vignolo's Token Test, and the Pyramids and Palm Trees test (see later and Video 9.13). Tasks of sentence ordering and narrative production may be helpful in detecting nonfluent/agrammatic variant primary progressive aphasia (Harris et al., 2019). To look for apraxia of speech, the features in Box 9.5 can be rated on a 0 to 4 scale, following Josephs et al. (2012). Note that patients with apraxia of speech may perform better on written tests than on oral ones, such as verbal fluency. Table 9.2 shows some of the common impairments observed in these disorders.

Testing for semantic variant primary progressive aphasia deserves special note. In this disorder impairments are prominent on tests of semantic memory, including verbal fluency to categories, picture naming, and single-word comprehension (defining words or pictures). The Pyramids and Palm Trees test was developed specifically to evaluate patients for this disorder; in this test patients are asked which of two pictures best go with a third picture (Fig. 9.1). In this way semantic information can be assessed in a nonverbal way, to help distinguish disorders that affect solely language from those affecting semantic information. (Very early patients with semantic variant primary progressive aphasia may perform normally on the Pyramids and Palm Trees test, but in later stages almost all patients show abnormalities.)

STRUCTURAL AND FUNCTIONAL IMAGING STUDIES

Although the structural imaging scan may be normal at the time of presentation, most of these communication disorders show focal atrophy at some point in the course of their disease. In general, functional studies such as single photon emission computed tomography (SPECT) and positron emission tomography (PET) typically show decreased function in the same regions as those that show atrophy on structural scans, often several years before the atrophy being noted. See Table 9.1 for the regions associated with cortical atrophy, hypoperfusion, or hypometabolism in these disorders. Fig. 9.2 provides an example of imaging in a patient with semantic variant primary progressive aphasia.

DIFFERENTIAL DIAGNOSIS

Table 9.3 shows the differential diagnosis of primary progressive aphasia and primary progressive apraxia of speech. Because these disorders are clinical syndromes with underlying neurodegenerative etiologies, the first row in the table shows likely underlying etiologies that may be the best characterization of the patient at

TABLE 9.3 **Differential Diagnosis of Primary Progressive Aphasia and Primary Progressive Apraxia of Speech**

	Logopenic Variant Primary Progressive Aphasia	Semantic Variant Primary Progressive Aphasia	Nonfluent/Agrammatic Variant Primary Progressive Aphasia	Primary Progressive Apraxia of Speech
Most likely underlying etiology	Alzheimer's disease	Frontotemporal lobar degeneration	Frontotemporal lobar degeneration, progressive supranuclear palsy, corticobasal degeneration	Progressive supranuclear palsy, corticobasal degeneration
Other possible disorders	Frontotemporal lobar degeneration, vascular cognitive impairment	Alzheimer's disease	Alzheimer's disease, vascular cognitive impairment	Vascular cognitive impairment

presentation or in the future. The second row shows other disorders that should be considered.

TREATMENTS

Treatment is supportive. Speech therapy may be beneficial for some patients, particularly those with apraxia of speech. Communication aids may be helpful, such as pictures on laminated pages or electronic devices that the patient can touch to communicate.

REFERENCES

Botha, H., & Josephs, K. A. (2019). Primary progressive aphasias and apraxia of speech. *Continuum (Minneapolis, Minn.),* *25*(1), 101–127.

Gorno-Tempini, M. L., Hillis, A. E., Weintraub, S., et al. (2011). Classification of primary progressive aphasia and its variants. *Neurology, 76,* 1006–1014.

Grossman, M. (2012). The non-fluent/agrammatic variant of primary progressive aphasia. *Lancet Neurology, 11,* 545–555.

Harris, J. M., Saxon, J. A., Jones, M., et al. (2019). Neuropsychological differentiation of progressive aphasic disorders. *Journal of Neuropsychology, 13*(2), 214–239.

Josephs, K. A., Duffy, J. R., Strand, E. A., et al. (2012). Characterizing a neurodegenerative syndrome: Primary progressive apraxia of speech. *Brain, 135,* 1522–1536.

Josephs, K. A., Duffy, J. R., Strand, E. A., et al. (2014). The evolution of primary progressive apraxia of speech. *Brain, 137,* 2783–2795.

Jung, Y., Duffy, J. R., & Josephs, K. A. (2013). Primary progressive aphasia and apraxia of speech. *Seminars in Neurology, 33,* 342–347.

Mesulam, M. M., & Weintraub, S. (2014). Is it time to revisit the classification guidelines for primary progressive aphasia? *Neurology, 82,* 1108–1109.

Santos-Santos, M. A., Rabinovici, G. D., Iaccarino, L., et al. (2018). Rates of amyloid imaging positivity in patients with primary progressive aphasia. *JAMA Neurology, 75*(3), 342–352.

Wicklund, M. R., Duffy, J. R., Strand, E. A., et al. (2014). Quantitative application of the primary progressive aphasia consensus criteria. *Neurology, 82,* 1119–1126.

Additional videos for this topic are available online at expertconsult.com.

10

Behavioral Variant Frontotemporal Dementia

QUICK START: BEHAVIORAL VARIANT FRONTOTEMPORAL DEMENTIA

Definition	• Behavioral variant frontotemporal dementia is a progressive neurodegenerative disorder with more than a dozen different pathologies.
Prevalence	• Behavioral variant frontotemporal dementia is found in about 5% of cases of dementia. • It most commonly presents in midlife, with a mean age of onset at 58 years, although it can present from the third to the tenth decade. • Its prevalence reaches about 13 per 100,000 in individuals in their early sixties. • Up to 10% to 15% of patients also show signs and symptoms of motor neuron disease (amyotrophic lateral sclerosis [ALS]).
Genetic risk	• Up to 40% of cases are familial with an autosomal dominant pattern.
Cognitive and behavioral symptoms	• Changes occur in personality and social conduct, including apathy, loss of insight, disinhibition, lack of empathy, inappropriate social remarks, abnormal eating behaviors, and neglect of self-care. • Neuropsychological testing may be normal or may show dysfunction of tests of attention, response inhibition, frontal/executive function, and language.

Diagnostic criteria	1. Required criterion—progressive deterioration of behavior and/or cognition by observation or history.
	2. Possible behavioral variant frontotemporal dementia—3 of 6 required:
	   a. Early behavioral disinhibition
	   b. Early apathy or inertia
	   c. Early loss of sympathy or empathy
	   d. Early perseverative, stereotyped, or compulsive/ritualistic behavior
	   e. Hyperorality and dietary changes
	   f. Neuropsychological profile: executive/generation deficits with relative sparing of memory and visuospatial functions.
	3. Probable behavioral variant frontotemporal dementia (all required):
	   a. Meets criteria for possible behavioral variant frontotemporal dementia
	   b. Significant functional decline
	   c. Imaging results consistent with behavioral variant frontotemporal dementia (frontal and/or anterior temporal atrophy on CT or MRI or hypoperfusion or hypometabolism on SPECT or PET).

(Continued)

QUICK START: BEHAVIORAL VARIANT FRONTOTEMPORAL DEMENTIA (*Continued*)

	4. Behavioral variant frontotemporal dementia with definite frontotemporal lobar degeneration pathology (a and either b or c required):
	  a. Meets criteria for possible or probable behavioral variant frontotemporal dementia
	  b. Histopathological evidence of frontotemporal lobar degeneration on biopsy or at postmortem
	  c. Presence of a known pathogenic mutation.
	5. Exclusion criteria for behavioral variant frontotemporal dementia—Criteria a and b must both be answered negatively; criterion c can be positive for possible but must be negative for probable:
	  a. Pattern of deficits is better accounted for by other nervous system or medical disorders.
	  b. Behavioral disturbance is better accounted for by a psychiatric diagnosis.
	  c. Biomarkers strongly indicative of Alzheimer's disease or other neurodegenerative process.

Treatment	• There are no U.S. Food and Drug Administration (FDA) approved medications to treat behavioral variant frontotemporal dementia. • Treatment consists of supportive management. • Many medications, including selective serotonin reuptake inhibitors (SSRIs) and atypical antipsychotics, can be used to treat the symptoms.
Top differential diagnoses	• Alzheimer's disease, vascular cognitive impairment, corticobasal degeneration, progressive supranuclear palsy, normal pressure hydrocephalus, Huntington's disease, brain sagging syndrome, primary psychiatric disorder, substance abuse, as well as other causes of frontal lobe dysfunction (such as a frontal tumor).

A 63-year-old man was brought to the clinic by his family because of his memory difficulties, apathy, and inappropriate behavior. They reported that the problems began 3 to 4 years ago; at that time he did not wash, dress, eat, or take his medications without prompting. Although he used to be very kind and caring, he now appeared unconcerned with others, and did not show any emotion over his wife's recent diagnosis of cancer and need for surgery. Overall, he seemed like a different person to them. Most recently they had to put a lock on the refrigerator because he began eating continually. They now do not feel comfortable leaving him at home alone for fear he would "get into something" that could be dangerous or cause damage.

PREVALENCE, PROGNOSIS, AND DEFINITION

Behavioral variant frontotemporal dementia (bvFTD) is a progressive neurodegenerative syndrome leading to changes in personality and social conduct. There are more than a dozen different underlying patterns of frontotemporal lobar degeneration (FTLD) pathology that can cause both behavioral variant frontotemporal dementia as well as the semantic and nonfluent/agrammatic variants of primary progressive aphasia (PPA) (see Chapter 9). Alzheimer's disease pathology can lead to the syndrome of behavioral variant frontotemporal dementia about 10% to 15% of the time (Perry et al., 2017).

Behavioral variant frontotemporal dementia is most common in midlife with a mean age of onset at 58 years, although it can present from the third to the tenth decade. Its prevalence reaches about 13 per 100,000 in individuals in their early sixties (Seeley, 2019). It may be as common as Alzheimer's disease in those with dementia aged younger than 65 years. It represents about 5% of patients in memory clinics. Although there is considerable variability, the average time from symptom onset to death in behavioral variant frontotemporal dementia is about 8 years.

CRITERIA

The International Behavioral Variant Frontotemporal Dementia Criteria were published in 2011 (Rascovsky

BOX 10.1   International Behavioral Variant Frontotemporal Dementia Criteria

1. Shows progressive deterioration of behavior and/or cognition by observation or history (as provided by knowledgeable informant)
2. Possible behavioral variant frontotemporal dementia: Three of the following behavioral/cognitive symptoms [a–f] must be present as persistent or recurrent events:
   a. [a]Early behavioral disinhibition (one of the following must be present):
      i. Socially inappropriate behavior
      ii. Loss of manners or decorum
      iii. Impulsive, rash, or careless actions
   b. Early apathy or inertia (one of the following must be present):
      i. Apathy: loss of interest, drive or motivation
      ii. Inertia: decreased initiation of behavior
   c. Early loss of sympathy or empathy (one of the following must be present):
      i. Diminished response to other people's needs or feelings: positive rating should be based on specific examples that reflect a lack of understanding or indifference to other people's feelings
      ii. Diminished social interest, interrelatedness or personal warmth: general decrease in social engagement
   d. Early perseverative, stereotyped, or compulsive/ritualistic behavior (one of the following must be present):
      i. Simple repetitive movements
      ii. Complex, compulsive, or ritualistic behaviors
      iii. Stereotypy of speech
   e. Hyperorality and dietary changes (one of the following must be present):
      i. Altered food preferences
      ii. Binge eating, increased consumption of alcohol or cigarettes
      iii. Oral exploration or consumption of inedible objects

   f. Neuropsychological profile: executive/generation deficits with relative sparing of memory and visuospatial functions (all of the following must be present):
      i. Deficits in executive tasks
      ii. Relative sparing of episodic memory (compared with degree of executive dysfunction)
      iii. Relative sparing of visuospatial skills (compared with degree of executive dysfunction)
3. Probable behavioral variant frontotemporal dementia: All criteria must be met:
   a. Meets criteria for possible behavioral variant frontotemporal dementia
   b. Exhibits significant functional decline (by caregiver report, clinician rating, or functional questionnaire)
   c. Imaging results consistent with behavioral variant frontotemporal dementia
      i. Frontal and/or anterior temporal atrophy on computed tomography or magnetic resonance imaging, and/or
      ii. Frontal and/or anterior temporal hypoperfusion or hypometabolism on single photon emission computed tomography or positron emission tomography
4. Behavioral variant frontotemporal dementia with definite frontotemporal lobar degeneration pathology. Criterion a and either b or c must be present:
   a. Meets criteria for possible or probable behavioral variant frontotemporal dementia
   b. Histopathological evidence of frontotemporal lobar degeneration on biopsy or at postmortem
   c. Presence of a known pathogenic mutation
5. Exclusionary criteria for behavioral variant frontotemporal dementia. Criteria a and b must be answered negatively. Criteria c can be positive for possible (but not probable) behavioral variant frontotemporal dementia.
   a. Pattern of deficits is better accounted for by other nondegenerative nervous system or medical disorders
   b. Behavioral disturbance is better accounted for by a psychiatric diagnosis
   c. Biomarkers strongly indicative of Alzheimer's disease or other neurodegenerative process

[a]Early refers to symptoms within the first 3 years.
Modified from Rascovsky, K., Hodges, J. R., Knopman, D., et al. (2011). Sensitivity of revised diagnostic criteria for the behavioural variant of frontotemporal dementia. *Brain, 134,* 2456–2477; LaMarre, A. K., Rascovsky, K., Bostrom, A., et al. (2013). Interrater reliability of the new criteria for behavioral variant frontotemporal dementia. *Neurology, 80,* 1973–1977.

et al., 2011) (Box 10.1) and are the gold standard; we use this version with the specificity added for several items by LaMarre et al. (2013). Diagnostic and Statistical Manual of Mental Disorders, 5th Edition also has criteria for Major or Mild Frontotemporal Neurocognitive Disorder (Box 10.2; see Chapter 3 for the general criteria for major and mild neurocognitive disorder).

BOX 10.2   **Diagnostic and Statistical Manual of Mental Disorders, 5th Edition Criteria for Major or Mild Frontotemporal Neurocognitive Disorder**

A. The criteria are met for major or mild neurocognitive disorder.

B. The disturbance has insidious onset and gradual progression.

C. Either (1) or (2)
1. Behavioral variant:
   a. Three or more of the following behavioral symptoms:
      i. Behavioral disinhibition
      ii. Apathy or inertia
      iii. Loss of sympathy or empathy
      iv. Perseverative, stereotyped, or compulsive/ritualistic behavior
      v. Hyperorality and dietary changes.
   b. Prominent decline in social cognition and/or executive abilities.
2. Language variant:
   a. Prominent decline in language ability, in the form of speech production, word-finding, object naming, grammar, or word comprehension.

D. Relative sparing of learning and memory and perceptual-motor function.

E. The disturbance is not better explained by cerebrovascular disease, another neurodegenerative disease, the effects of a substance, or another mental, neurological, or systemic disorder.

Probable frontotemporal neurocognitive disorder is diagnosed if either of the following is present; otherwise, **possible frontotemporal neurocognitive disorder** should be diagnosed:

1. Evidence of a causative frontotemporal neurocognitive disorder genetic mutation, from either family history or genetic testing.
2. Evidence of disproportionate frontal and/or temporal lobe involvement from neuroimaging.

Possible frontotemporal neurocognitive disorder is diagnosed if there is no evidence of a genetic mutation, and neuroimaging has not been performed.

From American Psychiatric Association. (2013). *Diagnostic and statistical manual of mental disorders* (*DSM-5*) (5th ed.). Arlington, VA: American Psychiatric Publishing, Inc.

RISK FACTORS, PATHOLOGY, AND PATHOPHYSIOLOGY

Other than family history there are no known risk factors for frontotemporal dementia. If a family history of dementia, psychiatric illness, Parkinson's disease, or amyotrophic lateral sclerosis are all considered positive indicators, one may conclude from various studies that up to 40% of cases of frontotemporal dementia are familial, and about 10% to 20% have a clear autosomal dominant pattern. The best studied familial frontotemporal dementia syndrome is that of familial frontotemporal dementia with parkinsonism linked to chromosome 17. Individuals with this disorder have a mutation in the microtubule-associated protein tau (MAPT) gene located in the chromosome 17q21-22 region, develop symptoms relatively younger, and may have more symmetric temporal lobe atrophy. Individuals with mutations of progranulin (GRN; chromosome 17q21) can develop behavioral variant frontotemporal dementia, nonfluent/agrammatic variant primary progressive aphasia, corticobasal syndrome, and Alzheimer's disease. Mutations of chromosome 9

open reading frame 72 (C9orf72) is the most common cause of inherited behavioral variant frontotemporal dementia, amyotrophic lateral sclerosis, and the combined frontotemporal dementia–motor neuron disease; psychotic features are relatively more common in these patients. Other genetic abnormalities that have been associated with frontotemporal dementia include those of the RNA-binding protein fused in sarcoma (FUS; chromosome 16), valosin-containing protein (VCP; chromosome 9p12-13), charged multivesicular body protein 2B (CHMP2B; chromosome 3), and TAR DNA-binding protein (TARDBP; chromosome 1), the gene that encodes TDP-43 (Perry & Miller, 2013).

Currently there are more than a dozen different pathologies that have been observed in patients diagnosed with behavioral variant frontotemporal dementia; we use the term frontotemporal lobar degeneration (FTLD) to refer to the underlying pathological entities that cause the frontotemporal dementias. Many frontotemporal dementias show tau-positive inclusions. These include classic Pick's disease which has tau- and ubiquitin-positive spherical cortical inclusions, familial frontotemporal dementia with characteristic tau-positive

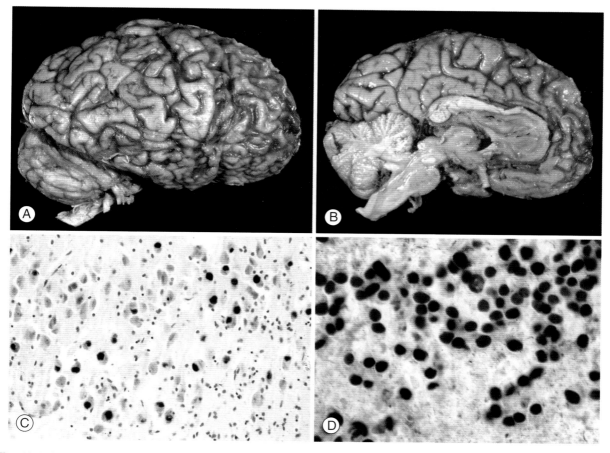

Fig. 10.1 Pathology of Pick's disease. Severe atrophy can be clearly seen in the frontal lobes and also the anterior portion of the temporal lobe **(A** and **B)**. Microscopically, Pick bodies—tau-immunoreactive rounded inclusions in neurons—can be seen **(C** and **D)**.

inclusions in neurons and glial cells, and argyrophilic grain disease. Many patients with frontotemporal dementias, particularly those with motor neuron disease but also those without it, also show ubiquitin-positive inclusions. TDP-43 immunoreactive inclusions are also common. Neuronal filament inclusions are sometimes observed. See Figs. 10.1 and 10.2 for two of the more common pathologies.

COMMON SIGNS, SYMPTOMS, AND STAGES (VIDEO 10.1)

In behavioral variant frontotemporal dementia there is insidious onset of gradual changes in personality and social conduct. Although changes in personality and social conduct can occur in many other dementias as well, in behavioral variant frontotemporal dementia these changes occur early in the disease process and are prominent. Apathy is probably one of the most common signs, although other dementias also commonly present with apathy. Insight is also generally lost very early. Early disinhibition is one of the more pathognomonic signs, and may manifest itself by inappropriate social remarks, improper remarks of a sexual nature, and poorly concealed use of pornography. Empathy for others is typically lacking. Abnormal eating behaviors can manifest in many different ways, ranging from dramatic changes in food preferences (particularly sweets), poor

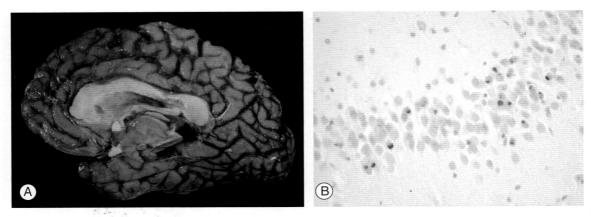

Fig. 10.2 Pathology of frontotemporal dementia with TDP-43 pathology. Note the atrophy of the front part of the brain (**A**, *left side* of figure), shrinking the gyri and making the vessels appear more prominent. **(B)** Phosphorylated TDP-43 cytoplasmic inclusions in neurons in the dentate gyrus of the hippocampus.

manners, gluttonous behavior, and eating inappropriate things. For example, one of our patients ate a raw steak and an entire jar of mayonnaise. Stereotypic and ritualistic behaviors such as pacing the same route, using the same verbal phrases, are common (e.g., another patient would repetitively walk right up to people and loudly state, "You're handsome!"). Neglect of self-care is common, and may be related to apathy. To reiterate, although all of these signs and symptoms could be present with Alzheimer's disease as well (as the frontal lobes become involved), they are early and prominent manifestations in behavioral variant frontotemporal dementia, but late and less prominent manifestations of Alzheimer's disease.

It is also interesting to note that the particular behavioral abnormalities that a patient presents with may relate to the different brain regions that are involved. For example, on a particular clinic day we happened to evaluate two very different patients with behavioral variant frontotemporal dementia. One patient showed signs and symptoms of ventromedial frontal lobe dysfunction: he was rude, disinhibited, and socially inappropriate, although he was perfectly able to achieve normal eye contact and relate to whomever he was speaking to. This patient came to the attention of his physicians because he began soliciting sexual acts from his daughter-in-law, quite an uncharacteristic thing for him to do! The second patient showed signs and symptoms of dorsolateral frontal lobe dysfunction: he was unable to make normal eye contact, he showed signs of apathy, slowness of movement, and performed no activity unless he was specifically asked (and he then was happy to comply). This second patient presented with extreme difficulty and slowness in doing simple things like shaving, and would walk out of the house holding items like shaving cream.

THINGS TO LOOK FOR IN THE HISTORY

As described earlier. there are different presentations of behavioral variant frontotemporal dementia (Fig. 10.3). Nevertheless, these different presentations share many common signs, and as a group, they differ from other dementias, such as Alzheimer's disease.

Incontinence is common early in frontotemporal dementia, and often presents in a very different manner than that of early Alzheimer's disease. Although in both disorders there is urgency, patients with Alzheimer's disease will rush to the bathroom and be embarrassed if they have an accident, whereas patients with frontotemporal dementia will often be indifferent to having an accident, allowing themselves to be soiled wherever they are. Many patients will subsequently refuse to be cleaned up. One patient we cared for with early behavioral variant frontotemporal dementia and a perfect score on the Mini-Mental State Examination (MMSE) refused to change his pants after a urinary accident, claiming "it will dry"! Another patient was found happily watching TV—despite there being feces all over the living room.

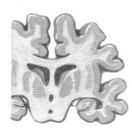

Atrophy of frontal and/or temporal areas

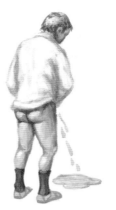

Bizarre, uninhibited socially inappropriate behavior

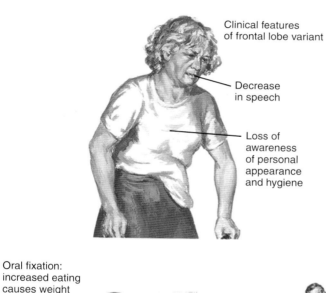

Clinical features of frontal lobe variant

Decrease in speech

Loss of awareness of personal appearance and hygiene

Oral fixation: increased eating causes weight gain

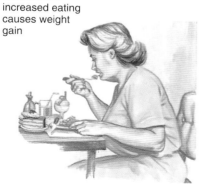

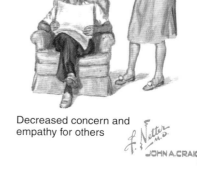

Decreased concern and empathy for others

Fig. 10.3 Frontotemporal dementia. (Netter illustration from www.netterimages.com. Copyright Elsevier Inc. All rights reserved.)

Problems in driving are common in frontotemporal dementia and also often present differently than in Alzheimer's disease. In Alzheimer's disease the first problem is invariably that the patient becomes lost, even when traveling familiar routes. In behavioral variant frontotemporal dementia the problem is more likely to be driving on the wrong side of the road, or other abnormal and risky behavior leading to accidents.

Sequencing problems are very common in frontotemporal dementia, making it difficult for patients to perform tasks like brushing their teeth, showering, making coffee, or preparing a sandwich. Often steps are missing or mixed up. One of our patients would make a sandwich with the bread on the inside and the meat on the outside. Another decided to paint the house upon returning from church, but did not change out of his suit and tie into appropriate painting clothes until after he had finished painting.

It is remarkable the number of patients with behavioral variant frontotemporal dementia who, when watching TV, believe that the persons or characters on it are either personally relevant for their life or actually talking directly to them. One patient we cared for thought that the events happening on a soap opera were events happening to her own children. Another patient believed that the political messages on the TV during a campaign season were all directed to him and he talked back to the TV.

Another characteristic behavior of behavioral variant frontotemporal dementia is sexual disinhibition. Many patients spend more time with pornography than previously. One patient we evaluated now showed more interest in sexual activity with his wife—making advances and requesting sexual activity—than in their 35+ years of marriage. Another patient began to try to pick up men from a restaurant—despite the fact that she was having dinner with her husband at the time! And we commented above about the patient who requested sexual favors from his daughter-in-law. Although patients with Alzheimer's disease will sometimes exhibit sexual disinhibition, in frontotemporal dementia it occurs earlier in the disease process and is typically more prominent than in Alzheimer's disease.

Memory problems are commonly mentioned by family, although they usually have a different flavor than memory problems in Alzheimer's disease (see Appendix C, for details). In frontotemporal dementia the memory problems tend to be related to poor frontal lobe function. Patients show difficulties in learning new information because they have difficulties paying attention, and thus information needs to be repeated a number of times to be learned. Once learned, information is generally retained in memory, although there is often difficulty accessing it because of poor frontally mediated memory search processes. Patients with frontotemporal dementia thus do much better on tests of multiple choice than free recall. Also related to their frontal lobe dysfunction, these patients show prominent distortions of memory, frequently mixing up details or confusing two or more memories.

THINGS TO LOOK FOR ON THE PHYSICAL AND NEUROLOGICAL EXAMINATION

There are no particular signs on the physical or neurological examination to suggest a frontotemporal dementia. Although one might suspect that frontal release signs such as the snout, grasp, and palmomental reflexes are more common in frontotemporal dementia, we have not found this to be the case.

The patient should be carefully examined for any signs of motor neuron disease because up to 10% to 15% of patients with motor neuron disease also show signs and symptoms of frontotemporal dementia. Thus so-called "mixed signs" of upper and lower motor neuron dysfunction should be sought for, including brisk reflexes, extensor plantars, fasciculations, and muscle wasting.

Some patients who begin with signs and symptoms of behavioral variant frontotemporal dementia end up having corticobasal syndrome (see Chapter 13) or progressive supranuclear palsy (see Chapter 12), and so signs of those disorders should also be looked for including parkinsonism, asymmetric or axial rigidity, apraxia, slowed saccades or vertical gaze restriction, dystonia, and gait or postural instability.

PATTERN OF IMPAIRMENT ON COGNITIVE TESTS

In many cases of behavioral variant frontotemporal dementia the standard cognitive testing may be normal until quite late in the disease. This point is particularly true for the MMSE; the Montreal Cognitive Assessment (MoCA) is more sensitive to frontotemporal dementia.

Thus additional tests specifically evaluating frontal lobe function should generally be performed when a frontotemporal dementia is suspected. And, perhaps because the frontal lobes are so large and mediate such a diverse group of cognitive and behavioral functions, different patients may show impairment on different tests, so (unfortunately) there is not a single frontal lobe test that can be used to make the diagnosis. Helpful tests include the Wisconsin Card Sorting Test, verbal fluency to letters, the Trailmaking Test Part B, the Delis–Kaplan Executive Function System (D-KEFS), and the Cambridge Neuropsychological Test Automated Battery (CANTAB).

When memory is impaired, it is usually secondary to problems with attention, encoding, retrieval, source memory, memory distortions, and other frontal aspects of memory (see Appendix C for details). However, there are some patients with behavioral variant frontotemporal dementia who exhibit severe memory loss including rapid forgetting; some of these patients have hippocampal sclerosis owing to TDP-43 pathology, similar to patients with limbic-predominant age-related TDP-43 encephalopathy (LATE, see Chapter 6) except that here the pathology is more widespread, and includes the frontal lobes.

LABORATORY STUDIES

There are no routine laboratory studies to support or refute the diagnosis of frontotemporal dementia. Genetic testing may be considered when there is a strong family history but should only be done when appropriate genetic counseling is available. Electromyogram and nerve conduction studies are essential when motor neuron disease is suspected.

STRUCTURAL AND FUNCTIONAL IMAGING STUDIES

Although the structural imaging scan may be normal at the time of presentation, most cases of behavioral variant frontotemporal dementia show frontal and/or anterior temporal lobe atrophy at some point in the course of their disease (Fig. 10.4). Functional imaging studies such as single photon emission computed tomography (SPECT) and positron emission tomography (PET) typically show decreased frontal hypofunction, often several years before the atrophy is noted on a structural image (Fig. 10.5), although they will sometimes be normal or ambiguous early in the course of the illness.

DIFFERENTIAL DIAGNOSIS

Because Alzheimer's disease is so common, when suspecting a frontotemporal dementia one must always consider the possibility that it is an atypical case of Alzheimer's disease (Table 10.1). Alzheimer's disease should be especially considered when the patient is over the age of 65 years because only one-quarter of cases of frontotemporal dementia (but most cases of Alzheimer's disease) present over age 65 years. Other disorders to consider are progressive supranuclear palsy (see Chapter 12), corticobasal degeneration (see Chapter 13), vascular dementia (see Chapter 7), normal-pressure hydrocephalus (see Chapter 14), and Huntington's disease. Brain sagging syndrome (see Chapter 17)—sometimes called frontotemporal brain sagging syndrome—should always be considered as it is a potentially treatable disorder (Vives-Rodriguez et al., 2020). Similarly, it is important to consider a primary psychiatric disease and/or substance abuse (see Chapter 17), particularly when the problems are longstanding over decades (Ducharme et al., 2015). Note that when it is clear that the patient is suffering from a frontotemporal dementia, it is always important to look for concomitant evidence of motor neuron disease.

TREATMENTS

Patients with behavioral variant frontotemporal dementias are difficult to manage, and treatment is supportive. Nonpharmacological measures include the use of redirection, music, and calm voices (see Chapter 26). Patients with frontotemporal dementia show deficits of serotonin, and it is therefore not surprising that selective serotonin reuptake inhibitors (SSRIs) are often of help (see Chapter 27). Studies have suggested that irritability, agitation, and abnormal eating behavior are improved by this class of medications (Table 10.2).

Unfortunately, as the disease progresses, patients with behavioral variant frontotemporal dementia almost always require additional medications to control agitation and aggression. Atypical antipsychotics are most often used to control these unwanted behaviors. Note: These medications are not approved by the U.S. Food and Drug Administration (FDA)

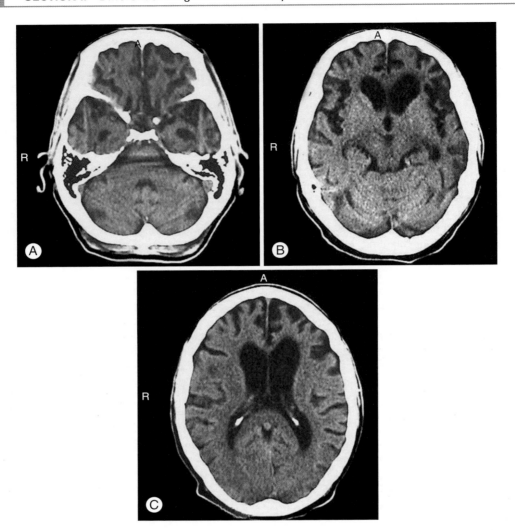

Fig. 10.4 Head computed tomography scan of a patient with behavioral variant frontotemporal dementia. The patient was a 70-year-old man whose family brought him in because he tried to cook on the stove with Tupperware and began driving on the wrong side of the road. He was passive and apathetic, but kept walking out of the office during the appointment. **(A–C)** Note the substantial atrophy of left > right frontal and anterior temporal lobes.

for any dementia and have very serious side effects; see Chapter 27 for important additional information before prescribing. Risperidone (Risperdal) may cause less sedation than others, and is often our first-line medication for daytime agitation, after the selective serotonin reuptake inhibitors. Quetiapine (Seroquel) is more sedating, and is therefore particularly useful for night-time agitation.

Other medications that may be useful include the sedating antidepressant trazodone. Although large clinical trials of memantine (Namenda; see Chapter 20) have not shown benefit, some smaller studies and our own experience suggest that some patients may show improvement in cognition and behavior with memantine; given the heterogeneity of the disorder we believe it is not unreasonable to try it—and to discontinue it if

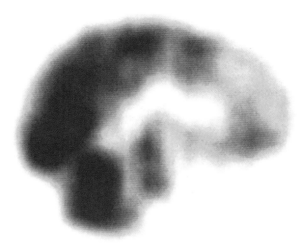

Fig. 10.5 Mid-sagittal slice of a single photon emission computed tomography scan in a patient with behavioral frontotemporal dementia. Note the reduced activity in the front of the brain (*right side* of image) relative to more posterior regions.

TABLE 10.1 **Similarities and Differences Between Alzheimer's Disease, Behavioral Variant Frontotemporal Dementia, Progressive Supranuclear Palsy, and Corticobasal Degeneration**

	Alzheimer's Disease	Behavioral Variant Frontotemporal Dementia	Progressive Supranuclear Palsy	Corticobasal Degeneration
Age of onset	Typically >65 years	Typically <70 years	Typically 55–75 years	Typically 45–75 years
Cognitive deficits	Memory deficits prominent, along with multiple other cognitive areas	Early none; executive function decline in the middle and late stages	Early none; slowing of processing and executive dysfunction later	May have executive, attention, visuospatial deficits
Behavioral symptoms	Absent early in the disease; apathy, agitation, and other symptoms as the disease progresses	Socially inappropriate behavior early in the disease	Absent early in the disease, but may become inappropriate as the disease progresses	Absent early in the disease, but may become inappropriate as the disease progresses
Examination findings	Generally none	Generally none	Eye movement abnormalities, parkinsonism, axial rigidity, gait abnormality	Asymmetric apraxia, myoclonus, dystonia, cortical sensory loss, and neglect

it doesn't show beneficial effects. We are quite cautious with cholinesterase inhibitors and stimulants, as these classes of medications can sometimes "activate" a patient with frontotemporal dementia and make behavior worse; nonetheless some patients do appear to show cognitive and behavioral improvement.

Lastly, note that caregivers of all dementia patients need support, but this is particularly true of those caring for individuals with behavioral variant frontotemporal dementia. Organizations such as The Association for Frontotemporal Dementia (www.theaftd.org) can be helpful for families.

TABLE 10.2   **Treatment of Behavioral Variant Frontotemporal Dementia**

Medication Class	Medication and U.S. Food and Drug Administration Approval Status	Summary of Benefits	Common Side Effects
Selective serotonin reuptake inhibitors (SSRIs)	Sertraline (Zoloft), citalopram (Celexa), and escitalopram (Lexapro); off-label use	Improvement of irritability, agitation, and abnormal eating behavior	Gastrointestinal upset and sexual dysfunction
Atypical antipsychotics	Risperidone (Risperidal) and quetiapine (Seroquel); off-label use	Control of agitation and aggression	Altered glucose metabolism, risk of cardiovascular disease, parkinsonism, sedation

REFERENCES

Ducharme, S., Price, B. H., Larvie, M., et al. (2015). Clinical approach to the differential diagnosis between behavioral variant frontotemporal dementia and primary psychiatric disorders. *The American Journal of Psychiatry, 172*(9), 827–837.

LaMarre, A. K., Rascovsky, K., Bostrom, A., et al. (2013). Interrater reliability of the new criteria for behavioral variant frontotemporal dementia. *Neurology, 80*, 1973–1977.

Perry, D. C., Brown, J. A., Possin, K. L., et al. (2017). Clinicopathological correlations in behavioural variant frontotemporal dementia. *Brain, 140*(12), 3329–3345.

Perry, D. C., & Miller, B. L. (2013). Frontotemporal dementia. *Seminars in Neurology, 33*, 336–341.

Rascovsky, K., Hodges, J. R., Knopman, D., et al. (2011). Sensitivity of revised diagnostic criteria for the behavioural variant of frontotemporal dementia. *Brain, 134*, 2456–2477.

Seeley, W. W. (2019). Behavioral variant frontotemporal dementia. *Continuum (Minneapolis, Minn.), 25*(1), 76–100.

Vives-Rodriguez, A., Turk, K. W., Vassy, E. A., et al. (2020). Reversible amnestic cognitive impairment in a patient with brain sagging syndrome. *Neurology: Clinical Practice*, May 2020, 10.1212/CPJ.0000000000000860; doi:10.1212/CPJ.0000000000000860

Additional videos for this topic are available online at expertconsult.com.

11

Posterior Cortical Atrophy

QUICK START: POSTERIOR CORTICAL ATROPHY

Definition and etiology	• Posterior cortical atrophy (PCA) is a clinical syndrome characterized by progressive visual and visuospatial dysfunction.
	• Most patients present between the ages of 50 and 65 years (mean age 59 years), although some present in their 70s and 80s.
	• Underlying Alzheimer's disease pathology is most common. Other common pathologies include Lewy body disease and corticobasal degeneration.
Prevalence	• Posterior cortical atrophy is rare, making up about 5% of patients in a specialty cognitive clinic.
Cognitive and behavioral symptoms	• Common visuospatial and perceptual deficits include: neglecting or not perceiving space (often on the left), difficulty perceiving objects and faces (prosopagnosia), difficulty reading, and Balint syndrome (ocular motor apraxia, optic ataxia, and simultanagnosia).
	• Common nonvisuospatial deficits include: apraxia and Gerstmann syndrome (acalculia, left-right disorientation, finger agnosia, and agraphia).
	• The following should all be relatively spared at onset: episodic memory, speech and nonvisual language, executive function, behavior, personality, and insight.

Diagnostic criteria	Core features of the posterior cortical atrophy clinico-radiological syndrome
	• Clinical features:
	  • All 3 must be present: insidious onset, gradual progression, prominent early disturbance of visual ± other posterior cognitive functions.
	• Cognitive features:
	  • At least 3 must be present as early or presenting features ± evidence of their impact on activities of daily living: space perception deficit, simultanagnosia, object perception deficit, constructional dyspraxia, environmental agnosia, oculomotor apraxia, dressing apraxia, optic ataxia, alexia, left/right disorientation, acalculia, limb apraxia, apperceptive prosopagnosia, agraphia, homonymous visual field defect, finger agnosia.
	  • All of the following must be relatively spared: anterograde memory, speech and nonvisual language, executive functions, behavior and personality.

(Continued)

QUICK START: POSTERIOR CORTICAL ATROPHY (*Continued*)

	• Neuroimaging: Predominant occipito-parietal or occipito-temporal atrophy/hypometabolism/hypoperfusion on MRI/FDG-PET/SPECT
	• Exclusion criteria: Evidence of: a brain tumor or other mass lesion sufficient to explain the symptoms, significant vascular disease including focal stroke sufficient to explain the symptoms, afferent visual cause (e.g., optic nerve, chiasm, or tract), or other identifiable causes for cognitive impairment (e.g., renal failure)
Treatment	• Most patients will benefit from cholinesterase inhibitors and all patients will benefit from nonpharmacological treatment approaches.
Top differential diagnoses	• Underlying Alzheimer's disease pathology is most common. Other common pathologies include Lewy body disease, corticobasal degeneration, and rarely, prion disease. Cerebrovascular disease may also produce similar symptoms.

A 62-year-old woman was referred for difficulty reading. She made several trips to her optometrist for new glasses over the last year without improvement. The optometrist could find no cause for her reading difficulty, although he documented a partial left lateral hemianopsia. The optometrist recommended she see her ophthalmologist who, upon finding no ocular problems, referred her to a general neurologist. After ruling out a strokes and mass lesions, the general neurologist referred her to us.

Her chief complaint was, "No one can get my eyeglass prescription right." In addition to difficulty reading, we learned that she had scraped the left side of her car backing out of her garage. Her examination showed that although she was impaired in reading paragraphs she had no difficulty reading single words, and she performed normally on tests of memory for visually or auditorily presented words. She was able to write sentences without difficulty. She was normal on tests of word fluency to letters and categories. Her naming of line drawings was impaired, but it was clear that it was owing to difficulties perceiving and comprehending the drawings, because when she was given a semantic cue (such as, "It's an ocean animal") she was usually able to say the correct name. She experienced difficulty finding the numbers on the Trailmaking Test Part A, resulting in an impaired, slow performance. She showed a similar impairment on the Trailmaking Test Part B. Subtracting serial 7s from 100 was also impaired. The elementary neurological examination showed the previously noted partial left lateral hemianopsia, which seemed to diminish with a stronger stimulus, making us wonder if it were actually left-sided neglect. Her magnetic

resonance imaging (MRI) scan showed prominent atrophy in right greater than left occipital and parietal cortices.

A diagnosis of the posterior cortical atrophy syndrome was made. We counseled her about not driving and provided her and her family with a home safety tips and recommendations handout for individuals with dementia and visual dysfunction. She was interested in both standard and experimental pharmacological treatments. After starting her on a cholinesterase inhibitor we screened her for a clinical trial, which included both amyloid and tau positron emission tomography (PET) scans. These revealed that although she had amyloid plaques throughout the brain, she had tau concentrated posteriorly in bilateral occipital and parietal cortices.

Visual problems are common in many dementias, including Alzheimer's disease, dementia with Lewy bodies, corticobasal syndrome, and vascular dementia. Some patients with progressive visual problems severe enough to compromise function do not meet criteria for any neurodegenerative diseases. These patients are best characterized as having posterior cortical atrophy (sometimes abbreviated as PCA).

PREVALENCE, DEFINITION, AND PATHOLOGY

Posterior cortical atrophy is not a disease. It is a clinical syndrome that patients may manifest, with varying underlying neurodegenerative disease etiologies. Alzheimer's disease (see Chapter 4) is by far the most common underlying pathology for posterior cortical atrophy, which is why other terms for this disorder include the "visual variant of Alzheimer's disease" and "biparietal Alzheimer's disease." In fact, one study showed that 14% of patients diagnosed with Alzheimer's disease had prominent visuospatial problems, suggesting that posterior cortical atrophy may be one end of a continuum of Alzheimer's signs and symptoms (Stopford et al., 2008). Other common pathologies underlying posterior cortical atrophy include Lewy body disease (see Chapter 8), corticobasal degeneration (see Chapter 13), and rarely, prion disease (see Chapter 16). Interestingly, according to the criteria, cerebrovascular disease (see Chapter 7) sufficient to cause the syndrome of posterior cortical atrophy is exclusionary, but the phenomenology and nonpharmacological treatment approaches outlined below would be equally relevant.

Most individuals with posterior cortical atrophy are young, presenting between 50 and 65 years of age, although some patients present in their 70s and 80s. In one study the mean age of onset was approximately 59 years, with almost 87% presenting before age 65 years (Schott et al., 2016). Posterior cortical atrophy is rare, making up about 5% of patients in a specialty cognitive clinic and up to 13% of cases of early-onset Alzheimer's disease (Schott & Crutch, 2019).

CRITERIA

Posterior cortical atrophy is described using a three-level classification framework. Level 1 establishes the clinical syndrome, based upon clinical, cognitive, and neuroimaging data (Box 11.1). Level 2 establishes whether the presentation is "pure" or whether the patient meets the criteria for posterior cortical atrophy plus another neurodegenerative disease syndrome (Box 11.2). Level 3 adds biomarker evidence of the underlying pathology (or pathologies) (Box 11.3).

COMMON SIGNS, SYMPTOMS, AND STAGES

There are two types of symptoms and signs that are commonly seen in posterior cortical atrophy. The first are visuospatial and perceptual deficits, including neglecting or not perceiving space (often on the left), difficulty perceiving objects and faces (prosopagnosia), difficulty reading, and Balint syndrome (ocular motor apraxia, optic ataxia, and simultanagnosia; see later). The second

---

BOX 11.1 Core Features of the Posterior Cortical Atrophy Clinico-Radiological Syndrome (Level 1)

Clinical features (all three must be present):
- Insidious onset
- Gradual progression
- Prominent early disturbance of visual ± other posterior cognitive functions

Cognitive features:
- At least three must be present as early or presenting features ± evidence of their impact on activities of daily living:
  - Space perception deficit
  - Simultanagnosia
  - Object perception deficit
  - Constructional dyspraxia
  - Environmental agnosia
  - Oculomotor apraxia
  - Dressing apraxia
  - Optic ataxia
  - Alexia
  - Left/right disorientation
  - Acalculia
  - Limb apraxia (not limb-kinetic)
  - Apperceptive prosopagnosia
  - Agraphia
  - Homonymous visual field defect
  - Finger agnosia
- All of the following must be evident:
  - Relatively spared anterograde memory function
  - Relatively spared speech and nonvisual language functions
  - Relatively spared executive functions
  - Relatively spared behavior and personality

Neuroimaging:
- Predominant occipito-parietal or occipito-temporal atrophy/hypometabolism/hypoperfusion on MRI/FDG-PET/SPECT

Exclusion criteria:
- Evidence of a brain tumor or other mass lesion sufficient to explain the symptoms
- Evidence of significant vascular disease including focal stroke sufficient to explain the symptoms
- Evidence of afferent visual cause (e.g., optic nerve, chiasm, or tract)
- Evidence of other identifiable causes for cognitive impairment (e.g., renal failure)

Clinical, cognitive, and neuroimaging features are rank ordered by frequency at first assessment as rated by online survey participants. *FDG-PET*, 18F-labeled fluorodeoxyglucose positron
(continued)

emission tomography; *MRI*, magnetic resonance imaging; *SPECT*, single-photon emission computed tomography.

Modified from Crutch, S. J., Schott, J. M., Rabinovici, G. D., et al. 2017. Consensus classification of posterior cortical atrophy. *Alzheimer's & Dementia: The Journal of the Alzheimer's Association, 13*(8), 870–884.

BOX 11.2 Classification of Posterior Cortical Atrophy-Pure and Posterior Cortical Atrophy-Plus (Level 2)

Posterior cortical atrophy-pure:
- Individuals must fulfill the criteria for the core clinico-radiological posterior cortical atrophy syndrome (level 1), and not fulfill core clinical criteria for any other neurodegenerative syndrome.

Posterior cortical atrophy-plus:
- Individuals must fulfill the criteria for the core clinico-radiological posterior cortical atrophy syndrome (level 1) and also fulfill core clinical criteria for at least one other neurodegenerative syndrome, such as:
  - Alzheimer's disease (see Chapter 4)
  - Dementia with Lewy bodies (see Chapter 8)
  - Corticobasal Syndrome (see Chapter 13)
  - Vascular dementia (see Chapter 7)
  - Prion disease (see Chapter 16)

Modified from Crutch, S. J., Schott, J. M., Rabinovici, G. D., et al. 2017. Consensus classification of posterior cortical atrophy. *Alzheimer's & Dementia: The Journal of the Alzheimer's Association, 13*(8), 870–884.

---

are nonvisuospatial deficits that arise with posterior cortical dysfunction including apraxia (see Chapter 13) and Gerstmann syndrome (acalculia, left-right disorientation, finger agnosia, and agraphia; see below). Importantly, the following should all be relatively spared at onset: episodic memory, speech and nonvisual language, executive function, behavior, personality, and insight. As with most neurodegenerative disorders, as the disease progresses many of these initially spared functions will become impaired.

Balint Syndrome

Named for the Hungarian neurologist and psychiatrist Rezső Bálint who described it in 1909, Balint syndrome—the combination of ocular motor apraxia, optic ataxia, and simultanagnosia—may occur whenever there is bilateral damage to parieto-occipital cortex. Ocular motor apraxia refers to the inability to voluntarily move the eyes to the relevant fixation.

BOX 11.3 Diagnostic Criteria for Posterior Cortical Atrophy Disease-Level Descriptions (Level 3)

Posterior cortical atrophy-Alzheimer's disease:
- Fulfillment of the posterior cortical atrophy syndrome (level 1) plus in vivo evidence of Alzheimer's pathology (at least one of the following):
  - Decreased $A\beta_{1-42}$ together with increased T-tau and/or P-tau in cerebrospinal fluid
  - Increased tracer retention on amyloid positron emission tomography (PET)
  - Alzheimer's disease autosomal-dominant mutation present (in PSEN1, PSEN2, or APP)
- If autopsy confirmation of Alzheimer's disease is available, the term definite posterior cortical atrophy-Alzheimer's disease would be appropriate.

Posterior cortical atrophy-Lewy body disease:
- Molecular biomarkers for Lewy body disease are currently unavailable; therefore an in vivo diagnosis of posterior cortical atrophy-Lewy body disease cannot be assigned at present.
- For individuals who are both:
  - classified as posterior cortical atrophy-plus by virtue of fulfilling dementia with Lewy bodies clinical criteria (see Chapter 8) and
  - shown to be Alzheimer's disease-biomarker negative, the term probable posterior cortical atrophy-Lewy body disease may be appropriate.
- If autopsy confirmation of Lewy body disease is available, the term definite posterior cortical atrophy-Lewy body disease would be appropriate.
- Other disease-level classifications may also be appropriate for individuals with mixed or multiple pathologies (e.g., posterior cortical atrophy-Alzheimer's/Lewy body diseases).

Posterior cortical atrophy-corticobasal degeneration:
- Molecular biomarkers for corticobasal degeneration are currently unavailable; therefore an in vivo diagnosis of posterior cortical atrophy-corticobasal degeneration cannot be assigned at present.
- For individuals who are both:
  - classified as posterior cortical atrophy-plus by virtue of fulfilling corticobasal syndrome criteria (see Chapter 13) and
  - shown to be Alzheimer's disease-biomarker negative, the term probable posterior cortical atrophy-corticobasal degeneration may be appropriate.
- If autopsy confirmation of corticobasal degeneration is available, the term definite posterior cortical atrophy-corticobasal degeneration would be appropriate.

(continued)

BOX 11.3 Diagnostic Criteria for Posterior Cortical Atrophy Disease-Level Descriptions (Level 3) (Continued)

- Other disease-level classifications may also be appropriate for individuals with mixed or multiple pathologies (e.g., posterior cortical atrophy-Alzheimer's disease/corticobasal degeneration).

Posterior cortical atrophy-prion disease:

- There are a number of promising biomarkers for prion disease; pending this process, an in vivo diagnosis of posterior cortical atrophy-prion may be feasible.
- If autopsy confirmation of prion disease is available or a known genetic form of prion disease has been determined, the term definite posterior cortical atrophy-prion would be appropriate.

Modified from Crutch, S. J., Schott, J. M., Rabinovici, G. D., et al. 2017. Consensus classification of posterior cortical atrophy. *Alzheimer's & Dementia: The Journal of the Alzheimer's Association, 13*(8), 870–884.

For example, although the patient can voluntarily move their eyes up, down, left, and right, they cannot look at the examiner's finger or nose when asked. Optic ataxia refers to the inability to accurately move a hand to an object using visual information. For example, although upper extremity strength and coordination is normal, the patient cannot accurately guide their hand to touch the examiner's finger by looking at it. Simultanagnosia refers to the inability to perceive more than one item at a time. It may be searched for by asking the patient to describe a complex scene (such as from a magazine or the "Cookie Theft" picture from the Boston Diagnostic Aphasia Examination, Lezak et al., 2012) or to circle letters of varying sizes on a page (from minute to enormous, taking up half the page). Note that in each case the entire stimulus (visual scene or paper with letters of varying sizes) should be as large as possible so as to require the healthy individual to make many fixations throughout their field of vision. The patient with simultanagnosia will not observe the entire scene or circle the larger letters.

Gerstmann Syndrome

Named for the Jewish Austrian-born American neurologist Josef Gerstmann who described it in 1924, Gerstmann syndrome—acalculia, left-right disorientation, finger agnosia, and agraphia—may be seen with damage to the inferior parietal lobule (angular and supramarginal gyri, Brodmann areas 39 and 40) of the dominant hemisphere. Acalculia refers to difficulty manipulating numbers and performing mathematical calculations. For example, the patient may not be able to put the numbers 6, 9, and 4 in numerical order, or calculate 11 minus 7. Left-right disorientation refers to the patient's difficulty distinguishing left from right both on themselves and on other people and objects. Finger agnosia refers to difficulty distinguishing, naming, and recognizing fingers, both on oneself and on other people or pictures. Agraphia refers to difficulty writing not due to problems with upper extremity strength or coordination.

THINGS TO LOOK FOR IN THE HISTORY

Probably the most common feature of the history we hear in patients with posterior cortical atrophy syndrome is repeated visits to optometrists or ophthalmologists, where new glasses and sometimes even surgical procedures are tried in unsuccessful attempts to improve vision. Sometimes occipital strokes or tumors are suspected when homonymous hemianopsia is present. We also often hear about minor damage to their cars owing to visuospatial impairments when parking. Reading difficulties are frequently present, but this is not a reliable sign because reading difficulties are common in other dementia syndromes as well. A more reliable sign of posterior cortical atrophy, however, is when reading actually improves when the text is made smaller. Difficulty finding items "in front of them" in cluttered environments (i.e., simultanagnosia) is common. Interestingly, items can be more difficult to find when they are still than when they are moving. Because of perceptual defects, crossing busy streets, going down stairs and escalators, using revolving doors, and even walking across shiny surfaces can all provoke disorientation and anxiety, and falls may occur (Schott & Crutch, 2019).

Nonvisual symptoms may include difficulties with calculations, using money, and writing checks. Spelling problems may develop. Apraxia is common, and may lead to difficulty dressing, including problems with buttons, zippers, neckties, finding sleeves, and putting clothes on backwards or inside out. Multistep complicated tasks that include vision such as cooking or using the computer are frequently impaired, and using television remote controls may be difficult (Schott & Crutch, 2019).

THINGS TO LOOK FOR ON THE PHYSICAL AND NEUROLOGICAL EXAMINATION

The most common features of the neurological examination are visual problems, including visual defects and visual neglect—which can be difficult to distinguish. Note that visual neglect is often most prominent on the left because whereas the right parietal lobe pays attention to both left and right space, the left parietal lobe only pays attention to right space. Thus a process which either affects both parietal lobes or just the right parietal lobe will produce greater neglect on left compared with right space.

Formal visual field testing often reveals somewhat unusual hemifield impairments or restrictions. Balance problems are common and, when combined with visual impairment, may lead to patients bumping into walls and doorframes when walking (Schott & Crutch, 2019). Other examination features which may be observed—regardless of the underlying pathology—include limb rigidity, myoclonus, and tremor (Ryan et al., 2014).

PATTERN OF IMPAIRMENT ON COGNITIVE TESTS

On a battery of standard neuropsychological tests there will be difficulty with visual and visuospatial tasks with relative preservation of episodic memory, semantic memory, simple and complex attention, and executive function—when these latter domains are tested without requiring vision. The Trailmaking Test Part B, for example, may be impaired because of visuospatial difficulties in finding the numbers and letters, rather than from executive dysfunction. The naming of line drawings may be impaired, and naming performance may improve considerably if an item (for example, a comb or harmonica) is touched and felt. Tests that specifically examine visuospatial function will generally be impaired, including clock drawing, dot counting (also called letter cancellation), line bisection, copying figures (such as intersecting pentagons), and tests for simultanagnosia. Reading will generally be impaired, and may improve when patients use their finger to keep their place and when the text is made smaller. When sending the patient for a formal neuropsychological evaluation, make sure that the psychologist understands the patient's difficulties so that they can evaluate performance of memory, attention, executive function, and so on, using nonvisual tests (Schott & Crutch, 2019).

STRUCTURAL AND FUNCTIONAL IMAGING STUDIES

Most patients with posterior cortical atrophy will, of course, have atrophy in their posterior cortex, namely in occipital and parietal lobes (see Fig. 11.1 for a visual rating scale). Having said this clearly, there are some patients who meet clinical and cognitive but not the MRI criteria for posterior cortical atrophy (Box 11.1). These patients may, however, show hypometabolism on fluorodeoxyglucose positron emission tomography (FDG PET) or technetium-99 single-photon emission computed tomography (SPECT), so one of these tests may be performed if there is clinical importance in confirming the diagnosis. Patients with posterior cortical atrophy as a result of Creutzfeldt-Jakob disease may show cortical ribboning in occipital lobes on diffusion-weighted imaging (DWI) MRI scans (see Chapter 16).

DIFFERENTIAL DIAGNOSIS

Because posterior cortical atrophy is a clinical syndrome with a number of possible underlying etiologies, the differential diagnosis is essentially these etiologies, as described in level 3 of the diagnostic criteria (Box 11.3). These are, in order of prevalence, Alzheimer's disease (see Chapter 4), Lewy body disease (see Chapter 8), corticobasal degeneration (see Chapter 13), and prion disease (see Chapter 16). Although not one of the usual etiologies, we would also add cerebrovascular disease (see Chapter 7) as either a singular or mixed etiology, as vascular dementia can also present with the clinical and cognitive signs and symptoms of posterior cortical atrophy.

TREATMENTS

Because most patients have either underlying Alzheimer's or Lewy body disease pathology, most patients will benefit from cholinesterase inhibitors (see Chapter 19) in the mild, moderate, and severe dementia stages, and may also benefit from memantine (see Chapter 20) in the moderate and severe stages. There are many nonpharmacological approaches that may be beneficial for patients with posterior cortical atrophy; see Schott and Crutch (2019).

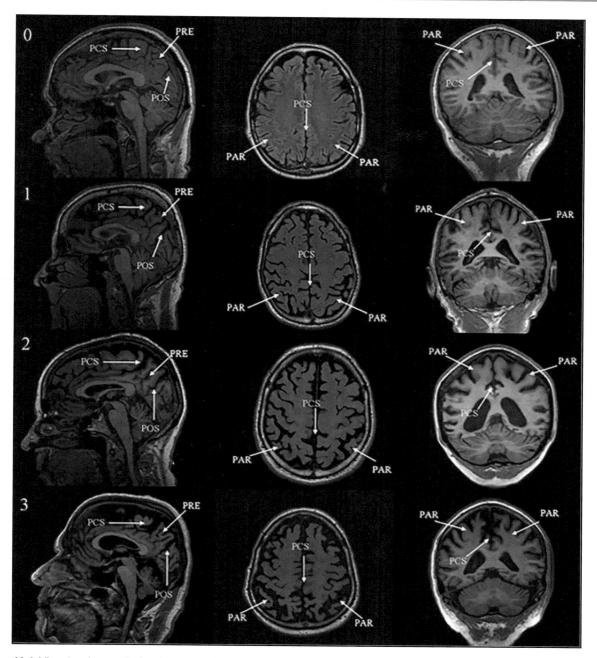

Fig. 11.1 Visual rating scale for the posterior brain regions. In sagittal, axial, and coronal orientation, this rating scale rates atrophy as follows: 0 = no atrophy, 1 = minimal atrophy, 2 = moderate atrophy, and 3 = severe atrophy. *PAR*, Parietal lobe; *PCS*, posterior cingulate sulcus; *POS*, parietooccipital sulcus; *PRE*, precuneus. (From Koedam, E. L., Lehmann, M., van der Flier, W. M., Scheltens, P., et al. (2011). Visual assessment of posterior atrophy development of a MRI rating scale. *European Radiology, 21*(12), 2618–2625. https://doi.org/10.1007/s00330-011-2205-4.)

REFERENCES

Lezak, M. D., Howieson, D. B., Bigler, E. D., et al. (2012). *Neuropsychological Assessment* (5th ed.). Oxford: Oxford University Press.

Ryan, N. S., Shakespeare, T. J., Lehmann, M., et al. (2014). Motor features in posterior cortical atrophy and their imaging correlates. *Neurobiology of Aging, 35*(12), 2845–2857.

Schott, J. M., & Crutch, S. J. (2019). Posterior cortical atrophy. *Continuum (Minneapolis, Minn.), 25*(1), 52–75.

Schott, J. M., Crutch, S. J., Carrasquillo, M. M., et al. (2016). Genetic risk factors for the posterior cortical atrophy variant of Alzheimer's disease. *Alzheimer's & Dementia: The Journal of the Alzheimer's Association, 12*(8), 862–871.

Stopford, C. L., Snowden, J. S., Thompson, J. C., et al. (2008). Variability in cognitive presentation of Alzheimer's disease. *Cortex; A Journal Devoted to the Study of the Nervous System and Behavior, 44*(2), 185–195.

12

Progressive Supranuclear Palsy

QUICK START: PROGRESSIVE SUPRANUCLEAR PALSY	
Definition	• Progressive supranuclear palsy (often abbreviated to PSP) is a neurodegenerative disease caused by the accumulation of hyperphosphorylated tau protein isoforms in the brain. • Main features include abnormalities of vertical eye movements (supranuclear palsy), along with postural instability with backwards falling, gait like "a drunken sailor," axial rigidity, frontal lobe signs and symptoms, and eventually difficulty talking and swallowing (pseudobulbar palsy).
Prevalence	• Progressive supranuclear palsy has a prevalence of 5 to 6 per 100,000. • The mean age of onset of the disease is 63 years. • The usual prognosis ranges from 5 to 10 years from diagnosis to death.
Cognitive and behavioral symptoms	• Early cognitive and affective symptoms may include slowing of all aspects of mental processing, executive dysfunction, dysarthria and/or apraxia of speech, irritability, irascibility, and apathy, introversion, and depression.

Diagnostic criteria (See text for additional elements)	• Sporadic occurrence
	• Age 40 years or older at onset
	• Gradual progression of symptoms
	• No clinical, imaging, laboratory, or genetic findings strongly suggestive of another disorder
	• Ocular motor dysfunction, consisting of either:
	  • Vertical supranuclear gaze palsy, or
	  • Slow velocity of vertical saccades
	• Plus one of the following core clinical features:
	  • Postural instability, consisting of either:
	    • Repeated unprovoked falls within 3 years, or
	    • Tendency to fall on the pull-test within 3 years
	  • Akinesia, consisting of either:
	    • Progressive gait freezing within 3 years, or
	    • Parkinsonism, akinetic-rigid, predominantly axial, and levodopa resistant, or
	    • Parkinsonism, with tremor and/or asymmetric and/or levodopa responsive
	  • Cognitive dysfunction, consisting of:
	    • Frontal cognitive/behavioral presentation

(Continued)

QUICK START: PROGRESSIVE SUPRANUCLEAR PALSY (*Continued*)	
Treatment	• Symptomatic treatments to consider include levodopa/carbidopa (Sinemet), memantine, amantadine, botulinum toxin, and desmopression.
Top differential diagnoses	• Corticobasal degeneration, dementia with Lewy bodies, vascular dementia, frontotemporal dementia, Creutzfeldt-Jakob disease, normal pressure hydrocephalus, Huntington's disease, multiple sclerosis, medication side effects.

A 62-year-old man presented to the clinic with a curious tale. The patient had been driving from California to Boston. When he stopped for gas, the attendant thought he was drunk and called the police. The police heard his slurred speech, found him unable to walk heel-to-toe in a straight line, and arrested him for driving under the influence. Ultimately, it was determined that he was not intoxicated, and he was released. In the clinic, the patient complained most that he had difficulty talking, and his speech was quite slow, hesitant, and dysarthric. His examination was notable for slow voluntary eye movements in all directions, including vertical gaze. Eye movements improved and became smooth by having the patient look straight ahead while his head was gently moved. He walked with a very wide-based gait and often staggered although he did not fall. He showed great difficulty with tests of executive function such as the Trail Making Test Part B and Digit Span Backwards; he was unable to correctly draw a clock.

PREVALENCE, PROGNOSIS, AND DEFINITION

Progressive supranuclear palsy (often abbreviated to PSP and sometimes referred to as the Steele–Richardson–Olszewski syndrome) is a neurodegenerative disease of the brain caused by the accumulation of hyperphosphorylated tau protein isoforms in the brain. Its main feature is an abnormality of vertical eye movements (supranuclear palsy), along with postural instability with falls, axial rigidity, frontal lobe signs and symptoms, and difficulty swallowing and talking (pseudobulbar palsy). It has a prevalence of 5 to 6 per 100,000, with approximately only 1.5 per 100,000 being accurately diagnosed. The mean age of onset of the disease is 63 years, with a usual prognosis ranging from 5 to 10 years from diagnosis to death; median 7 (Golbe, 2014). More rarely patients have been observed to succumb as quickly as 2 years or as slowly as 28 years (Greene, 2019). The disease received increased attention in the popular press when the comedian Dudley Moore was diagnosed with it in 1999.

TERMINOLOGY

Supranuclear Palsy

A "supranuclear palsy" causing eye movement abnormalities means that there is dysfunction of the part of the brain that controls voluntary eye movements above (*supra* in Latin) the level of the oculomotor nucleus (in the midbrain, the upper part of the brainstem). This type of palsy affects mainly voluntary eye movements, while involuntary movements are relatively spared. (Involuntary movements may be controlled by a group of neurons called the superior colliculus.) Testing for a supranuclear palsy involves comparing eye movements for voluntary and involuntary gaze. Testing for voluntary gaze may be easily accomplished by having the patient look rapidly between two points (often called "saccades"), usually between the thumb on one hand and the index finger on the other ("Look at my thumb, look at my finger," and so on). Testing for involuntary gaze is best performed by having the patient stare at a stationary point while you gently move their head up and down and back and forth, thus moving their eyes in their head. In a supranuclear palsy the rapid, voluntary eye movements will be abnormal while the involuntary movements will be normal (or relatively normal) demonstrating that the eye movement problem is in the voluntary gaze centers, above the oculomotor nucleus.

Pseudobulbar Palsy

If a patient has a "pseudobulbar palsy," it indicates that there is dysfunction of part of the brain that mimics dysfunction of the lower part of the brainstem, the medulla. A "pseudobulbar palsy" refers to dysfunction of the part of the brain above the medulla that controls movements of the tongue, pharynx, and larynx. Thus the patient with a pseudobulbar palsy typically exhibits slurred and otherwise abnormal speech (dysarthria), and difficulty eating and swallowing (dysphagia).

CRITERIA AND DIAGNOSIS

The cardinal feature of progressive supranuclear palsy is an abnormality of vertical eye movements. Because up-gaze is sometimes impaired in normal aging, abnormalities of down-gaze are particularly sought for as confirmatory clinical signs when this diagnosis is being considered. Diagnostic criteria developed by the Movement Disorder Society not only provide a for a diagnosis of progressive supranuclear palsy but also of eight different clinical phenotypes. Boxes 12.1 and 12.2 provide a summary of the criteria for a clinical diagnosis of progressive supranuclear palsy; those who are interested in the phenotypes are referred to the original paper (Höglinger et al. 2017) as well others which have tried to streamline the issue of multiple phenotypes (Ali, Botha, & Whitwell, 2019).

RISK FACTORS, PATHOLOGY, AND PATHOPHYSIOLOGY

There are no known risk factors for developing progressive supranuclear palsy. The disorder is associated with the accumulation of hyperphosphorylated tau protein isoforms in the brain. Neuropathological diagnostic criteria for progressive supranuclear palsy include the presence of numerous neurofibrillary tangles and neuropil threads in a number of subcortical regions, such as globus pallidus, subthalamic nucleus, substantia nigra, pons, corpus striatum, oculomotor nucleus, medulla oblongata, and dentate cerebellar nuclei. The tangles are composed of 12- to 20-nm straight filaments, tend to be rounded, and have been termed "globose." Tau immunostaining has shown that tau in progressive supranuclear palsy is primarily made up of a four-repeat tau, whereas in frontotemporal dementia the tau is predominantly composed of a three-repeat tau. Atrophy of midbrain, pontine tegmentum, and globus pallidus is common in progressive supranuclear palsy (Fig. 12.1).

COMMON SIGNS, SYMPTOMS, AND STAGES

One useful way to think about progressive supranuclear palsy is that it is a disorder of several aspects of

---

BOX 12.1   Diagnostic Criteria for the Clinical Diagnosis of Progressive Supranuclear Palsy

Mandatory Inclusion Criteria
- Sporadic occurrence
- Age 40 years or older at onset of first progressive supranuclear palsy-related symptom
- Gradual progression of progressive supranuclear palsy-related symptoms

Mandatory Exclusion Criteria
- No clinical, imaging, laboratory, or genetic findings strongly suggestive of Alzheimer's disease, multiple system atrophy, Lewy body disease, dementia with Lewy bodies, amyotrophic lateral sclerosis, vascular etiology, prion disease, encephalitis, or any other cause of cognitive and/or motor dysfunction.

Definite Progressive Supranuclear Palsy (Gold Standard)
- Neuropathological diagnosis

Probable Progressive Supranuclear Palsy (Specific but Not Very Sensitive)
- Ocular motor dysfunction, consisting of either:
  - Vertical supranuclear gaze palsy, or
  - Slow velocity of vertical saccades
- Plus one of the following core clinical features:
  - Postural instability, consisting of either:
    - Repeated unprovoked falls within 3 years, or
    - Tendency to fall on the pull-test within 3 years
  - Akinesia, consisting of either:
    - Progressive gait freezing within 3 years, or
    - Parkinsonism, akinetic-rigid, predominantly axial, and levodopa resistant, or
    - Parkinsonism, with tremor and/or asymmetric and/or levodopa responsive
  - Cognitive dysfunction, consisting of:
    - Frontal cognitive/behavioral presentation

Possible Progressive Supranuclear Palsy (More Sensitive but Less Specific)
- One of the following:
  - Vertical supranuclear gaze palsy
  - Slow velocity of vertical saccades + more than two steps backward on the pull-test within 3 years
  - Progressive gait freezing within 3 years
  - Speech/language disorder (nonfluent/agrammatic variant of primary progressive aphasia or progressive apraxia of speech) + ocular motor dysfunction, consisting of either:

(Continued)

BOX 12.1   Diagnostic Criteria for the Clinical Diagnosis of Progressive Supranuclear Palsy (*Continued*)

- - Vertical supranuclear gaze palsy, or
  - Slow velocity of vertical saccades
- Corticobasal syndrome + ocular motor dysfunction, consisting of either:
  - Vertical supranuclear gaze palsy, or
  - Slow velocity of vertical saccades

Suggestive of Progressive Supranuclear Palsy

- One of the following:
- Ocular motor dysfunction, consisting of either:
  - Slow velocity of vertical saccades, or
  - Frequent macro square wave jerks or "eyelid opening apraxia"
- Postural instability, consisting of either:
  - Repeated unprovoked falls within 3 years, or
  - Tendency to fall on the pull-test within 3 years
- Cognitive dysfunction, consisting of either:
  - Speech/language disorder (nonfluent/agrammatic variant of primary progressive aphasia or progressive apraxia of speech), or
  - Corticobasal syndrome
- Frontal cognitive/behavioral presentation + more than two steps backward on the pull-test within 3 years
- Both:
  - Akinesia, consisting of either:
    - Parkinsonism, akinetic-rigid, predominantly axial, and levodopa resistant, or
    - Parkinsonism, with tremor and/or asymmetric and/or levodopa responsive
  - Plus one of the following other clinical features:
    - Frontal cognitive/behavioral presentation
    - Levodopa-resistance
    - Hypokinetic, spastic dysarthria
    - Dysphagia
    - Photophobia

Supportive Imaging Findings

- Predominant midbrain atrophy or hypometabolism
- Postsynaptic striatal dopaminergic degeneration

See Box 12.2 for operationalized definitions.
Modified from Höglinger, G. U., Respondek, G., Stamelou, M., et al. (2017). Clinical diagnosis of progressive supranuclear palsy: the Movement Disorder Society criteria. *Movement Disorders, 32*(6), 853–864.

BOX 12.2   Operationalized Definitions of Core Clinical Features, Supportive Clinical Clues, and Supportive Imaging Findings

Ocular Motor Dysfunction

- Vertical supranuclear gaze palsy: A clear limitation of the range of voluntary gaze in the vertical more than in the horizontal plane, affecting both up- and downgaze, more than expected for age, which is overcome by activation with the vestibulo-ocular reflex; at later stages, the vestibulo-ocular reflex may be lost, or the maneuver prevented by nuchal rigidity.
- Slow velocity of vertical saccades: Decreased velocity (and amplitude) of vertical greater than horizontal saccadic eye movements; gaze should be assessed by command ("Look at the flicking finger") rather than by pursuit ("Follow my finger"), with the target >20 degrees from the position of primary gaze; to be diagnostic, saccadic movements are slow enough for the examiner to see their movement (eye rotation), rather than just initial and final eye positions in normal subjects; a delay in saccade initiation is not considered slowing; findings are supported by slowed or absent fast components of vertical optokinetic nystagmus (i.e., only the slow following component may be retained).
- Frequent macro square wave jerks: Rapid, involuntary saccadic intrusions during fixation, displacing the eye horizontally from the primary position, and returning it to the target after 200–300 milliseconds; most square wave jerks are <1 degree in amplitude and rare in healthy controls, but up to 3–4 degrees and more frequent (>10 per minute) in progressive supranuclear palsy.
- "Eyelid opening apraxia": An inability to voluntarily initiate eyelid opening after a period of lid closure in the absence of involuntary forced eyelid closure (i.e., blepharospasm).

Postural Instability

- Repeated unprovoked falls within 3 years: Spontaneous loss of balance while standing, or history of more than one unprovoked fall, within 3 years after onset of progressive supranuclear palsy-related features.
- Tendency to fall on the pull-test within 3 years: Tendency to fall on the pull-test if not caught by examiner, within 3 years after onset of progressive supranuclear palsy-related features.
- More than two steps backward on the pull-test within 3 years: More than two steps backward, but unaided recovery, on the pull-test, within 3 years after onset of progressive supranuclear palsy-related features.

(*Continued*)

BOX 12.2 Operationalized Definitions of Core Clinical Features, Supportive Clinical Clues, and Supportive Imaging Findings (*Continued*)

- The pull-test: The response to a quick, forceful pull on the shoulders with the examiner standing behind the patient and the patient standing erect with eyes open and feet comfortably apart and parallel.

Akinesia

- Progressive gait freezing within 3 years: Sudden and transient motor blocks or start hesitation are predominant within 3 years after onset of progressive supranuclear palsy-related symptoms, progressive, and not responsive to levodopa; in the early disease course, akinesia may be present, but limb rigidity, tremor, and dementia are absent or mild.
- Parkinsonism, akinetic-rigid, predominantly axial, and levodopa resistant: Bradykinesia and rigidity with axial predominance, and levodopa resistance.
- Parkinsonism, with tremor and/or asymmetric and/or levodopa responsive: Bradykinesia with rigidity and/or tremor, and/or asymmetric predominance of limbs, and/or levodopa responsiveness.
- Levodopa resistance: Improvement of the Movement Disorders Society Unified Parkinson's Disease Rating Scale (MDS-UPDRS) motor scale by $\leq$30%; to fulfill this criterion patients should be assessed having been given at least 1000 mg (if tolerated) at least 1 month or once patients have received this treatment they could be formally assessed following a challenge dose of at least 200 mg.
- The MDS-UPDRS can be found here: https://www.movementdisorders.org/MDS/MDS-Rating-Scales/MDS-Unified-Parkinsons-Disease-Rating-Scale-MDS-UPDRS.htm.

Cognitive Dysfunction

- Speech/language disorder: At least one of the following features, which has to be persistent (rather than transient) (see Chapter 9):
  1. Nonfluent/agrammatic variant of primary progressive aphasia (nfaPPA): Loss of grammar and/or telegraphic speech or writing, or
  2. Progressive apraxia of speech: Effortful, halting speech with inconsistent speech sound errors and distortions or slow syllabically segmented prosodic speech patterns with spared single-word comprehension, object knowledge, and word retrieval during sentence repetition.

- Frontal cognitive/behavioral presentation: at least three of the following features, which have to be persistent (rather than transient):
  1. Apathy: Reduced level of interest, initiative, and spontaneous activity; clearly apparent to informant or patient.
  2. Bradyphrenia: Slowed thinking; clearly apparent to informant or patient.
  3. Dysexecutive syndrome: e.g., reverse digit span, Trails B or Stroop test, Luria sequence (at least 1.5 standard deviations below mean of age- and education-adjusted norms).
  4. Reduced phonemic verbal fluency: e.g., "D, F, A, or S" words per minute (at least 1.5 standard deviations below mean of age- and education-adjusted norms).
  5. Impulsivity, disinhibition, or perseveration: e.g., socially inappropriate behaviors, overstuffing the mouth when eating, motor recklessness, applause sign, palilalia, echolalia.
- Applause sign: Patients are asked to clap three times. If they clap more than three times, it is considered positive.
- Corticobasal syndrome (see also Chapter 13): At least one sign each from the following two groups (may be asymmetric or symmetric):
  1. Cortical signs:
     a. Orobuccal or limb apraxia.
     b. Cortical sensory deficit.
     c. Alien limb phenomena.
  2. Movement disorder signs:
     a. Limb rigidity.
     b. Limb akinesia.
     c. Limb myoclonus.

Other Clinical Features

- Hypokinetic, spastic dysarthria: Slow, low volume and pitch, harsh voice.
- Dysphagia: Otherwise unexplained difficulty in swallowing, severe enough to request dietary adaptations.
- Photophobia: Intolerance to visual perception of light due to adaptive dysfunction.

Imaging Findings

- Predominant midbrain atrophy or hypometabolism relative to pons, as demonstrated, e.g., by MRI or [^{18}F]DG-PET.
- Postsynaptic striatal dopaminergic degeneration as demonstrated, e.g., by [^{123}I]IBZM-SPECT or [^{18}F]-DMFP-PET.

Modified from Höglinger, G. U., Respondek, G., Stamelou, M., et al. (2017). Clinical diagnosis of progressive supranuclear palsy: the Movement Disorder Society criteria. *Movement Disorders, 32*(6), 853–864.

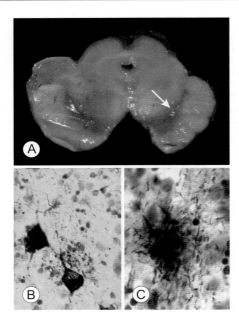

Fig. 12.1 Pathology in progressive supranuclear palsy. **(A)** Pallor of the substantia nigra (*arrow;* should be black) and atrophy of the midbrain, particularly in the anterior–posterior dimension (up and down in this figure). Tangles **(B)** and a tufted astrocyte **(C)**.

the nervous system, any or all of which may be affected depending upon the relative distribution of pathology. All clinical diagnoses of probable progressive supranuclear palsy must include some abnormality of eye movements. Other signs and symptoms of the disorder will be present in varying degrees; these include disorders of movement (postural instability with backwards falls, axial rigidity and dystonia, bradykinesia and rigidity), pseudobulbar palsy (difficulty swallowing and talking), and speech/language and/or frontal/executive cognitive deficits. Over time, the features that the patient presents with typically worsen, and other symptoms may occur (but not invariably).

Some more common signs and symptoms that are seen as the disorder progresses are as follows:
- The gait, sometimes described as that of a drunken sailor, becomes more abnormal.
- Impulsiveness may lead to suddenly rising from sitting, increasing risk of falls.
- Balance becomes more impaired.
- Fractures and bruises are common resulting from falls.

- Sloppy eating is due to the combination of loss of dexterity, swallowing difficulties, and difficulty looking down at the plate of food.
- Dysarthria and/or apraxia of speech may be the presenting symptom (Josephs et al., 2014; see Chapter 9)
- In the severe stages the patient is typically confined to a wheelchair, incontinent, and more severe chewing and swallowing difficulties, drooling, coughing, spluttering, and choking are common.
- Death is typically as a result of aspiration pneumonia.

THINGS TO LOOK FOR IN THE HISTORY

Testimony to the fact that progressive supranuclear palsy is a difficult disorder to diagnose is the common occurrence of a delay in diagnosis of 3 years or more. The most important feature to look for in the history is that of falls. Early cognitive and affective symptoms may include irritability, irascibility, apathy, introversion, and depression. Disruption of speech due to dysarthria or apraxia may be an early sign. Inappropriate sexual behavior may also be present. The patient may complain of visual symptoms including blurred vision, difficulty focusing, dry eyes, photophobia, and double vision. Navigating stairs is usually difficult. These visual symptoms frequently lead to appointments with optometrists or ophthalmologists, often resulting in new eyeglasses prescriptions (which of course do not alleviate symptoms). The patient may also note difficulties walking, speaking, or swallowing, as well as fatigue, dizziness, and clumsiness.

THINGS TO LOOK FOR ON THE PHYSICAL AND NEUROLOGICAL EXAMINATION

The most important feature to look for on the neurological examination is a supranuclear vertical gaze disturbance, as described above. It should be emphasized that, although there must be at least a slowing or disruption of vertical or horizontal eye movements, an actual reduction in the degree of downward gaze is not necessary (Video 12.1). Other common ocular abnormalities include spontaneous involuntary eyelid closure, reduced spontaneous blink rate (0–4 per minute), and a mild drooping of the eyelid (ptosis). It is likely from these latter symptoms that patients with progressive

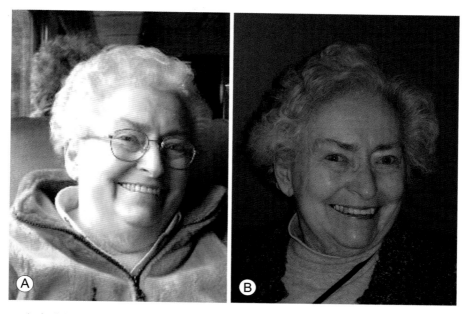

Fig. 12.2 Changes in facial expression due to progressive supranuclear palsy. Note the somewhat astonished look of the patient after she was diagnosed with progressive supranuclear palsy **(B)**, compared with how she looked several years earlier **(A)**.

supranuclear palsy are often described as having a slightly astonished and worried look, felt to be due to the patient compensating for the mild drooping of the eyelids by raising their eyebrows, in combination with the decreased blink rate (Fig. 12.2).

Other features to look for on the neurological examination are abnormalities of speech (Video 12.2), gait (Video 12.3), postural reflexes (often tested with the "pull test," see Video 12.4), axial and limb rigidity, apraxia (Video 12.5), tremor, axial and limb dystonia, and myoclonus. Impairment of gait and postural reflexes leads to loss of balance and staggering when walking, with frequent falls. On rising from a chair the patient may extend the neck and trunk and spontaneously topple backwards. Axial rigidity can be assessed by passively and gently moving the head and bending the neck forward and backward. One useful tool assessing patients with possible progressive supranuclear palsy and following them over time is the clinical rating scale by Golbe and Ohman-Strickland (2007).

PATTERN OF IMPAIRMENT ON COGNITIVE TESTS (VIDEOS 12.6–12.8)

The first thing that should be noted is that not all patients with progressive supranuclear palsy demonstrate cognitive deficits. One study found that approximately one-third of patients examined showed moderate cognitive impairment, one-third showed mild impairment, and one-third showed no clinically significant cognitive impairment (Maher, Smith, & Lees, 1985).

Two main aspects of cognition are commonly impaired in patients with progressive supranuclear palsy. First there is a slowing of mental processing, often termed "bradyphrenia." This slowing will obviously produce impairment on any timed test, including verbal fluency to letters and categories, the Trailmaking Tests parts A and B, and others.

The second aspect of cognition that is impaired is executive function. As described in detail in Chapter 2 there are a number of tests available to measure executive function. Patients with progressive supranuclear palsy have been observed to show impairment on many of these, including the Tower of London Task, the Addenbrookes Cognitive Examination, the Frontal Assessment Battery, and tests such as the Trailmaking Test part B, which require the patient to shift back and forth between two or more cognitive sets (going up the alphabet and counting forwards). Tests of memory, by contrast, will be either normal (in the early stages) or abnormal owing to poor executive function, showing poor encoding and free recall with relatively normal recognition. When executive function becomes severely impaired, other aspects of cognition will also show impairment.

LABORATORY STUDIES

There are no routine, readily available laboratory, genetic, or cerebrospinal fluid studies that are helpful in either confirming or ruling out progressive supranuclear palsy.

STRUCTURAL IMAGING STUDIES

Atrophy of the midbrain has been observed on magnetic resonance imaging (MRI) in many patients with progressive supranuclear palsy at some point in their disease course. Although not an obligatory part of the diagnostic criteria, if such atrophy is present it adds the label of "imaging supported diagnosis" (Höglinger et al., 2017). However, we wish to state clearly that if the midbrain size is normal, it does not "rule out" progressive supranuclear palsy, as one study found that 14% of patients with autopsy-confirmed progressive supranuclear palsy did not have midbrain atrophy (Whitwell et al., 2017). Another study found that whereas the average midbrain area of healthy individuals was 117 mm², the average midbrain area was significantly smaller in progressive supranuclear palsy (56 mm²). Patients with Parkinson's disease and the parkinsonian syndrome multiple system atrophy also showed smaller midbrains than healthy individuals on average (103 and 97 mm², respectively), although their size was still much larger than those with progressive supranuclear palsy (Oba et al., 2005). When viewed from a midline sagittal perspective, the shrunken midbrain with a relatively normal pons leads to what has been called the "hummingbird" sign. Warmuth-Metz, Naumann, and Csoti (2001) found that patients with progressive supranuclear palsy had midbrain anterior–posterior diameters ranging from 11 to 15 mm (average 13.4 mm), much smaller than both controls (range 17–20 mm, average 18.2 mm) and patients with Parkinson's disease (range 17–19 mm, average 18.5 mm). Although midbrain measurement does not have 100% sensitivity or specificity, it should always be obtained as supportive data if the diagnosis of progressive supranuclear palsy is suspected. In our experience, anterior–posterior midbrain measurement can be performed by the radiologist if requested, and it is also fairly easily measured using the viewing software. The midbrain is usually present on two MRI slices, and we measure both (Fig. 12.3).

FUNCTIONAL IMAGING STUDIES

Fluorodeoxyglucose positron emission tomography (FDG PET) studies have found hypometabolism in midbrain, basal ganglia, thalamus, and frontal lobes (premotor, precentral, prefrontal regions) in patients with the classic progressive supranuclear palsy syndrome with both prominent eye movement abnormalities and postural instability. Patterns of hypometabolism were more variable, however, when other symptoms were predominant (Whitwell et al., 2017). That such differences in imaging would be present between different patients with different patterns of signs and symptoms of course makes sense; both reflect where in the brain the underlying tau pathology is most prominent. From a practical standpoint, however, this means that the FDG PET scan will provide clear results when the patient presents in a classic manner and the diagnosis can usually be made on clinical grounds alone. When the clinical picture is less certain, the imaging study is less useful.

Dopamine active transporter (DAT) imaging using [¹²³I]IBZM-SPECT or [¹⁸F]-DMFP-PET will help differentiate patients with progressive supranuclear palsy from those with non-parkinsonian dementias, such as behavioral variant frontotemporal dementia or primary progressive aphasia due to a frontotemporal lobar degeneration. These DAT scans will not differentiate patients with progressive supranuclear palsy from those with other parkinsonian disorders, such as Parkinson's disease, dementia with Lewy bodies, or corticobasal degeneration (Whitwell et al., 2017).

DIFFERENTIAL DIAGNOSIS

The differential diagnosis of progressive supranuclear palsy, from the standpoint of a patient presenting with a cognitive impairment, involves considering other etiologies that can cause some combination of cognitive impairment (especially executive dysfunction), behavioral changes, eye movement abnormalities, slurred

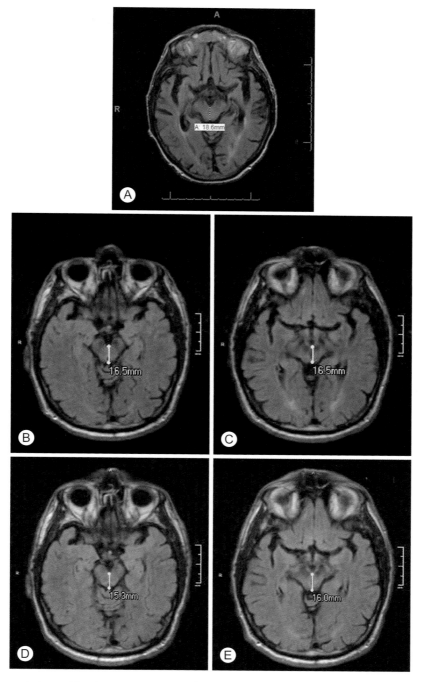

Fig. 12.3 Anterior–posterior midbrain measurements in a patient with progressive supranuclear palsy compared with a patient with Alzheimer's disease. **(A)** An 81-year-old patient with Alzheimer's disease, with notable temporal lobe atrophy but normal midbrain measurement. **(B–C)** A patient with progressive supranuclear palsy when he first presented to an outside neurologist at age 69 years. **(D–E)** The same patient imaged on the same MRI scanner one year later at age 70 years, showing remarkable midbrain shrinkage within 1 year.

TABLE 12.1　Comparison Between Progressive Supranuclear Palsy and Other Conditions With Cognitive and Sensory/Motoric Symptoms

	Progressive Supranuclear Palsy	Corticobasal Degeneration	Dementia With Lewy Bodies
Cognitive deficits	Early cognitive and affective symptoms may include slowing of all aspects of mental processing and executive dysfunction. Cognitive symptoms are rarely the first symptoms. Speech may be disrupted owing to apraxia or nonfluent aphasia	Cognitive testing demonstrates frontal and parietal cognitive dysfunction with relative preservation of memory. Speech may be disrupted owing to apraxia or nonfluent aphasia	More prominent deficits in visuospatial, attentional, and executive function with memory deficits as a less prominent complaint. Speech is normal
Behavioral symptoms	Irritability, irascibility, apathy, introversion, and depression	Insight and accompanying depression	Visual hallucinations often present early in the disease
Motor and sensory symptoms	Backward falls, postural instability, and disrupted voluntary gaze are present early in the disease	Focal and asymmetric signs and symptoms are the cardinal features of corticobasal degeneration, including asymmetric apraxia, cortical sensory loss, and unilateral visual or sensory neglect	Parkinsonian symptoms often present early in the disease

speech (dysarthria), difficulty swallowing (dysphagia), rigidity, dystonia, or parkinsonism (Table 12.1). Such disorders include the following:

- corticobasal degeneration (see Chapter 13)
- dementia with Lewy bodies (see Chapter 8)
- vascular dementia (see Chapter 7)
- frontotemporal dementia (see Chapter 10) including
  - frontotemporal dementia with parkinsonism linked to chromosome 17
  - frontotemporal dementia with amyotrophic lateral sclerosis
- prion disease including Creutzfeldt-Jakob disease (see Chapter 16)
- hydrocephalus including normal pressure hydrocephalus (see Chapter 14)
- Huntington's disease
- multiple sclerosis
- medication side-effects including those of neuroleptics and antiemetics
- Rare disorders such as Whipple disease, Niemann-Pick disease type C, Gaucher disease.

TREATMENTS

There are no U.S. Food and Drug Administration–approved treatments for progressive supranuclear palsy. Symptomatic treatments that are worth trying include levodopa/carbidopa (Sinemet), memantine, and amantadine. Atropine 1% eye drops can be administered sublingually to help reduce drooling. Botulinum toxin may be used to treat spasms, dystonia, blepharospasm, apraxia of eyelid opening, and drooling. Desmopression at bedtime may reduce nocturnal incontinence (Greene, 2019). Management of dysphagia to prevent choking and aspiration is critical.

REFERENCES

Ali, F., Botha, H., Whitwell, J. L., et al. (2019). Utility of the Movement Disorders Society criteria for progressive supranuclear palsy in clinical practice. *Movement Disorders Clinical Practice*, 6(6), 436–439.

Golbe, L. I., & Ohman-Strickland, P. A. (2007). A clinical rating scale for progressive supranuclear palsy. *Brain*, *130*(6), 1552–1565.

Golbe. L. I. (2014). Progressive supranuclear palsy. *Seminars in Neurology, 34,* 151–159.

Greene. P. (2019). Progressive supranuclear palsy, corticobasal degeneration, and multiple system atrophy. *Continuum (Minneapolis, Minn.), 25*(4), 919–935.

Höglinger, G. U., Respondek, G., Stamelou, M., et al. (2017). Clinical diagnosis of progressive supranuclear palsy: The Movement Disorder Society criteria. *Movement Disorders, 32*(6), 853–864.

Maher, E. R., Smith, E. M., & Lees, A. J. (1985). Cognitive deficits in the Steele-Richardson-Olszewski syndrome (progressive supranuclear palsy). *Journal of Neurology, Neurosurgery, and Psychiatry, 48,* 1234–1239.

Josephs, K. A., Duffy, J. R., Strand, E. A., et al. (2014). The evolution of primary progressive apraxia of speech. *Brain, 137,* 2783–2795.

Oba, H., Yagishita, A., Terada, H., et al. (2005). New and reliable MRI diagnosis for progressive supranuclear palsy. *Neurology, 64,* 2050–2055.

Warmuth-Metz, M., Naumann, M., & Csoti, I. (2001). Measurement of the midbrain diameter on routine magnetic resonance imaging: A simple and accurate method of differentiating between Parkinson disease and progressive supranuclear palsy. *Archives of Neurology, 58,* 1076–1079.

Whitwell, J. L., Höglinger, G. U., Antonini, A., et al. (2017). Radiological biomarkers for diagnosis in PSP: Where are we and where do we need to be? *Movement Disorders, 32*(7), 955–971. doi:10.1002/mds.27038.

Additional videos for this topic are available online at expertconsult.com.

13

Corticobasal Degeneration and Corticobasal Syndrome

(Continued)

QUICK START: CORTICOBASAL DEGENERATION AND CORTICOBASAL SYNDROME (*Continued*)

- plus two of:
  - d. orobuccal or limb apraxia
  - e. cortical sensory deficit
  - f. alien limb phenomena
- Frontal behavioral-spatial syndrome:
  - Two of:
    - a. executive dysfunction
    - b. behavioral or personality changes
    - c. visuospatial deficits
  - plus at least one corticobasal feature (a–f, above)
- Nonfluent/agrammatic variant of primary progressive aphasia
  - Effortful, agrammatic speech plus at least one of:
    - a. impaired grammar/sentence comprehension with relatively preserved single word comprehension
    - b. groping, distorted speech production (apraxia of speech)
  - plus at least one corticobasal feature (a–f, above)
- Exclusion criteria: evidence of other neurological disorder that could explain signs and symptoms.

Treatment	• There are no U.S. Food and Drug Administration-approved medications to treat corticobasal degeneration; treatment is supportive. • Antidepressants should be used to treat depression, which is often present. • Dystonia may be relieved with botulinum toxin. • Physical and occupational therapy is important for range of motion in affected limbs so that contractures do not develop.
Top differential diagnoses	• Frontotemporal dementia, primary progressive aphasia or apraxia of speech, progressive supranuclear palsy, dementia with Lewy bodies, Alzheimer's disease, vascular dementia.

A 73-year-old woman was brought in by her daughter for functional decline. The patient did not notice anything wrong. Per her daughter, memory problems were prominent, but there was also trouble with her movements. Her daughter noted that she did not have control of the left hand or foot; they had "a mind of their own." She reported that these difficulties came out when her mother dressed and undressed, and when she ate using utensils; she was unable to cut up anything. On examination a paucity of spontaneous speech was evident. She had almost continuous myoclonus and asterixis evident in both upper extremities, which her family described as "shaking" and another clinician described as "tremor." She veered off to the left when walking and sometimes bumped into the hallway wall. She did not use the left hand spontaneously. She attempted to untie her shoes with her right hand only—the left hand stayed gripping the arm of the chair. She demonstrated multiple apraxias, all worse with the left hand, including an inability to pantomime use of objects such as a comb or

a knife, which improved markedly when imitating the examiner or using the actual object. She was unable to identify coins placed in either hand or identify any number (except 1) drawn in either hand.

PREVALENCE, PROGNOSIS, AND DEFINITION

Corticobasal degeneration is a neurodegenerative disease of the brain caused by the accumulation of hyperphosphorylated 4-repeat tau isoforms. Corticobasal syndrome is a clinical diagnosis characterized by asymmetric cortical dysfunction, often affecting motor control of a limb, along with executive dysfunction, rigidity, a jerky postural tremor, myoclonus, dystonia, and a gait disorder; speech may be disrupted owing to apraxia or nonfluent aphasia. We now recognize that not all patients with corticobasal syndrome have underlying corticobasal degeneration pathology, and not all patients with corticobasal degeneration pathology present with corticobasal syndrome (Ali & Josephs, 2018); see Chapter 3 for a more general discussion of the issue of separating degenerative diseases from dementia syndromes. Corticobasal degeneration is a relatively rare disorder with a prevalence of about 2 per 100,000. From one literature review, the mean age of onset was 64 years, ranging from 45 to 77 years, with an average prognosis from diagnosis to death of about 6.6 years, ranging from 2 to 12.5 years (Armstrong et al., 2013).

CRITERIA

Based on the clinical phenotypes of 129 autopsy-proven cases, a 2013 paper presented two sets of criteria for corticobasal degeneration: more specific clinical research criteria for sporadic probable corticobasal degeneration and broader, more inclusive criteria for possible corticobasal degeneration that may overlap with other tau-based pathologies (Table 13.1) (Armstrong et al., 2013).

TABLE 13.1   Diagnostic Criteria for Corticobasal Degeneration

	Clinical Research Criteria for Probable Sporadic Corticobasal Degeneration	Clinical Criteria for Possible Corticobasal Degeneration
Presentation	Insidious onset and gradual progression	Insidious onset and gradual progression
Minimum duration of symptoms	1 year	1 year
Age at onset	≥50 years	No minimum
Family history (≥2 or more relatives)	Exclusion	Permitted
Permitted phenotypes (see Table 13.2)	1. Probable corticobasal syndrome or 2. Frontal behavioral-spatial syndrome plus at least one corticobasal feature (a–f in Table 13.2) or 3. Nonfluent/agrammatic variant of primary progressive aphasia plus at least one corticobasal feature (a–f in Table 13.2)	1. Possible corticobasal syndrome or 2. Frontal behavioral-spatial syndrome or 3. Nonfluent/agrammatic variant of primary progressive aphasia or 4. Progressive supranuclear palsy syndrome plus at least one corticobasal feature (b–f in Table 13.2)
Genetic mutation affecting tau (e.g., microtubule-associated protein tau)	Exclusion	Permitted
Exclusion criteria (same for both)	1. Evidence of Lewy body disease: classic 4-Hz Parkinson disease resting tremor, excellent and sustained levodopa response, or hallucinations. 2. Evidence of multiple system atrophy: dysautonomia or prominent cerebellar signs. 3. Evidence of amyotrophic lateral sclerosis: presence of both upper and lower motor neuron signs. 4. Semantic- or logopenic-variant primary progressive aphasia. 5. Structural lesion suggestive of focal cause. 6. Granulin mutation or reduced plasma progranulin levels; TDP-43 mutations; fused in sarcoma mutations. 7. Evidence of Alzheimer's disease (this will exclude approximately 14% of cases of corticobasal degeneration with coexisting amyloid): laboratory findings strongly suggestive of Alzheimer's disease such as low cerebral spinal fluid Aβ42 to tau ratio or positive amyloid positron emission tomography, or genetic mutation suggesting Alzheimer's disease (e.g., presenilin, amyloid precursor protein).	

Modified from Armstrong, M. J., Litvan, I., Lang, A. E., et al. (2013). Criteria for the diagnosis of corticobasal degeneration. *Neurology, 80,* 496–503.

Both criteria are based on five clinical phenotypes that have been proven to be associated with the pathology of corticobasal degeneration (Table 13.2). Definitions and explanations for many of the terms used in these criteria can be found in the Common Signs, Symptoms, and Stages section. Unfortunately, studies have found that these criteria are not highly sensitive or specific (Alexander et al., 2014; Greene, 2019).

It is worth noting that one of the clinical phenotypes associated with corticobasal degeneration is "progressive supranuclear palsy syndrome." That this syndrome is one of the clinical phenotypes does not mean that progressive supranuclear palsy is a subset of corticobasal degeneration or that the two disorders are really the same. It does mean that some patients with underlying corticobasal degeneration pathology look very similar to patients with underlying progressive supranuclear palsy pathology.

RISK FACTORS, PATHOLOGY, AND PATHOPHYSIOLOGY

There are no known risk factors for developing corticobasal degeneration. A characteristic of this disorder is that the distribution of pathology and atrophy is asymmetric. Cortical regions affected are around the main sulci of the brain: parasagittal, peri-Rolandic, and peri-Sylvian. Subcortical structures affected include substantia nigra, and variably the globus pallidus, subthalamic nucleus, and thalamus. Under the microscope,

TABLE 13.2 Clinical Phenotypes Associated With the Pathology of Corticobasal Degeneration	
Probable corticobasal syndrome	Asymmetric presentation of two of: a. limb rigidity or akinesia b. limb dystonia c. limb myoclonus plus two of: d. orobuccal or limb apraxia e. cortical sensory deficit f. alien limb phenomena (more than simple levitation)
Possible corticobasal syndrome	May be symmetric: one of: a. limb rigidity or akinesia b. limb dystonia c. limb myoclonus plus one of: d. orobuccal or limb apraxia e. cortical sensory deficit f. alien limb phenomena (more than simple levitation)
Frontal behavioral-spatial syndrome	Two of: a. executive dysfunction b. behavioral or personality changes c. visuospatial deficits
Nonfluent/agrammatic variant of primary progressive aphasia	Effortful, agrammatic speech plus at least one of: a. impaired grammar/sentence comprehension with relatively preserved single word comprehension b. groping, distorted speech production (apraxia of speech)
Progressive supranuclear palsy syndrome	Three of: a. axial or symmetric limb rigidity or akinesia b. postural instability or falls c. urinary incontinence d. behavioral changes e. supranuclear vertical gaze palsy or decreased velocity of vertical saccades (see Chapter 12 for description)

Modified from Armstrong, M. J., Litvan, I., Lang, A. E., et al. (2013). Criteria for the diagnosis of corticobasal degeneration. *Neurology, 80,* 496–503.

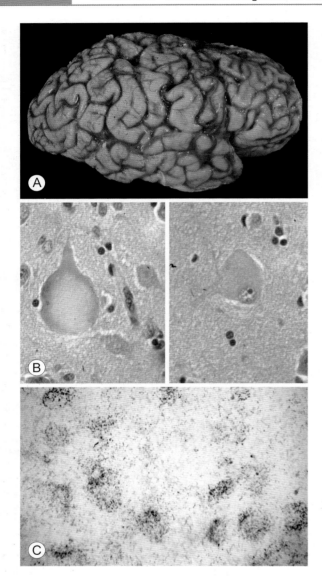

Fig. 13.1 Pathology of corticobasal degeneration. **(A)** Atrophy of the frontal lobe. **(B)** Swollen and ballooned achromatic neurons. **(C)** Astrocytic plaques.

the pathology consists of swollen achromatic neurons in amygdala and limbic structures, as well as ballooned neocortical achromatic neurons in specific layers (III, V, and VI) in frontal and parietal lobes (Fig. 13.1). Hippocampal and temporal lobe regions are least affected. Corticobasal degeneration is associated with the accumulation of hyperphosphorylated 4-repeat tau protein isoforms in neurons and glia.

COMMON SIGNS, SYMPTOMS, AND STAGES

Corticobasal syndrome classically starts with an impaired limb, which may present as an "alien limb," but more often it presents as a stiff, clumsy, and useless hand. Retrospective autopsy studies show, however, that more patients actually present with cognitive, speech, behavioral, or gait abnormalities than those who present with limb abnormalities. Limb abnormalities are likely relatively specific for corticobasal degeneration but are not sensitive enough to allow one to rely upon this sign to detect the disorder. Presenting and early symptoms may include the following:

- Alien limb (not common but pathognomonic when it occurs): The affected limb is described as "having a mind of its own," and patients report having little or no control over it. It may grasp, grope, wander, or take hold of objects, clothes, and people. Occasionally it may interfere with the function of the unaffected limb.
- Useless limb (common): The limb is not able to participate in functional activities, often because of varying combinations of rigidity, akinesia, dystonia, myoclonus, and apraxia.
- Focal/limb apraxias: Inability to perform skilled and/ or learned movements unexplained by abnormalities such as weakness, incoordination, language difficulties, and so on. See Box 13.1 and Videos 13.1–13.3.
- Rigidity: An increase in muscle tone causing resistance to movement of the joint.
- Akinesia: An inability to initiate movement owing to difficulty selecting and/or activating motor programs.
- Dystonia: Occurs when sustained muscle contractions cause abnormal postures or movements.
- Asterixis: A sudden involuntary loss of tone in a muscle group.
- Myoclonus: A brief, involuntary twitching of a muscle group.
- A jerky postural tremor: A "tremor" typically caused by frequent asterixis and myoclonus.
- Sensory symptoms: Includes numbness and tingling.
- Cortical sensory loss: Primary sensory abilities are normal, but there are deficits in the ability to use this information to make appropriate judgments. Patients can feel a touch, distinguish sharp from dull, warm from cold, and so on, but they are unable to identify a coin by feeling it (stereognosis, see Video 13.4) or a number when it is drawn in their hand (graphesthesia, see Video 13.5).

BOX 13.1 Apraxia (see Videos 13.1–13.3)

A patient is said to have an apraxia when he or she is unable to perform a purposeful, coordinated movement despite normal strength and sensation. The patient's actions often appear clumsy and uncoordinated. Apraxias come in a variety of types. Some of the more common are as follows.

- Limb-kinetic apraxia refers to the loss of the ability to make precise independent finger movements, such as the pincer grasp that is needed to pick up a small coin off a flat surface.
- Patients with ideomotor apraxia make errors in spatial movement, orientation, and/or timing of previously learned skilled movements. For example, when pantomiming cutting paper with scissors, he or she may not keep the scissors correctly oriented to the paper.
- In conduction apraxia, patients show more difficulty imitating a skilled movement (such as a salute) than performing the movement to command.
- Dissociation apraxia refers to the inability to pantomime to command, despite the ability to imitate and use objects perfectly.
- Although the term ideational apraxia has been used to describe a variety of apraxias, its current meaning is an inability to correctly sequence a series of acts that lead to a goal (such as making a sandwich).
- Patients with conceptual apraxia show errors in trying to use or pantomime using tools correctly, such that they may show hammering when asked to demonstrate the use of a screwdriver. Many of these patients also show deficits in semantic memory, having lost the meaning of these items.

- Visuospatial deficits: Impairment in one or more visuospatial functions such as copying a cube or intersecting pentagons, left/right discrimination, neglect, simultagnosia (difficulty perceiving multiple objects at the same time), or directing limb movement via visual guidance. (See Chapter 11.)
- Neglect: Ignoring one side of space. Often tested by presenting stimuli on both sides of the body simultaneously and ascertaining whether patients ignore stimuli on one side of the body in the absence of a primary sensory deficit. Left neglect is much more common than right. (See Chapter 11.)
- Apraxia of speech: Abnormality of speech including slow speaking rate, abnormal prosody (some of the nonlinguistic aspects of speech such as emotion and intonation), and distorted sound substitutions. (See Chapter 9.)
- Speech disturbance: The disturbance in speech can include orobuccal apraxia (apraxia of the mouth, lips, and tongue), apraxia of speech, halting and/or effortful speech. (See Chapter 9.)
- Executive dysfunction: Impairments in planning, abstraction, problem solving, judgment, working memory, and goal-directed behavior.
- Behavioral disorder: Symptoms may include apathy, bizarre or antisocial behavior, personality changes, irritability, disinhibition, and hypersexuality. (See Chapter 10.)

Over time the affected limbs become more rigid, with rapid movements such as pronation/supination and alternating finger tapping becoming impaired. Eventually even passive stretch may not be possible. Dystonia may become prominent, with the hand often becoming a clenched fist or having hyperextension of one or more fingers. Myoclonus is often seen in the fingers, which may increase with sensory stimulation and finger movements. Although all four limbs are commonly involved in the later stages, asymmetry is usually maintained.

THINGS TO LOOK FOR IN THE HISTORY

The characteristic feature of corticobasal syndrome that should be sought in the history is that of asymmetric limb dysfunction. The limb dysfunction may consist of rigidity, apraxia, dystonia, myoclonus, alien limb phenomena, or some combination thereof. By history, the apraxia will often present as a loss of a previously acquired function, such as being unable to fold laundry or use a screwdriver (see Box 13.1). A speech disturbance, usually of the nonfluent variety, is common and often includes word-finding difficulties and decreased fluency of speech. Some families have reported that patients often confuse yes/no responses, nodding their head when they mean "no," and shaking their head when they mean "yes." The most common neuropsychiatric symptoms in corticobasal syndrome are depression, fatigue, and irritability—symptoms all too common in many kinds of dementia. Memory complaints are common, but when recognition memory is tested in the clinic it is found to be relatively preserved. Thus complaints of memory are very consistent with corticobasal syndrome, whereas impairment of recognition memory on testing is unusual in this syndrome.

However, patients with underlying corticobasal degeneration pathology may present with clinical phenotypes other than corticobasal syndrome. When patients with corticobasal degeneration present with frontal behavioral-spatial syndrome, nonfluent/agrammatic primary progressive aphasia, or progressive supranuclear palsy syndrome, the history will reflect those other phenotypes.

THINGS TO LOOK FOR ON THE PHYSICAL AND NEUROLOGICAL EXAMINATION (VIDEOS 13.6 AND 13.7)

The examination of the limbs, and in particular the hands, is critical when suspecting corticobasal syndrome. Asymmetry of findings in the limbs should be expected. In addition to looking for signs of alien limb, the arms and hands should be examined for signs of rigidity, dystonia, myoclonus, asterixis, and jerky action tremor. (A pill-rolling rest tremor suggesting Parkinson's disease or dementia with Lewy bodies is exclusionary.) Eye movement abnormalities, including supranuclear gaze palsies, may be found in up to one-third of patients (Murray et al., 2007), particularly those who show the progressive supranuclear palsy syndrome clinical phenotype, making it often difficult to differentiate corticobasal degeneration from progressive supranuclear palsy. Cortical sensory loss is often present, making it difficult for patients to identify a coin by feeling it (stereognosis, see Video 13.4) or a number when it is drawn in their hand (graphesthesia, see Video 13.5), despite normal primary sensory function. Naming and other aspects of language should be tested, looking for a pattern of nonfluent aphasia. Comprehension difficulties, when present, are most likely to be due to difficulty understanding grammatically complex sentences. When looking for corticobasal syndrome, praxis should be carefully tested (see Box 13.1). Ideomotor apraxia is most common, such that patients are often unable to correctly pantomime using tools such as scissors, hammer, or screwdriver (see Videos 13.1–13.3).

PATTERN OF IMPAIRMENT ON COGNITIVE TESTS

The dementia of corticobasal syndrome differs from that of Alzheimer's disease. In Alzheimer's disease, medial temporal lobe dysfunction is most prominent, leading to memory difficulties, whereas in corticobasal syndrome, frontal and parietal dysfunction are common, thus leading to difficulties with executive function, visuospatial function, language, and praxis. Difficulties with calculations are common; caregivers report that patients are impaired at handling money. Neglect may also occur. Episodic memory is relatively preserved. Neuropsychological tests that show prominent impairment include reverse digit span, word fluency to letters and animals, Stroop test, Pyramid and Palm Trees test, and visuospatial constructions. One aspect of corticobasal syndrome that may help to distinguish it from frontotemporal dementia is that insight is sometimes preserved in corticobasal syndrome, leading to frequent depression.

LABORATORY STUDIES

There are no laboratory, genetic, or cerebrospinal fluid studies that are helpful in either confirming or ruling out corticobasal degeneration.

STRUCTURAL IMAGING STUDIES

Structural imaging of corticobasal degeneration typically shows asymmetric posterior frontal and parietal atrophy. A meta-analysis found that atrophy in premotor and supplementary-motor areas and the posterior midcingulate and fronto-median cortex can be specific for corticobasal syndrome and corticobasal degeneration (Albrecht et al., 2017). Another study found that atrophy in corticobasal degeneration was greater than that observed in Alzheimer's disease, dementia with Lewy bodies, frontotemporal dementia, and progressive supranuclear palsy (Whitwell et al., 2007). Fig. 13.2 shows the asymmetric cortical atrophy, right greater than left, of the patient presented in the beginning of the chapter.

FUNCTIONAL AND MOLECULAR IMAGING STUDIES

Functional imaging studies, such as single photon emission computed tomography (SPECT) or fluorodeoxyglucose positron emission tomography (FDG PET), can help to differentiate corticobasal syndromes from other clinical syndromes such as those associated with Alzheimer's disease and frontotemporal dementia. Typically, the patient with corticobasal syndrome will show marked asymmetry of motor and premotor blood

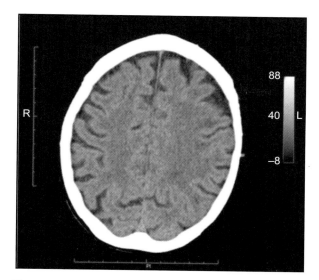

88

40 L

−8

R

Fig. 13.2 Structural imaging of corticobasal syndrome. Note the asymmetric atrophy, right greater than left, in this head computed tomography scan of a patient with corticobasal syndrome. (Note that the right side of the brain is on the left side of the image.)

flow and metabolism on SPECT and FDG PET imaging. There may also be asymmetric prefrontal, posterior parietal, lateral temporal, cingulate gyrus, basal ganglia, and thalamic hypometabolism. These studies may also give a clue as to the underlying pathology: parietal lobule and posterior cingulate hypometabolism suggests Alzheimer's disease, anterior cingulate and associated frontal cortex hypometabolism suggests frontotemporal lobar degeneration or progressive supranuclear palsy (Nobili et al., 2018). Amyloid PET scans (see Chapter 2) can be useful to evaluate for Alzheimer's pathology in patients with corticobasal syndrome. Several tau PET ligands, currently only available in research studies, have been found to detect tau in patients with corticobasal degeneration (Ali & Josephs, 2018). These tau PET scans may be clinically useful in the future.

DIFFERENTIAL DIAGNOSIS

It is worth stating that it is difficult to correctly diagnose this disorder. Autopsy studies have shown that, on average, only half of those patients premorbidly diagnosed with corticobasal degeneration meet pathological criteria for the disorder, and, conversely, only half of those patients with pathologically confirmed corticobasal degeneration were correctly diagnosed premorbidly. In a study published in 2007 only six of 15 pathologically proven cases were suspected of having corticobasal degeneration (Murray et al., 2007). The most common misdiagnoses were frontotemporal dementia, primary progressive aphasia, and progressive supranuclear palsy. Alzheimer's disease was less likely to be mistaken for corticobasal degeneration. A study of the new diagnostic criteria found that only 9/19 patients with pathologically confirmed corticobasal degeneration met criteria for probable corticobasal degeneration at presentation, rising to only 13/19 at the last clinical assessment. Moreover, all 14/14 patients with corticobasal syndrome without corticobasal degeneration pathology met clinical criteria for possible or probable corticobasal degeneration (Alexander et al., 2014).

The primary differential diagnosis when considering corticobasal degeneration includes frontotemporal dementia (see Chapter 10), primary progressive aphasia (see Chapter 9), progressive supranuclear palsy (see Chapter 12), and dementia with Lewy bodies (see Chapter 8). Other conditions to consider include Alzheimer's disease (see Chapter 4), vascular dementia (see Chapter 7), prion disease (see Chapter 16), spinocerebellar atrophy 8, progressive multifocal leukodystrophy, sudanophilic leukodystrophy (Pelizaeus–Merzbacher disease), neurosyphilis, familial idiopathic basal ganglia calcification, and Marchiafava–Bignami disease.

TREATMENTS

There are no U.S. Food and Drug Administration–approved treatments for corticobasal degeneration. Antidepressants should be used to treat depression, which is often present. Dystonia may be relieved with botulinum toxin. Clonazepam may be helpful for myoclonus, but will cause cognitive impairment. Physical and occupational therapy is important for range of motion in affected limbs so that contractures do not develop.

REFERENCES

Albrecht, F., Bisenius, S., Schaack, R. M., et al. (2017). Disentangling the neural correlates of corticobasal syndrome and corticobasal degeneration with systematic and quantitative ALE meta-analyses. *NPJ Parkinson's Disease*, *3*, 12.

Alexander, S. K., Rittman, T., Xuereb, J. H., et al. (2014). Validation of the new consensus criteria for the diagnosis of corticobasal degeneration. *Journal of Neurology, Neurosurgery, and Psychiatry, 85*(8), 923–927.

Ali, F., & Josephs, K. A. (2018). Corticobasal degeneration: Key emerging issues. *Journal of Neurology, 265*(2), 439–445.

Armstrong, M. J., Litvan, I., Lang, A. E., et al. (2013). Criteria for the diagnosis of corticobasal degeneration. *Neurology, 80*, 496–503.

Greene, P. (2019). Progressive supranuclear palsy, corticobasal degeneration, and multiple system atrophy. *Continuum (Minneapolis, Minn.), 25*(4), 919–935.

Murray, R., Neumann, M., Forman, M. S., et al. (2007). Cognitive and motor assessment in autopsy-proven corticobasal degeneration. *Neurology, 68*, 1274–1283.

Nobili, F., Arbizu, J., Bouwman, F., et al. (2018). European Association of Nuclear Medicine and European Academy of Neurology recommendations for the use of brain 18 F-fluorodeoxyglucose positron emission tomography in neurodegenerative cognitive impairment and dementia: Delphi consensus. *European Journal of Neurology, 25*(10), 1201–1217.

Whitwell, J. L., Jack, C. R., Jr., Parisi, J. E., et al. (2007). Rates of cerebral atrophy differ in different degenerative pathologies. *Brain, 130*, 1148–1158.

14

Normal Pressure Hydrocephalus

QUICK START: NORMAL PRESSURE HYDROCEPHALUS	
Definition	• Normal pressure hydrocephalus (often referred to as NPH) is a relatively rare disorder characterized by enlargement of the ventricles, a gait disorder, cognitive impairment, and incontinence. • It is thought to result from low-grade scarring or obstruction of the ventricular system or subarachnoid pathways.
Prevalence	• It is a relatively rare disorder, making up between 1% and 5% of patients referred to a memory clinic.
Cognitive and behavioral symptoms	• The most common cognitive and behavioral presentation is that of a frontal subcortical disturbance including apathy, abulia, poor attention, and slowing of processing.
Diagnostic criteria	• Normal pressure hydrocephalus should be suspected when the triad of symptoms of cognitive impairment, gait disorder, and urinary urge incontinence are present in the setting of enlarged ventricles. • The frontal gait disturbance in normal pressure hydrocephalus, also called a "magnetic gait" or "marche à petits pas" (walk of little steps), is typically the most prominent symptom and earliest in onset. • Although incontinence generally occurs late, urinary urgency and frequency may be early symptoms. • A CT or MRI scan showing enlargement of the ventricles, rounding of the ventricular contours, and a tight high convexity is essential to making the diagnosis. • Lumbar puncture to withdraw 30 mL of cerebral spinal fluid with pre- and post-lumbar puncture gait evaluations can help to determine both diagnosis and response to treatment.
Treatment	• A ventricular–peritoneal shunt provides the definitive treatment.
Top differential diagnoses	• Because many disorders can cause cognitive impairment, a gait disorder, and urinary incontinence, and virtually all dementias lead to dilatation of the ventricles, the differential diagnosis must be carefully considered.

A 76-year-old woman presented to the clinic with poor cognition over 6 to 12 months. She had poor memory and was easily distracted. After finding several bills unpaid, her daughter took over the management of her finances. She would also forget to take her pills if her daughter did not call to remind her twice each day. She used to walk for several miles each day but now she could only walk a block or two. Review of systems was remarkable for urinary urge incontinence. Her physical examination was notable for a frontal or "magnetic" gait disorder with stiff legs and short steps, brisk reflexes, as well as grasp and palmomental reflexes bilaterally. Her ability to pay attention was so impaired that she was frequently distracted during our interview and examination. Tests of attention and executive function were impaired. Memory was impaired secondarily because of poor attention. Her head computed tomography (CT) scan is shown in Fig. 14.2.

PREVALENCE, PROGNOSIS, AND DEFINITION

Normal pressure hydrocephalus is a relatively rare disorder characterized by enlargement of the ventricles, a gait disorder, incontinence, and cognitive impairment. Although some studies have suggested that up to 5% of patients with dementia have normal pressure hydrocephalus, other studies have found the prevalence to be closer to 1%, which is consistent with our experience of patients referred to a memory disorders clinic (for a review see Tanaka et al., 2009). It may, however, be underdiagnosed in the general population; one study showed that 5.9% of individuals 80 years and older met criteria for normal pressure hydrocephalus (Jaraj et al., 2014). In Norway, the overall prevalence was found to be 21.9 per 100,000 and the incidence was 5.5 per 100,000 (Graff-Radford & Jones, 2019). The Mayo Clinic Study of Aging found magnetic resonance imaging (MRI) scans consistent with normal pressure hydrocephalus in 5% of their study population (Graff-Radford et al., 2017).

CRITERIA

Normal pressure hydrocephalus should be suspected when the so-called "triad" of symptoms (cognitive impairment, gait disorder, and urinary incontinence) is present in the setting of enlarged ventricles. However, it cannot be stated strongly enough that many disorders can cause cognitive impairment, a gait disorder, and urinary incontinence, and virtually all neurodegenerative diseases lead to ex vacuo dilatation of ventricles (enlarged ventricles caused by loss of brain tissue), so the differential diagnosis of these symptoms and signs must be carefully considered. Frequently used criteria for diagnosing normal pressure hydrocephalus are shown in Box 14.1.

RISK FACTORS, PATHOLOGY, AND PATHOPHYSIOLOGY

Normal pressure hydrocephalus may result from low-grade scarring or obstruction of the ventricular system or subarachnoid pathways. Thus, although most cases are idiopathic, other causes include subarachnoid hemorrhage, head trauma, tumor, prior surgery, aqueductal stenosis, meningitis, and even lumbar puncture. The basic idea is that one of these etiologies causes enough scarring and/or obstruction to increase pressure and to damage the myelinated fibers surrounding the ventricles, but an equilibrium is reached such that the pressure is not raised enough to present as high-pressure hydrocephalus (Fig. 14.1). Periventricular frontal cortical-basal ganglia-thalamocortical circuitry is disrupted in normal pressure hydrocephalus, which may be related to the observed cognitive deficits (Townley et al., 2018).

COMMON SIGNS, SYMPTOMS, AND STAGES

The gait disturbance in normal pressure hydrocephalus is typically the most prominent symptom and is usually the earliest in onset. The gait disorder is of a frontal type, and has been described as a "magnetic gait" or a "marche à petits pas" (walk of little steps), and is somewhat different from shuffling. It is very unsteady. There are a number of different problems that can occur with a frontal gait, including a gait apraxia, spasticity, and unsteadiness. Patients may describe a loss of strength in their legs that may not be the result of weakness of any individual muscles. Some patients may complain of difficulty lifting their feet off the ground, feeling like their feet are stuck to the floor.

BOX 14.1 Criteria For Probable Normal Pressure Hydrocephalus

1. History must include:
   a. Insidious onset
   b. Age 40 years or older
   c. Duration of symptoms greater than three months
   d. No evidence of an antecedent event known to cause hydrocephalus
   e. Progression of symptoms over time
   f. No other neurological, psychiatric, or medical condition that can explain the presenting signs and symptoms
2. Brain imaging:
   a. (computed tomography [CT] or magnetic resonance imaging [MRI]) must show
      i. Ventricular enlargement not solely attributed to atrophy or congenital enlargement
      ii. No visible obstruction of cerebrospinal fluid flow
      iii. Callosal angle of 40 degrees or greater (rounding of the ventricular contours)
      iv. Evidence of periventricular trans-ependymal flow of cerebrospinal fluid
      v. Aqueductal or fourth ventricular flow void on MRI
   b. Supportive brain imaging (CT or MRI) findings include
      i. Prior brain imaging study showing smaller ventricular size
      ii. Radionuclide cisternogram showing delayed clearance of radiotracer
      iii. Cine MRI showing increased ventricular flow
      iv. SPECT-acetazolamide challenge showing decreased perfusion not altered by acetazolamide
3. Clinical findings of gait/balance disturbance plus either cognitive impairment or urinary symptoms or both:
   a. Gait disturbance that includes at least two of the following (not entirely attributable to other conditions)
      i. Decreased step height
      ii. Decreased step length
      iii. Decreased cadence (speed of walking)
      iv. Increased trunk sway during walking
      v. Widened standing base
      vi. Toes turned outward on walking
      vii. Spontaneous or provoked retropulsion
      viii. En bloc turning (needing 3+ steps for turning 180 degrees)
      ix. Impaired walking balance, tested by 2+ corrections needed for tandem gait of eight steps
   b. Cognitive impairment that includes at least two of the following (not entirely attributable to other conditions)
      i. Psychomotor slowing (increased latency of response)
      ii. Decreased fine motor speed
      iii. Decreased fine motor accuracy
      iv. Difficulty dividing or maintaining attention
      v. Impaired memory recall, especially for recent events
      vi. Executive dysfunction, including impairment in multistep procedures, working memory, abstractions, similarities, and insight
      vii. Behavioral or personality changes
   c. Urinary incontinence not entirely attributable to other conditions consisting of either
      i. Episodic urinary incontinence
      ii. Persistent urinary incontinence
      iii. Urinary and fecal incontinence
      Or any two of the following
      iv. Frequent perception of the need to void
      v. Urinary frequency
      vi. Nocturia greater than two times per night
4. Physiological
   a. Cerebrospinal fluid (CSF) opening pressure of 70–245 mm H_2O (5–18 mm Hg)

Modified from Relkin, N., Marmarou, A., Klinge, P., et al. (2005). Diagnosing idiopathic normal-pressure hydrocephalus. *Neurosurgery, 57*, S4–S16.

Cognitive impairment generally presents next. A number of cognitive disturbances can occur, but the most common presentation is that of a frontal subcortical disturbance. Normal pressure hydrocephalus puts pressure on, and ultimately damages, periventricular white matter tracts. Because most of the brain's white matter is involved in transferring information to or from the frontal lobes, patients with normal pressure hydrocephalus usually show signs and symptoms of frontal subcortical dysfunction. Attention is often severely affected. Most cognitive processes are slow, and some, such as memory, require additional trials to reach normal performance. Changes in behavior, including a slowing of thought and action that may progress to apathy and abulia, are often observed.

Although urinary urgency and frequency may be present early, frank incontinence generally occurs late in normal pressure hydrocephalus. Urge incontinence is usually seen, such that the patient only has a very short time between when he or she feels the need to empty

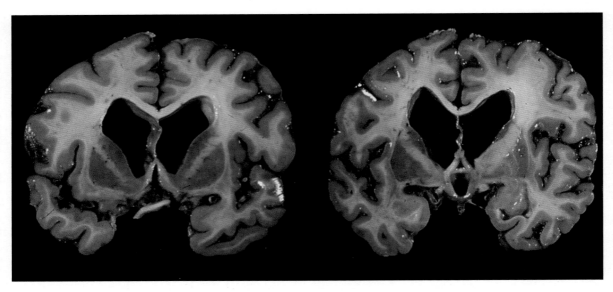

Fig. 14.1 Gross pathology of a patient with normal pressure hydrocephalus. Note the large ventricles but little hippocampal or cortical atrophy (compare with Fig. 4.5 see how it looks like the normal brain except for the enlarged ventricles).

their bladder and when it empties. Fecal incontinence may also be seen.

THINGS TO LOOK FOR IN THE HISTORY

The history will typically be that of a progressive gait disorder of the type described above, followed by changes in behavior and cognition including apathy, abulia, slowness, and poor attention. Patients are generally very easily distracted and may have difficulty focusing on tasks. Memory problems will typically be secondary to poor attention. Urinary urgency, frequency, or incontinence are the third major symptom.

THINGS TO LOOK FOR ON THE PHYSICAL AND NEUROLOGICAL EXAMINATION

Observation of the gait is the most important aspect of the neurological examination. As discussed above it will usually present as a frontal, unsteady, apraxic, and/or spastic gait. The deep tendon reflexes are generally increased, and an extensor plantar (Babinski's sign) may be present in one or both feet. Frontal release signs may also be present such as the snout,

grasp, and palmomental reflexes (see Chapter 2 for details). Hand tremors, poor fine-finger movements, and poor handwriting may also be seen. To distinguish normal pressure hydrocephalus from other disorders, efforts should also be made to look for signs of other disorders, such as Parkinson's disease and progressive supranuclear palsy (see Chapter 12).

PATTERN OF IMPAIRMENT ON COGNITIVE TESTS

Because of the disruption of frontal subcortical white matter tracts and cortical-basal ganglia-thalamocortical circuitry, normal pressure hydrocephalus causes impairment on a variety of cognitive tests. In general, the pattern is similar to that described for vascular dementia (see Chapter 7). Attention is invariably impaired. Working memory tasks, such as keeping information in mind and/or manipulating it, are also commonly impaired. Cognition tends to be generally slow. Word-finding difficulties are common, but true aphasia is not. Episodic memory performance shows a frontal pattern: encoding is often impaired, as is free recall, whereas recognition is relatively preserved. Visuospatial tasks may or may not be impaired.

STRUCTURAL IMAGING STUDIES

A structural imaging study supportive of a diagnosis of normal pressure hydrocephalus is essential in making the diagnosis (Fig. 14.2). The imaging study, either a CT or magnetic resonance imaging (MRI) scan, will invariably show enlargement of the ventricles and rounding of the ventricular contours, with the superior portion of the ventricles often looking like sausages on axial images—the shape an elastic tube assumes under pressure (see Fig. 14.2B). Periventricular abnormalities, particularly around the frontal horns, may be present because of transependymal flow of cerebrospinal fluid, that is, cerebrospinal fluid that has pushed into the white matter.

The Evans index should be measured by dividing the maximal ventricular width in the frontal horns by the largest distance between the inner tables of the skull measured on the same axial slice (see Fig. 14.2A). An Evans index of greater than 0.3 suggests that the ventricles are in the top fifth in size of individuals over 70 years of age.

Because normal pressure hydrocephalus is usually communicating hydrocephalus (meaning that there is no observable anatomical blockage of the ventricular system), the subarachnoid space around the brain is also increased in volume. Spinal fluid often collects in the sylvian and other major fissures in the brain, compressing adjacent sulci and leading to a tight high convexity. This characteristic pattern has been termed disproportionately enlarged subarachnoid space hydrocephalus (DESH) (Fig. 14.3). This pattern in general and the tight high convexity in particular should always be looked for as they are predictive of improvement after shunt placement (Graff-Radford & Jones, 2019; Narita et al., 2016). Do not confuse this pattern with cerebral atrophy!

LUMBAR PUNCTURE

After a structural imaging study, the most important test is a lumbar puncture. Measuring the opening pressure is important, as some patients with suspected normal pressure hydrocephalus will actually have high-pressure hydrocephalus.

The next step is to withdraw about 30 mL of cerebrospinal fluid and see if the gait improves. Have the patient walk approximately 30 feet, turn around, and return to the starting point. A number of trials should be undertaken both before and after the lumbar puncture until several reliable measurements are obtained for each, which can then be averaged. A video recording of

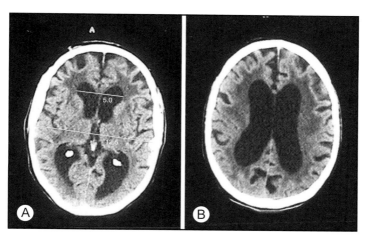

Fig. 14.2 Computed tomography scan from a patient with normal pressure hydrocephalus. In this example there is some cortical atrophy, but note the overly large, "ballooned-out" expansion of the ventricular system in both slices. Note also the trans-ependymal cerebrospinal fluid that appears hypodense anterior to the frontal horns of the lateral ventricles **(A)** and surrounding the ventricles **(B)**. This patient improved dramatically after a diagnostic lumbar puncture, and subsequently received a ventricular–peritoneal shunt. Maximal ventricular width in the frontal horns (5.0 cm) divided by the largest distance between the inner tables of the skull (12.5 cm) yielded an Evans index of 0.40 (see text for details).

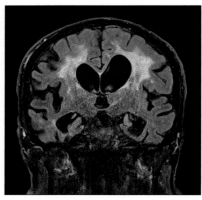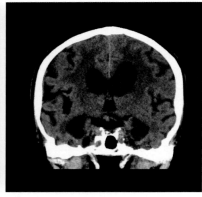

Fig. 14.3 Disproportionately enlarged subarachnoid space hydrocephalus (DESH). Coronal slices of magnetic resonance imaging (MRI) *(left)* and computed tomography (CT) *(right)* scans in the same patient with normal pressure hydrocephalus showing the high tight convexity and enlarged sylvian fissures caused by DESH. The majority of the MRI T2 hyperintensity and CT hypodensity is due to transependymal cerebrospinal fluid. Note that we find it somewhat easier to diagnose normal pressure hydrocephalus on CT than MRI scans.

the gait pre- and postlumbar puncture provides both a record of the timing and also a valuable way to evaluate other aspects of gait, such as stride length, apraxia, and the number of steps needed to turn. If the gait improves after a single large-volume lumbar puncture, the diagnosis is confirmed, and, more importantly, the patient will likely respond to treatment by shunting (see Treatments later). If there is no definite response from a single large-volume lumbar puncture, additional large-volume lumbar punctures can be performed on two successive days. Improvement of gait after three successive days of lumbar punctures also predicts a good response to shunting.

Note that if some of the cerebrospinal fluid drawn off is sent for measurements of Aβ, total tau, and phospho tau, the results may be difficult to interpret. Studies have found both low Aβ and tau in normal pressure hydrocephalus (Graff-Radford & Jones, 2019). The reason for these decreases is unknown but they resolve after shunting. Thus cerebrospinal fluid Aβ may be low in both Alzheimer's disease and normal pressure hydrocephalus. Elevated tau would suggest a neurodegenerative disease.

OTHER STUDIES

If the lumbar puncture is nondiagnostic, a number of other tests can be used to work toward confirming the diagnosis and predicting response to treatment, although none are particularly reliable. MRI has been used to measure the flow of cerebrospinal fluid through

the sylvian aqueduct; increased flow has been reported in those who ultimately had a good response to shunting. Continuous pressure monitoring for 24 to 48 hours can be performed using a frontal ventricular catheter, lumbar catheter, or epidural transducer; elevated baseline cerebrospinal fluid pressure or pressure waves also suggest a good response to shunting. Improvement in gait with a lumbar drain also predicts a good response to shunting. Cisternography (in which an intrathecal injection of either a radioactive isotope or contrast material is performed and the flow pattern of cerebrospinal fluid is observed) is less frequently performed.

DIFFERENTIAL DIAGNOSIS AND COMORBID DISORDERS

The differential diagnosis of normal pressure hydrocephalus is quite broad. Any disorder that damages the periventricular frontal subcortical white matter tracts can lead to the clinical triad of gait disorder, cognitive impairment, and urinary incontinence. Vascular dementia (see Chapter 7) and multiple sclerosis should always be considered, as these disorders frequently damage these periventricular frontal subcortical white matter tracts. Lyme disease (see Chapter 17) can also damage this region of the brain. Other disorders that should be considered include disorders that affect gait and cognition, such as Parkinson's disease, dementia with Lewy bodies (see Chapter 8), progressive supranuclear palsy (see Chapter 12), and corticobasal degeneration (see Chapter 13). Behavioral variant frontotemporal dementia (see Chapter 10) (with or without motor neuron disease/amyotrophic lateral sclerosis) and Huntington's disease should also be considered. Alzheimer's disease (see Chapter 4) must be considered; because it is so common unusual presentations may occur. Any cause of preexisting enlarged ventricles (e.g., from congenital hydrocephalus, cerebral palsy, traumatic brain injury) plus a degenerative disease, such as Alzheimer's, can mimic normal pressure hydrocephalus. Other causes of hydrocephalus, such as carcinomatous meningitis, should be considered. Lastly, it should be noted that approximately 30% of patients with normal pressure hydrocephalus also have Alzheimer's disease simply because of the prevalence of Alzheimer's in an elderly population.

TREATMENTS

The treatment for normal pressure hydrocephalus is a shunt to help remove excess cerebrospinal fluid from the ventricular system. The most common type shunts fluid from the lateral ventricle (usually on the right to avoid language centers on the left) to the peritoneum. The typical approach is either right frontal or right parieto-occipital. A meta-analysis found that of patients shunted for normal pressure hydrocephalus 82% were improved at one year and 73% were improved at three or more years. The most common complications were subdural hematomas (4.5%) and infection (3.5%); a total of 13% required shunt revision (Graff-Radford & Jones, 2019). For patients with normal pressure hydrocephalus without Alzheimer's or other comorbid disease, gait, continence, and cognition may all improve with shunting (Peterson et al., 2016).

Many studies have been performed in an attempt to determine whether patients with both normal pressure hydrocephalus and Alzheimer's disease should be shunted. Our reading of this literature is that whereas the chances of improvement in gait and continence are the same for patients with normal pressure hydrocephalus with and without Alzheimer's disease, those with concomitant Alzheimer's disease are unlikely to show improvement in cognition (Hiraoka et al., 2015; Kazui et al., 2016).

In addition, whereas shunted patients with normal pressure hydrocephalus alone may be stable for some time, shunted patients with Alzheimer's disease will, of course, show cognitive decline. Each patient and family will need to come to their own decision as to whether a shunt makes sense in this situation. Often it depends upon how severe the Alzheimer's disease is. A patient with mild cognitive impairment due to Alzheimer's disease plus normal pressure hydrocephalus may do well for many years following a shunt, whereas a patient with Alzheimer's disease in the moderate dementia stage will likely soon become incontinent from the Alzheimer's even if the shunt is successful in treating the normal pressure hydrocephalus.

REFERENCES

Graff-Radford, N., Gunter, J., Thomas, C., et al. (2017). Ventriculomegaly is a biomarker of gait and cognitive decline. *Alzheimer's & Dementia: The Journal of the Alzheimer's Association, 13*(7 suppl), 1092.

Graff-Radford, N. R., & Jones, D. T. (2019). Normal pressure hydrocephalus. *Continuum (Minneapolis, Minn.), 25*(1), 165–186.

Hiraoka, K., Narita, W., Kikuchi, H., et al. (2015). Amyloid deposits and response to shunt surgery in idiopathic normal-pressure hydrocephalus. *Journal of the Neurological Sciences, 356*(1–2), 124–128.

Jaraj, D., Rabiei, K., Marlow, T., et al. (2014). Prevalence of idiopathic normal-pressure hydrocephalus. *Neurology, 82*, 1449–1454.

Kazui, H., Kanemoto, H., Yoshiyama, K., et al. (2016). Association between high biomarker probability of Alzheimer's disease and improvement of clinical outcomes after shunt surgery in patients with idiopathic normal pressure hydrocephalus. *Journal of the Neurological Sciences, 369*, 236–241.

Narita, W., Nishio, Y., Baba, T., et al. (2016). High-convexity tightness predicts the shunt response in idiopathic normal pressure hydrocephalus. *American Journal of Neuroradiology, 347*(10), 1831–1837.

Peterson, K. A., Savulich, G., Jackson, D., et al. (2016). The effect of shunt surgery on neuropsychological performance in normal pressure hydrocephalus: A systematic review and meta-analysis. *Journal of Neurology, 263*(8), 1669–1677.

Tanaka, N., Yamaguchi, S., Ishikawa, H., et al. (2009). Prevalence of possible idiopathic normal-pressure hydrocephalus in Japan: The Osaki-Tajiri project. *Neuroepidemiology, 32*, 171–175.

Townley, R. A., Botha, H., Graff-Radford, J., et al. (2018). 18F-FDG PET-CT pattern in idiopathic normal pressure hydrocephalus. *NeuroImage: Clinical, 18*, 897–902.

15

Chronic Traumatic Encephalopathy

Definition and etiology	• Chronic traumatic encephalopathy is a progressive neurodegenerative disease associated with repetitive brain trauma. Pathology includes perivascular tau deposition.
Cognitive and behavioral symptoms, in order of prevalence at presentation	• Memory impairment • Executive dysfunction • Attention and concentration difficulties • Sadness/depression • Hopelessness • Explosivity • Language impairment • Visuospatial difficulties • "Out of control" • Physically violent • Verbally violent • Impulse control problems • Suicidal ideation/attempts

Summary of diagnostic criteria	**Primary Criteria for the National Institute of Neurological Disorders and Stroke Consensus Diagnostic Criteria for Traumatic Encephalopathy Syndrome**: Components I, II, and III are required. Component IV grades the level of function.
	
	I. Substantial Exposure to Repetitive Head Impacts including:
	   • Involvement in 'high exposure' contact or collision sports for at least 5 years
	   • Military service involving repetitive head impacts
	   • Other sources involving multiple head impacts over an extended time
	II. Cognitive Impairment or Neurobehavioral Dysregulation or both, plus a progressive course over at least 1 year
	III. Not Fully Accounted for by Other Disorders
	IV. Level of Functional Dependence/Dementia
	   • Independent
	   • Subtle/Mild Functional Limitation
	   • Mild Dementia
	   • Moderate Dementia
	   • Severe Dementia

(Continued)

QUICK START: CHRONIC TRAUMATIC ENCEPHALOPATHY (*Continued*)

Imaging findings	• Cavum septum pellucidum is commonly seen on MRI or CT. Patchy atrophy and hypofunction are typically observed in medial temporal and in frontal lobes.
Treatment	• Treatment is supportive. Cholinesterase inhibitors, memantine, and selective serotonin reuptake inhibitors can be tried.
Top differential diagnoses	• Alzheimer's disease, dementia with Lewy bodies, frontotemporal dementia, vascular dementia, progressive supranuclear palsy, corticobasal degeneration, and normal pressure hydrocephalus.

A 63-year-old man presented with progressive memory, concentration, mood, and behavior problems over several years. He was a veteran of the army for six years in his twenties, and reported being "knocked out" or "dazed" more than a dozen times while in combat. In the army he also boxed competitively for several years and frequently had his "bell rung," although he reported only being knocked unconscious five times. After the army he married and owned a successful small business. For the past 4 to 5 years his wife noted that he became increasingly withdrawn and moody. After making several poor financial decisions he closed down his business. In the last three years he began very uncharacteristic behaviors including yelling and "flying off the handle" over minor issues. His primary care physician referred him to a psychiatrist who prescribed fluoxetine, which improved his mood and anger. Two years ago, his mood and anger worsened, and increasing doses of fluoxetine and other selective serotonin reuptake inhibitors (SSRIs) could not control the symptoms; after an episode of physical aggression toward his wife risperidone was prescribed. In the past year he had clear-cut impairment of his concentration, memory, and function. His wife notes that he now has "no short-term memory" and that he "does nothing" all day long. Neurological examination revealed mild bilateral 3–4 Hz tremor present at rest and with action. He scored 15 on the Montreal Cognitive Assessment (MoCA), making errors on the visuospatial/executive, attention, delayed recall, and orientation sections. Head computed tomography (CT) scan revealed atrophy (most notably in hippocampi and frontal lobes, bilaterally) and a cavum septum pellucidum.

PREVALENCE, DEFINITION, PATHOLOGY, AND PATHOPHYSIOLOGY

There is increasing evidence that head trauma may be associated with encephalopathy and dementia later in life. The exact pathogenesis of how head trauma at one point in life can cause dementia decades later is complex and is still being determined. We do know that, in addition to causing an encephalopathy that is maximal at the time of the head injury and generally improves (though not necessarily back to baseline), repetitive head injury has been associated with chronic traumatic encephalopathy, a progressive tauopathy with distinctive clinical and pathological features (McKee et al., 2013) (see Table 15.1 and Fig. 15.1).

In one series McKee and colleagues analyzed the brains of 85 individuals with a history of repetitive mild traumatic brain injury and found evidence of chronic traumatic encephalopathy (CTE) in 68 (80%) of them, including 64 athletes, 21 military veterans (most of whom were also athletes), and one individual with self-injurious head-banging behavior. The athletes included those who played football, hockey, boxing, rugby, soccer, and wrestling; the veterans included those who fought in World War II, Vietnam, Gulf War, Iraq, and Afghanistan (McKee et al., 2013). Another series showed that multiple pathologies are common; of 177 football players who came to autopsy, 55% had pure chronic traumatic encephalopathy and 45% had additional pathologies, the most common being Lewy body disease (19%) (Fig. 15.2) (Mez et al., 2017; Turk & Budson, 2019). CTE has also been observed in individuals who regularly engaged in bull riding and mixed martial arts. Because of the selection bias of cases referred to autopsy, the exact prevalence of chronic traumatic encephalopathy in athletes,

TABLE 15.1   Pathologic and Clinical Stages of Chronic Traumatic Encephalopathy

Stage	Pathology	Clinical Symptoms and Signs
I	Perivascular phospho-tau neurofibrillary tangles in focal epicenters at the depths of the sulci in frontal cortex	Headache, loss of attention and concentration
II	Stage I plus neurofibrillary tangles in superficial cortical layers adjacent to the focal epicenters and in the nucleus basalis of Meynert and locus coeruleus	Depression and mood swings, explosivity, loss of attention and concentration, headache, and short-term memory loss
III	Stage II plus mild cerebral atrophy, septal abnormalities, ventricular dilatation, concave third ventricle, depigmentation of locus coeruleus and substantia nigra, dense phospho-tau pathology in the cortex, medial temporal lobe, diencephalon, brainstem, and spinal cord	Cognitive impairment with memory loss, executive dysfunction, loss of attention and concentration, depression, explosivity, and visuospatial abnormalities
IV	Stage III plus further cerebral, medial temporal lobe, hypothalamic, thalamic, and mammillary body atrophy, septal abnormalities, ventricular dilatation, and pallor of substantia nigra and locus coeruleus; phospho-tau in widespread regions including white matter, with prominent neuronal loss, gliosis of cortex, and hippocampal sclerosis	Dementia with profound short-term memory loss, executive dysfunction, attention and concentration loss, explosivity, and aggression. Most also show paranoia, depression, impulsivity, and visuospatial abnormalities. Many also have parkinsonism, speech, and gait abnormalities

From McKee, A. C., Stern, R. A., Stein, T. D., et al. (2013). The spectrum of disease in chronic traumatic encephalopathy. *Brain*, 136, 43–64.

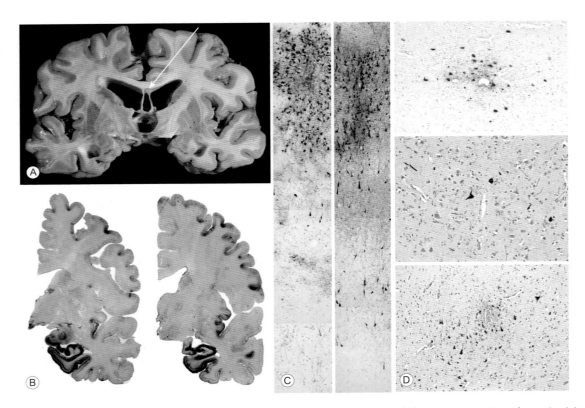

Fig. 15.1 Pathology of chronic traumatic encephalopathy. Gross pathology **(A)** shows atrophy of cerebral hemispheres, medial temporal lobes, ventricular dilatation, and a fenestrated cavum septum pellucidum *(arrow)*. Whole-mount 50-mm-thick coronal sections show dense deposition of tau protein in medial temporal lobe structures, with less dense deposition elsewhere in the cortex in two cases **(B)**. Microscopic views of the same two cases showing prominent perivascular collections of neurofibrillary and astrocytic tangles evident in the superficial cortical layers with lesser involvement of the deep laminae **(C)**. Note that this pathology is different from that of Alzheimer's disease (see Chapter 4). Perivascular deposition of tau pathology is pathognomonic for chronic traumatic encephalopathy **(D)**.

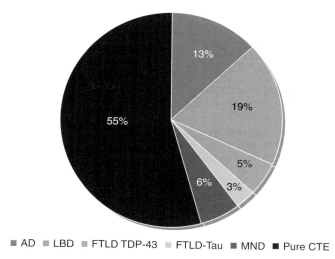

■ AD   ■ LBD   ▨ FTLD TDP-43   ▨ FTLD-Tau   ■ MND   ■ Pure CTE

Fig. 15.2 Neuropathologic diagnoses among a cohort of 177 football players from the Veterans Affairs-Boston University-Concussion Legacy Foundation brain bank who were diagnosed with chronic traumatic encephalopathy (CTE), Alzheimer's disease *(AD)*, Lewy body disease *(LBD)*, frontotemporal lobar degeneration from TDP-43 *(FTLD TDP-43)*, frontotemporal lobar degeneration from tau *(FTLD-Tau)*, and motor neuron disease *(MND)* by autopsy. Some 55% exhibited pure CTE pathology, and the remaining cases exhibited overlap with other neurodegenerative conditions, including Alzheimer's disease, Lewy body disease, frontotemporal lobar degeneration with transactive response DNA binding protein 43, frontotemporal lobar degeneration with tau pathology (FTLD-Tau), and motor neuron disease. (Modified from Turk, K. W., & Budson, A. E. (2019). Chronic traumatic encephalopathy. *Continuum (Minneapolis, Minn.), 25*(1), 187–207 using data from Mez, J., Daneshvar, D. H., Kiernan, P. T., et al. (2017). Clinicopathological evaluation of chronic traumatic encephalopathy in players of American football. *JAMA, 318*(4), 360–370.)

veterans, and the general population is unknown. Three studies of American professional football players, each with more than 1000 subjects, have found the risk of all types of neurodegenerative disease between three and five times greater than that of the general United States population (Lehman, 2013).

CRITERIA

Katz and colleagues have developed research criteria for traumatic encephalopathy syndrome (Katz et al., 2021). See the Quick Start for a summary of the primary criteria and Box 15.1 for an abbreviated version of the primary criteria.

COMMON SIGNS, SYMPTOMS, AND STAGES

McKee et al. (2013) have defined four pathological stages of chronic traumatic encephalopathy and the common symptoms and signs associated with each (Table 15.1). There has also been the recognition that there are two common

clinical presentations of chronic traumatic encephalopathy (Box 15.1; Katz et al., 2021; Stern et al., 2013):
- A behavioral/mood variant whose initial features develop at a younger age with behavioral and/or mood disturbance, and
- A cognitive variant whose initial features develop at an older age and involve more cognitive impairment.

THINGS TO LOOK FOR IN THE HISTORY

There are two main things to look for in the history of a patient who may have chronic traumatic encephalopathy. The first is a history of repetitive head trauma of some type, such as contact sports, military service, domestic abuse, head banging, motor vehicle accidents, etc. Note that a history of clinical concussion (also referred to as mild traumatic brain injury) is not necessary to develop chronic traumatic encephalopathy, as asymptomatic subconcussive impacts are associated with CTE pathology (Tagge et al., 2018; Turk & Budson, 2019). The second is the constellation of behavioral, mood, cognitive, and sometimes motor features that are common

BOX 15.1 Primary Criteria for the National Institute of Neurological Disorders and Stroke Consensus Diagnostic Criteria for Traumatic Encephalopathy Syndrome

Components I, II, and III are required. Component IV grades the level of function.

I. Substantial Exposure to Repetitive Head Impacts
Impacts may or may not have been associated with concussion or traumatic brain injury (TBI). Examples include:
- **Involvement in 'high exposure' contact or collision sports** such as boxing, American football, ice hockey, soccer, rugby, professional wrestling, mixed martial arts, as well as others.
  - For American football, minimum of 5 years organized play is required, including 2 or more years at the high school level or beyond.
  - Exposure risk thresholds for other contact or collision sports should involve a substantial number of years, such as 5 or more.
- **Military service** involving repetitive head impacts, including combat exposure to multiple blast and other explosions, non-combat exposure to explosions (including blasting and forced opening of lock doors), or multiple blows to the head over an extended period of time (such as repeated blows with a padded military training weapon).
- **Other sources** involving multiple head impacts over an extended time including domestic/intimate partner violence, head banging, and vocational activities such as breaching locked doors and other barriers by first responders.

II. Cognitive Impairment or Neurobehavioral Dysregulation or both, plus a progressive course
- **Cognitive Impairment** (all 4 are required)
  - As reported by self or informant, or by clinician's report.
  - Representing a significant decline from baseline functioning.
  - With deficits in episodic memory and/or executive functioning (+/- additional domains).
  - Substantiated by impaired performance:
    - At least 1.5 standard deviations below appropriate norms on formal neuropsychological testing.
    - If formal neuropsychological testing is not available, substantial evidence of impairment below a person's estimated baseline in episodic memory and/or executive functioning on a standardized mental status examination (e.g., Montreal Cognitive Assessment [MoCA], Mini-Mental State Examination [MMSE]) by a clinician experienced in the evaluation of cognition.
- **Neurobehavioral Dysregulation** (all 3 are required)
  - As reported by self or informant, or by clinician's report.

- Representing a significant change from baseline functioning.
- With symptoms and/or observed behaviors representing poor regulation or control of emotions and/or behavior, including explosiveness, impulsivity, rage, violent outbursts, "short fuse," or emotional lability.
  - Preferably substantiated by standardized measures.
  - Not from a transient response to life events, e.g., divorce, death of loved one, financial problems.
- **Progressive Course**
  - Progressive worsening of these clinical features over at least 1 year in the absence of continued repetitive head impacts or TBI. Supported by:
    - Serial standardized testing (if available), or
    - Clear history supporting a change in functioning over time (e.g., clinician reports, job performance evaluations, or self- or informant-report).

III. Not Fully Accounted for by Other Disorders
- **The pattern of the cognitive deficits** is not fully accounted for by other pre-existing, established, or acquired non-degenerative nervous system, medical, or psychiatric disorders and conditions.
- **The Core Clinical Feature of Neurobehavioral Dysregulation**, if present, is not fully accounted for by other pre-existing, established, or acquired non-degenerative nervous system, medical, or psychiatric disorders and conditions.
- **Comorbid diagnosis of another neurodegenerative disease** does not exclude a TES diagnosis.
  - However, TES may be excluded if the clinical features and any available biomarkers are fully accounted for by another neurodegenerative disorder.
- **Comorbid diagnosis of substance use disorder, posttraumatic stress disorder (PTSD), mood or anxiety disorders**, or a combination of these, can be present and do not exclude a TES diagnosis, unless they are determined to account for all Core Clinical Features.

IV. Level of Functional Dependence/Dementia
The level of functional dependence should be based on the impact of Cognitive Impairment and/or Neurobehavioral Dysregulation and not on physical limitations or medical illness.
- **Independent**. Independent at usual level in job, household responsibilities, or family, social, and community roles. Able to engage in hobbies and intellectual activities at usual levels; fully independent instrumental and basic activities of daily living (ADLs, see *Box 2.2*).

- **Subtle/Mild Functional Limitation**. Slightly reduced performance in job, household responsibilities, or family, social and community roles; slight problems in hobbies and intellectual interests reported; mostly independent but may be more challenged in some instrumental ADLs and fully independent in basic ADLs.
- **Mild Dementia**. Definite impairment of instrumental ADLs; may be engaged in some home, family, social, and community activities; more difficult activities abandoned; needs *cues* for some basic ADLs.
- **Moderate Dementia**. Not independent but can be taken to some functions outside the home; only simple chores preserved; very restricted interests; needs *assistance* with basic ADLs.
- **Severe Dementia**. Cannot participate in functions outside the home; no significant function in home; impaired basic ADLs; not independent with self-care; frequently incontinent.

Modified from Katz, D. I., Bernick, C., Dodick, D. W., et al. (2021). National Institute of Neurological Disorders and Stroke Consensus Diagnostic Criteria for Traumatic Encephalopathy Syndrome. *Neurology*, 10.1212/WNL.0000000000011850. Please see Katz et al. for full research criteria.

with the disorder. See Box 15.1 for additional details. See Box 15.2 for some of the features that are most common at presentation.

THINGS TO LOOK FOR ON THE PHYSICAL AND NEUROLOGICAL EXAMINATION

The physical and neurological examination in most patients with chronic traumatic encephalopathy will be normal. Patients who have concomitant Lewy body pathology, however, show signs and symptoms of parkinsonism including tremor, abnormal gait, and falls. Other patients can show frontal signs and symptoms indistinguishable from a frontotemporal dementia (Video 15.1).

PATTERN OF IMPAIRMENT ON COGNITIVE TESTS

Following the cognitive domains commonly affected (Box 15.2), tests that most often show abnormalities in patients with chronic traumatic encephalopathy include those for memory, executive function, and simple and complex attention, followed by language and visuospatial function.

STRUCTURAL AND FUNCTIONAL IMAGING STUDIES

There are two types of imaging abnormalities to look for in patients who may have chronic traumatic encephalopathy. The first are abnormally enlarged cavum septum pellucidum and/or cavum vergae; these are anterior and posterior, respectively, fluid-filled spaces between the

> ### BOX 15.2   Specific Clinical Features Present at Initial Clinical Presentation
>
> - Memory impairment (85%)
> - Executive dysfunction (79%)
> - Attention and concentration difficulties (73%)
> - Sadness/depression (64%)
> - Hopelessness (64%)
> - Explosivity (58%)
> - Language impairment (58%)
> - Visuospatial difficulties (55%)
> - "Out of control" (52%)
> - Physically violent (52%)
> - Verbally violent (49%)
> - Impulse control problems (46%)
> - Suicidal ideation/attempts (30%)
> - Motor symptoms (parkinsonism, tremor, gait abnormalities, falls) (30%)
>
> Note: "%" indicates the percentage of individuals with autopsy proven chronic traumatic encephalopathy who had each feature at presentation.
> From Stern, R. A., Daneshvar, D. H., Baugh, C. M., et al. (2013). Clinical presentation of chronic traumatic encephalopathy. *Neurology, 81*, 1122–1129.

leaflets of the septum pellucidum (see Figs. 15.1 and 15.3 for examples of cavum septum pellucidum). Although these spaces may be present in up to 15% of healthy individuals, the theory is that during head trauma fluid waves produce fenestrations or holes in the septum pellucidum, allowing fluid to enter between the leaflets, creating the cavum septum pellucidum and/or cavum vergae. Thus the cavum suggests the possibility of repetitive head trauma, not chronic traumatic encephalopathy directly. The second type of abnormality to look for on imaging studies is atrophy (on magnetic resonance

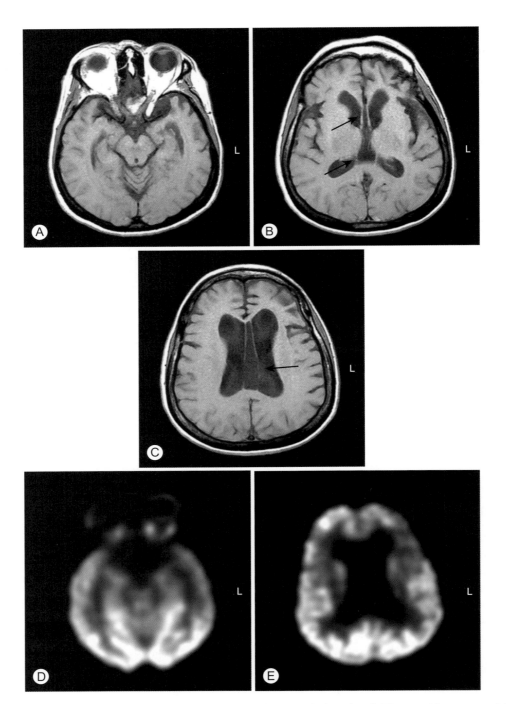

Fig. 15.3 Imaging studies of a patient with chronic traumatic encephalopathy. A 59-year-old woman with a history of multiple episodes of mild traumatic brain injury from domestic abuse starting in late childhood. Axial T1-magnetic resonance imaging slices showing **(A)** bilateral medial temporal and left > right anterior temporal lobe atrophy; **(B)** cavum septum pellucidum *(upper arrow)* and cavum vergae *(lower arrow)* as well as left > right frontal and temporal lobe atrophy; and **(C)** cavum septum pellucidum and cavum vergae with multiple fenestrations at the level of the arrow, as well as left > right frontal lobe atrophy. A fluorodeoxyglucose positron emission tomography scan shows **(D)** left > right medial and anterior temporal lobe hypometabolism, and **(E)** patchy left > right frontal hypometabolism. (Note that left side of brain is right side of image.)

imaging [MRI] or CT scans), hypometabolism (on fluorodeoxyglucose positron emission tomography [FDG PET) scans), and/or hypoperfusion (on technetium-99 [⁹⁹Tc] single photon emission computed tomography [SPECT] scans) of the cortex, particularly in medial temporal and frontal lobes (Fig. 15.3). Abnormalities in the frontal lobes are frequently patchy, mirroring the pathology.

DIFFERENTIAL DIAGNOSIS

Head trauma does not always cause chronic traumatic encephalopathy. McKee et al. (2013) found that of the 85 individuals studied with a history of repetitive mild traumatic brain injury, 17 (20%) did not show changes of chronic traumatic encephalopathy. Epidemiological studies have suggested that head trauma is a risk factor for other causes of dementia—especially Alzheimer's disease—as well as amyotrophic lateral sclerosis and Parkinson's disease.

Depending upon the specific signs and symptoms the patient is presenting with, other disorders to think about when considering chronic traumatic encephalopathy include Alzheimer's disease (see Chapter 4), dementia with Lewy bodies (see Chapter 8), and behavioral variant frontotemporal dementia (see Chapter 10), as well as disorders that can cause executive dysfunction and/or parkinsonism, such as vascular dementia (see Chapter 7), progressive supranuclear palsy (see Chapter 12), corticobasal degeneration (see Chapter 13), and normal-pressure hydrocephalus (see Chapter 14).

TREATMENTS

Treatment is supportive. There are no U.S. Food and Drug Administration–approved medications to treat chronic traumatic encephalopathy. Cholinesterase inhibitors (see Chapter 19) can be tried for those with memory problems. SSRIs (see Chapter 27) can be tried to help with behavior and mood symptoms. Memantine (Namenda) (see Chapter 20) can be tried to improve attention in patients who are in the moderate to severe stage of dementia. Treatment with atypical antipsychotic medications may be tried in those who are explosive and physically violent (see Chapter 27 for more information, including important warnings regarding the use of these medications).

REFERENCES

Katz, D. I., & Bernick, C., Dodick, D. W., et al. (2021). National Institute of Neurological Disorders and Stroke Consensus Diagnostic Criteria for Traumatic Encephalopathy Syndrome. *Neurology*, 10.1212/WNL.0000000000011850.

Lehman. E. J. (2013). Epidemiology of neurodegeneration in American-style professional football players. *Alzheimer's Research & Therapy, 5*, 34.

McKee, A. C., Stern, R. A., Stein, T. D., et al. (2013). The spectrum of disease in chronic traumatic encephalopathy. *Brain, 136*, 43–64.

Mez, J., Daneshvar, D. H., Kiernan, P. T., et al. (2017). Clinicopathological evaluation of chronic traumatic encephalopathy in players of American football. *The Journal of the American Medical Association, 318*(4), 360–370.

Stern, R. A., Daneshvar, D. H., Baugh, C. M., et al. (2013). Clinical presentation of chronic traumatic encephalopathy. *Neurology, 81*, 1122–1129.

Tagge, C. A., Fisher, A. M., Minaeva, O. V., et al. (2018). Concussion, microvascular injury, and early tauopathy in young athletes after impact head injury and an impact concussion mouse model. *Brain, 141*(2), 422–458.

Turk, K. W., & Budson, A. E. (2019). Chronic traumatic encephalopathy. *Continuum (Minneapolis, Minn.), 25*(1), 187–207.

Additional video for this topic are available online at expertconsult.com.

16

Creutzfeldt–Jakob Disease

QUICK START: CREUTZFELDT–JAKOB DISEASE	
Definition	• Creutzfeldt–Jakob disease (CJD) is one of several prion transmissible neurodegenerative diseases characterized by a rapid cognitive decline that can progress to akinetic mutism over weeks.
	• Creutzfeldt–Jakob disease is the most common type of prion disease; prion diseases are also called transmissible spongiform encephalopathies.
	• Prion diseases have a specific neuropathology characterized by spongiform changes, neuronal death, astrocytosis, and accumulation of a pathological protein (PrP^{Sc}) in the brain and sometimes other organs.
	• Other forms of Creutzfeldt–Jakob disease include genetic and acquired. Acquired forms include iatrogenic and variant.
	• Variant Creutzfeldt–Jakob disease is similar biochemically and histopathologically to bovine spongiform encephalopathy (aka "mad cow disease").
Prevalence	• Sporadic Creutzfeldt–Jakob disease has an incidence of approximately 1 to 2 per million.
	• The usual age of onset of sporadic Creutzfeldt–Jakob disease is from 55 to 75 years; variant Creutzfeldt–Jakob disease often presents in younger individuals.
Genetic and transmission risk	• Prion diseases are transmissible, meaning an inoculation with the pathological protein can cause the disease in another individual.
	• There are a number of mutations of the gene PRNP (located on the short arm of chromosome 20), which codes for the pathological protein (PrP^{Sc}), leading to familial, autosomal dominant Creutzfeldt–Jakob disease, Gerstmann–Sträussler–Scheinker syndrome, and fatal familial insomnia.
Cognitive, behavioral, and other symptoms	• Cognitive and behavioral changes include impairment of memory and executive function, as well as depression and sometimes personality changes.
	• Cerebellar signs and myoclonus are frequent, and can worsen over a period of days.

(Continued)

QUICK START: VASCULAR COGNITIVE IMPAIRMENT AND VASCULAR DEMENTIA (*Continued*)

Diagnostic criteria	1. Rapid cognitive decline
	2. Two of the following six signs/symptoms:
	  • Myoclonus
	  • Pyramidal/extrapyramidal dysfunction
	  • Visual dysfunction
	  • Cerebellar dysfunction
	  • Akinetic mutism
	  • Focal cortical signs (e.g., neglect, aphasia, acalculia, apraxia)
	3. Typical electroencephalogram and/or magnetic resonance imaging (MRI)
	  • MRI shows diffusion-weighted imaging (DWI) brighter than fluid-attenuated inversion recovery (FLAIR) hyperintensity in the cingulate, striatum, and/or greater than one neocortical gyrus, ideally with sparing of the precentral gyrus and apparent diffusion coefficient map supporting restricted diffusion
	4. Other investigations should not suggest an alternative diagnosis

Treatment	• Treatment for Creutzfeldt–Jakob disease is supportive.

Top differential diagnoses	• Slow progression: common degenerative diseases
	  • Dementia with Lewy bodies
	  • Frontotemporal dementia
	  • Corticobasal degeneration
	  • Progressive supranuclear palsy
	  • Alzheimer's disease (particularly when associated with cerebral amyloid angiopathy)
	• Rapidly progressing dementias
	  • Cerebrovascular disease
	  • Vasculitis
	  • Autoimmune encephalopathies
	  • Collagen vascular and granulomatous disease
	  • Infectious disease
	  • Malignancies
	  • Paraneoplastic disorders
	  • Toxic and metabolic disorders
	  • Psychiatric disorders

A 68-year-old man presented to our clinic for evaluation of a 5-month history of memory problems. Memory loss, feeling "funny," and loss of appetite were initial symptoms. At the first visit the daughter reported that the problems appeared to be accelerating, and were much worse over the last two weeks. He now had difficulty getting dressed, using the toilet, and finding his way around his own house. He had emotional lability and paranoia. He complained of blurry vision and was noted to be very drowsy at times.

His neurologic examination was notable for myoclonus and a coarse intention tremor in both upper extremities due to ataxia. He had perseveration, anomia, and apraxia. He was unable to complete the Montreal Cognitive Assessment (MoCA) because of perseveration. Cerebrospinal fluid 14-3-3 was within normal limits. Electroencephalogram (EEG) showed diffuse slowing and occasional triphasic complexes. Magnetic resonance imaging (MRI) showed significant atrophy, along with abnormal diffusion signal in the thalami and bilateral parietal lobes. He died seven months after symptom onset.

PREVALENCE, PROGNOSIS, AND DEFINITION

Creutzfeldt–Jakob disease (CJD) (also known as Jakob-Creutzfeldt disease, JCD) is the most common type of prion disease. Prion diseases, also called transmissible spongiform encephalopathies, are progressive neurodegenerative diseases characterized by a specific neuropathology and a rapid cognitive decline that can progress to akinetic mutism over weeks. Cerebellar signs and myoclonus are frequent. EEG recordings often show a characteristic periodic sharp-wave complex. Sporadic Creutzfeldt–Jakob disease (making up 85%–90% of prion diseases) has an incidence of approximately 1 to 2 per million, with a usual age of onset from 55 to 75 years (average 67 and median 64 years) (Geschwind, 2015; Hermann et al., 2018). Average survival is about six months. Other forms of Creutzfeldt–Jakob disease include genetic (gCJD; 10%–15% of prion diseases) and acquired (1%–3% of prion diseases). Acquired forms include iatrogenic (iCJD) and variant (vCJD). Age of onset of variant Creutzfeldt–Jakob disease is generally younger, sometimes presenting in the second decade of life. Creutzfeldt–Jakob disease can be confirmed neuropathologically by biopsy or at autopsy, although these are rarely performed given the risk of transmission.

CRITERIA

Two commonly used sets of criteria are the University of California, San Francisco (UCSF) Criteria (Box 16.1; Geschwind, 2015) and those of the Diagnostic and Statistical Manual of Mental Disorders, 5th Edition (Box 16.2).

RISK FACTORS, PATHOLOGY, AND PATHOPHYSIOLOGY

Prions are unconventional agents that consist of proteinaceous infectious particles that produce transmissible diseases characterized by spongiform changes, neuronal death, astrocytosis, and accumulation of a pathological protein (PrP^{Sc}) in the brain as well as other organs to a lesser extent (Fig. 16.1). Prion diseases are transmissible, meaning an inoculation with the pathological protein can cause the disease in another individual. Iatrogenic cases have been due to transplantation of human brain tissues or human pituitary hormones from individuals with unrecognized prion diseases. Patients with familial Creutzfeldt–Jakob disease have been found to have mutations in the gene that codes for the PrP^{Sc} protein.

Variant Creutzfeldt–Jakob disease is similar biochemically and histopathologically to bovine spongiform encephalopathy, often referred to in the lay press

---

BOX 16.1   University of California, San Francisco Creutzfeldt–Jakob Criteria

1. Rapid cognitive decline
2. Two of the following six signs/symptoms:
   a. Myoclonus
   b. Pyramidal/extrapyramidal dysfunction
   c. Visual dysfunction
   d. Cerebellar dysfunction
   e. Akinetic mutism
   f. Focal cortical signs (e.g., neglect, aphasia, acalculia, apraxia)
3. Typical electroencephalogram and/or magnetic resonance imaging (MRI)
   a. MRI shows diffusion-weighted imaging brighter than fluid-attenuated inversion recovery hyperintensity in the cingulate, striatum, and/or greater than one neocortical gyrus, ideally with sparing of the precentral gyrus and apparent diffusion coefficient map supporting restricted diffusion.
4. Other investigations should not suggest an alternative diagnosis.

Modified from Geschwind, M. D. (2015). Prion diseases. *Continuum (Minneapolis, Minn.), 21*(6 Neuroinfectious Disease),1612–1638.

BOX 16.2   Diagnostic and Statistical Manual of Mental Disorders, 5th Edition Criteria for Major or Mild Neurocognitive Disorder Caused by Prion Disease

A. The criteria are met for major or mild neurocognitive disorder.
B. There is insidious onset, and rapid progression of impairment is common.
C. There are motor features of prion disease, such as myoclonus or ataxia, or biomarker evidence.
D. The neurocognitive disorder is not attributable to another medical condition and is not better explained by another mental disorder.

From American Psychiatric Association. (2013). *Diagnostic and Statistical Manual of Mental Disorders (DSM-5)* (5th ed.). Arlington, VA: American Psychiatric Publishing, Inc.

---

as "mad cow disease." A number of these cases in the United Kingdom have been attributed to ingesting beef contaminated with bovine spongiform encephalopathy. Other prion diseases have been described including kuru, Gerstmann–Sträussler–Schenker disease, and fatal familial insomnia.

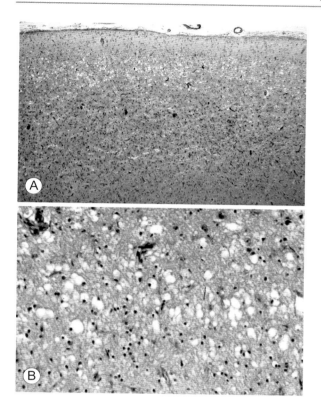

Fig. 16.1 Pathology of Creutzfeldt–Jakob disease. Note spongiform changes (i.e., the clear spaces), which can be visualized at both low power **(A)** and high power **(B)**.

CLINICAL PRESENTATION

Patients with Creutzfeldt–Jakob disease present with a rapid cognitive and motor decline that can progress to akinetic mutism within weeks. Myoclonus and cerebellar signs (such as ataxia), as well as pyramidal abnormalities (such as weakness), may all occur. Myoclonus occurring as a heightened startle response to sound or light is often present in the middle to late stages. The vast majority of patients show a significant cognitive decline, including abnormalities of memory and executive function in addition to depression and/or other changes in personality (Geschwind, 2015).

LABORATORY STUDIES AND ELECTROENCEPHALOGRAPHY

The EEG in Creutzfeldt–Jakob disease classically shows diffuse slowing with periodic triphasic complexes; however, this is a nonspecific sign of generalized brain dysfunction and is not always present until the disease is evident clinically. Similarly, the elevation of the 14-3-3 protein in the cerebral spinal fluid is a nonspecific sign of rapid neuronal injury, but in a review of cases in which there was a strong suspicion of Creutzfeldt–Jakob disease, the sensitivity was 92% and the specificity was 80%. Cerebrospinal fluid total tau is another useful marker; when higher than 1150 pg/mL there is reported sensitivity and specificity of greater than 90%. Combining these markers may increase their diagnostic accuracy (Takada & Geschwind, 2013).

A newer diagnostic test, the real-time quaking-induced conversion assay (RT-QuIC), can detect the presence of the prion protein scrapie in cerebrospinal fluid. When combined with other criteria, the addition of this assay can provide a sensitivity of 97% and specificity of 99% (Hermann et al., 2018).

Brain biopsy can often provide a definitive diagnosis. However, the diagnostic specificity of MRI now rivals that of brain biopsy. Moreover, brain biopsy poses the risk of transmission to operating room personnel and other patients because standard surgical sterilization methods do not remove prion proteins.

STRUCTURAL IMAGING STUDIES

Because of the rapid death of neurons, an MRI scan showing restricted diffusion in the cortical or deep nuclei gray matter resulting in diffusion-weighted imaging (DWI) hyperintensities greater than fluid-attenuated inversion recovery (FLAIR) hyperintensities has a sensitivity 92% to 96%, specificity 93% to 94%, and accuracy of about 97% (Geschwind, 2015) (Fig. 16.2).

DIFFERENTIAL DIAGNOSIS

When suspecting a case of Creutzfeldt–Jakob disease that is progressing relatively slowly over months, the differential diagnosis includes common degenerative diseases such as dementia with Lewy bodies (see Chapter 8), frontotemporal dementia (see Chapter 10), corticobasal degeneration (see Chapter 13), progressive supranuclear palsy (see Chapter 12), and Alzheimer's disease (see Chapter 4) (particularly when associated with cerebral amyloid angiopathy). Vascular dementia (see Chapter 7) can also be confused with Creutzfeldt–Jakob disease. See Box 16.3 for the differential diagnosis of rapidly progressing dementias (for review, see Geschwind, 2016).

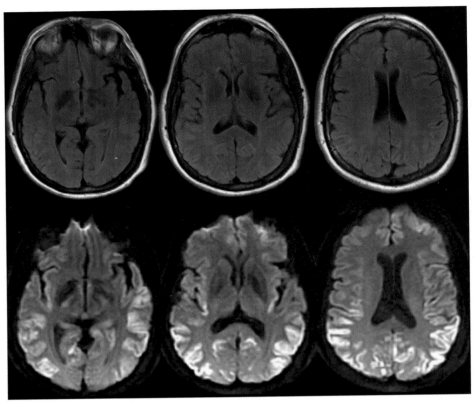

Fig. 16.2 Note characteristic diffusion-weighted imaging *(bottom row)* hyperintensities greater than fluid-attenuated inversion recovery *(top row)* hyperintensities in temporal, parietal, and frontal lobes. (From Puoti, G, Bizzi, A., Forloni, G., et al. (2012). Sporadic human prion diseases: molecular insights and diagnosis [published correction appears in *Lancet Neurology*, 2012; *11*(10), 841]. *Lancet Neurology, 11*(7), 618–628.)

BOX 16.3   Differential Diagnosis of Rapidly Progressing Dementias

- Cerebrovascular disease
- Autoimmune encephalopathy (e.g., Hashimoto's encephalopathy)
- Vasculitis
- Collagen vascular and granulomatous diseases (e.g., sarcoid)
- Infectious disease
  - Human immunodeficiency virus (HIV)
  - Opportunistic infections in HIV and other immunocompromised states
  - Cryptococcus
  - JC virus
  - Mycobacteria
  - Syphilis
- Lyme disease
- Subacute sclerosing panencephalitis
- Whipple's disease
- Malignancies
  - Primary central nervous system lymphoma
  - Intravascular lymphoma
  - Lymphomatoid granulomatosis
- Paraneoplastic disorders (e.g., limbic encephalitis)
- Toxic metabolic disorders
  - Heavy metals (e.g., bismuth from Pepto-Bismol)
  - Vitamin deficiencies (e.g., Wernicke's encephalopathy)
- Metabolic disorders (e.g., metachromatic leukodystrophy)
- Psychiatric disorders

TREATMENTS

Treatment for Creutzfeldt–Jakob disease is supportive. Selective serotonin reuptake inhibitors (SSRIs) are commonly used to treat depression and agitation, atypical antipsychotics (particularly quetiapine) have been used to treat agitation and psychosis, and clonazepam has been used to treat severe myoclonus. Note: These medications are not approved by the U.S. Food and Drug Administration (FDA) for any dementia and have very serious side effects; see Chapter 27 for important additional information before prescribing. Although a number of therapies aimed at ameliorating the underlying disorder have been tried, none has proved to be effective. In the majority of cases Creutzfeldt–Jakob disease is rapidly fatal, with most patients dying from the disease within a year of diagnosis, often within weeks to months.

REFERENCES

Geschwind, M. D. (2015). Prion diseases. *Continuum (Minneapolis, Minn.)*, *21*(6 Neuroinfectious Disease), 1612–1638.

Geschwind, M. D. (2016). Rapidly progressive dementia. *Continuum (Minneapolis, Minn.)*, *22*(2 Dementia), 510–537.

Hermann, P., Laux, M., Glatzel, M., et al. (2018). Validation and utilization of amended diagnostic criteria in Creutzfeldt-Jakob disease surveillance. *Neurology*, *91*(4), e331–e338.

Takada, L. T., & Geschwind, M. D. (2013). Prion diseases. *Seminars in Neurology*, *33*, 348–356.

17

Other Disorders That Cause Memory Loss or Dementia

(Continued)

QUICK START: OTHER DISORDERS THAT CAUSE MEMORY LOSS OR DEMENTIA (*Continued*)

Subdural and epidural hematomas	• Subdural and epidural hematomas may cause a number of symptoms, including drowsiness, inattention, hemiparesis, or seizures, depending upon the size, age, and composition of the fluid collection.
Vitamin B12 deficiency	• Symptoms of B12 deficiency include memory loss, psychosis including hallucinations and delusions, fatigue, irritability, depression, and personality changes.
	• B12 deficiency should be suspected when the patient is elderly, a vegetarian, taking certain medications (e.g., metformin), or has had intestinal infections.
Seizures	• Seizures are an uncommon cause of memory problems but must be considered both because they are treatable and because they can lead to disability and death if they were to occur, for example, while driving a car.
	• Focal impaired awareness seizures should be suspected in patients of any age in whom there is a history of "episodes" of memory loss that may be quite profound in the setting of otherwise good memory and normal cognitive testing.
Human immunodeficiency virus (HIV)-associated neurocognitive disorder	• HIV can cause cognitive impairment, including apathy, slow processing speed, and executive dysfunction, with or without extrapyramidal motor features.
	• Consider this disorder in the patient with these cognitive signs and symptoms who has HIV-risk factors, as well as in the patient with known HIV disease.
Brain sagging syndrome	• Spontaneous intracranial hypotension causing brain sagging syndrome is treatable and can mimic behavioral variant frontotemporal dementia and Alzheimer's disease.
Hashimoto's encephalopathy (steroid-responsive encephalopathy associated with autoimmune thyroiditis)	• Hashimoto's encephalitis is a rare, rapidly progressing, treatable, autoimmune disorder associated with chronic lymphocytic Hashimoto's thyroiditis.
	• It often begins with psychiatric symptoms such as depression, personality changes, or psychosis, and then progresses with cognitive decline and one or more of a variety of signs and symptoms including myoclonus, ataxia, pyramidal and extrapyramidal signs, stroke-like episodes, altered levels of consciousness, confusion, and seizures.
	• Patients with Hashimoto's encephalitis can be euthyroid, hypothyroid, or hyperthyroid.

In this chapter we present additional disorders that can cause memory loss and other cognitive impairment. Although some of these disorders are common, because none are causes of dementia per se, we touch on them here just briefly to round out the differential diagnosis of memory loss and dementia. These disorders are presented in the order that roughly corresponds to how often we see them in our clinic.

DEPRESSION AND ANXIETY

It is quite common that we will see a patient with memory loss or mild dementia who was treated with an antidepressant rather than a cholinesterase inhibitor by their primary care physician. The typical scenario is that the patient noticed that they were beginning to lose their memory, were concerned that they might be developing Alzheimer's disease, and understandably felt quite concerned, anxious, and depressed about their memory loss. The physician, correctly picking up on their anxiety and depression, prescribed an antidepressant. In our experience it is much more likely that a patient who is over the age of 65 and presents with both memory loss and depression has depression because of the memory loss, rather than the other way around. In fact, studies suggest that 20% to 40% of patients with dementia also have major depression, and up to 70% of patients have some depressive symptoms (Cummings et al., 1995; Kuring, Mathias, & Ward, 2018; Tractenberg et al., 2003).

It used to be a rule of thumb that patients who do not think that they have memory problems have Alzheimer's disease, whereas patients who are worried about their memory problems are aging normally or are depressed. Now we believe that it is much more likely that patients who are worried about their memory problems actually have mild cognitive impairment or very early Alzheimer's disease dementia (see Chapters 3 and 4).

The relationship between Alzheimer's disease and depression is both complex and controversial (for review see Bennett & Thomas, 2014). Studies have suggested that (1) a history of depression earlier in life is a risk factor for Alzheimer's disease and (2) symptoms of depression are common in the few years preceding the diagnosis of Alzheimer's disease, prompting some researchers to hypothesize that it is an early symptom of Alzheimer's disease, especially in individuals with no lifetime history of depression (Van der Mussele et al., 2014).

The history is one important clue to help determine whether the memory loss or the depression is primary. It would be extremely unlikely that a 75-year-old patient without a prior history of major depression would now develop a first episode of major depression severe enough to cause memory problems. On the other hand, a patient with a lifelong history of major depression severe enough to lead to multiple hospitalizations and medication trials may certainly be experiencing another episode of depression at age 75 years, causing his or her memory loss.

Some of the most common cognitive disturbances caused by depression include poor energy, motivation, and attention (Fig. 17.1). Frontal/executive and speed of processing deficits are often found on neuropsychological testing. Memory problems are typically secondary to these disturbances. Depression and anxiety disrupt the "file clerk" of the memory system, whereas Alzheimer's disease disrupts the "file cabinet." In other words, the patient with depression has difficulty placing (storing, encoding) information in the memory (the file clerk isn't doing its job), but, once it is stored, the brain mechanisms that maintain the memory are intact (the file cabinet is fine). (See Appendix C for more on the filing analogy of memory.) Thus patients with depression may appear to have a "frontal pattern" of memory loss, often performing poorly in learning (encoding) and freely recalling information off the top of their head, while performing relatively normally when choosing previously studied items from a list. Another pattern that is sometimes present in patients with depression is that they experience more difficulty remembering things in the past than the present. This pattern is thought to occur because it is more effortful for a person whose memory is normal to recall items from the distant past than to recall events that occurred yesterday. This pattern is just the opposite of that of most patients with Alzheimer's disease, in which the patient recalls the past easily but cannot remember what happened yesterday.

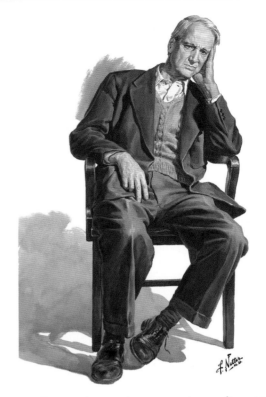

Fig. 17.1 Depression and memory loss often occur together. (Netter illustration from www.netterimages.com. Copyright Elsevier Inc. All rights reserved.)

In treating a patient who has both memory loss and depression, we always recommend treating the underlying disorder first. This recommendation may seem obvious, but many clinicians suggest treating the depression first regardless of whether it is primary or secondary. In our experience the depression secondary to awareness of memory loss typically improves when the memory improves. Similarly, the cognitive impairments secondary to depression generally improve when the depression is treated. Each patient may still benefit from a medication to treat the secondary symptom. For example, the patient with memory loss and secondary depression may still benefit from an selective serotonin reuptake inhibitor medication, sertraline (Zoloft) and escitalopram (Lexapro) being our favorites. Each of these medications has been approved for the treatment of both depression and anxiety. See Chapter 27 for more on the pharmacological treatment of depression.

Latrogenic

Overmedication

Side effects

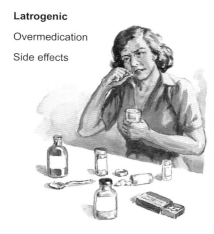

Fig. 17.2 Medication side effects are a common cause of cognitive dysfunction. (Netter illustration from www. netterimages.com. Copyright Elsevier Inc. All rights reserved.)

MEDICATION SIDE EFFECTS

Medication side effects are one of the most common causes of cognitive dysfunction (Fig. 17.2). In our experience, attention is the most common cognitive function to become affected, followed by memory, and then language. There are too many medications that interfere with cognition to individually list them all. Note that even a relatively safe class of medication from a cognitive perspective may still contain a few individual drugs that can cause confusion. Boxes 17.1 and 17.2 list some classes and properties of medications that can lead to cognitive dysfunction.

DISRUPTED SLEEP

Disrupted sleep is one of the most common causes of memory problems we see in patients younger than age 60 years. Poor sleep can disrupt memory in two main ways. First, sleep is necessary for good attention. To encode or learn new information, being able to focus and sustain attention is critical. Second, consolidation of memory—memories going from temporary to more long-term storage—requires sleep (Hennies et al., 2016). Thus poor sleep makes it difficult to learn new information and to retain that information in long-term storage.

> **BOX 17.1 Common Classes or Properties of Medications Causing Cognitive Dysfunction**
>
> - **Allergy/antihistamines/common cold medications**
> - **Analgesics including migraine medications**
> - Anesthetics
> - Antiarrhythmics
> - **Anticholinergics**
> - Anticonvulsants
> - Antidiarrheals
> - Antiemetics
> - **Antipsychotics/dopamine antagonists**
> - **Antispasmodics/incontinence medications**
> - Asthma/pulmonary medications
> - **Barbiturates**
> - **Benzodiazepines**
> - Beta-blockers
> - **Cancer chemotherapy**
> - **Corticosteroids**
> - Digoxin
> - Dopamine (Sinemet)/dopamine agonists
> - **Muscle relaxants**
> - **Opioids (narcotics)**
> - **Sedating medications of any class**
> - **Sleeping medications of any class**
> - Stimulants/stimulating medications of any class
> - Tricyclic antidepressants

Note: Worst offenders are in **bold**. This is not an exhaustive list. Please consult the Physicians Desk Reference or other source when determining whether a particular medication may be causing cognitive impairment in your patient.

Disrupted sleep may be the result of a sleep disorder such as insomnia, sleep apnea, periodic limb movements of sleep, and restless leg syndrome. Sleep may be disrupted by depression. And sleep may be commonly disrupted by poor sleep cycle or hygiene—that is, poor scheduling or management of sleep.

Shift workers, including nurses, factory workers, and others, are one group that is prone to memory disorders because of poor sleep hygiene. However, in our experience even more common than shift workers are individuals of any age who simply have too many things to do in their day to allow enough time for adequate sleep. When we are referred individuals with memory problems who are in their 30s or 40s, we always ask about sleep problems in several different ways. When asked, "Do you have any problems with sleep?" the response

---

BOX 17.2   The Incontinence Medications

The incontinence medications deserve special mention. Virtually all of the medications used to control incontinence, such as hyoscyamine and oxybutynin, are anticholinergic not as a side effect, but as their primary mode of action.

- Should these medications be discontinued in a patient with dementia who is on a cholinesterase inhibitor? The simple answer requires one question:
- Is the medication working to control the patient's incontinence such that he or she does not need to wear Depends (or similar absorbent underwear)?
  - If the answer is "yes," the medication would appear to be working and should be continued, despite any possible worsening of cognition. The reason being is that incontinence, being distressing, inconvenient, and burdensome for caregivers, is one of the major causes of patients being placed in long-term care facilities. It is therefore worth enduring cognitive side effects if incontinence can be eliminated.
  - If the answer is "no"—as it often is—then the medication is unlikely to be doing anything to improve the patient's quality of life and should most likely be discontinued.

---

is usually no. But when asked to briefly take us through their day, a common response often goes something like the following. *"I'm up at 5 AM to exercise, shower, and get myself ready for work at 6, get the kids up and get them ready for school at 7, and then leave for work at 8. I come home from work around 6 PM, make dinner, help the kids with their homework, and get them ready for bed by 9. Then I usually spend an hour or two finishing up work for the office, and then at 10 or 11 I have an hour or two to spend some time with my spouse talking or watching TV, till we go to bed after the evening news around 11:30 or 12."* Although this may sound like a perfectly normal schedule, this individual is only allowing themselves between 5 and 5½ hours of sleep a night. For the average individual, who is best with 8 hours of sleep, one can often get away with 7 hours without noticeable cognitive consequences. But trying to reduce sleep further often causes difficulty with attention and memory.

HORMONES?

Another possible cause of memory problems in individuals younger than age 60 years is a decrease in gonadotropin hormones. For women this is most commonly because of perimenopausal status; for either women or men this can be secondary to treatment for cancer or other disorders. The literature on this topic is quite mixed, with some studies demonstrating memory impairment and other studies not, and at least one literature review suggests that the natural transition to menopause is not associated with objective change in episodic memory (Henderson, 2009). Nonetheless, many individuals who come to us in the clinic are quite clear about their subjective experience that their memory is not as good as it was previously, which they relate to a change in their hormone status.

Regarding treatment, the literature again shows mixed results, with some studies finding improvement with hormone replacement therapy and others not, and literature reviews suggest that there is no improvement (Gava et al., 2019; Henderson, 2009). Most importantly, however, large randomized controlled trials have now shown no evidence for improvement and instead worsening of cognition and increased risk for dementia with hormone replacement therapy (Bojar et al., 2013; Coker et al., 2010; Craig, Maki, & Murphy, 2005; Henderson, 2009).

In summary, despite historical claims that hormone replacement therapy has cognitive benefit, we now know from randomized controlled trials that there is no evidence for this claim, and indeed there are increased risks for dementia and other disorders. As such, we do not recommend hormone replacement therapy for postmenopausal women solely as a treatment for memory problems.

METABOLIC DISORDERS

Almost any medical disorder that makes a patient ill can cause memory loss and/or impair other aspects of cognition. Common disorders that impair cognition include renal failure, liver failure, congestive heart failure, hypercapnia from chronic obstructive pulmonary disease, hypercalcemia, and many others (Fig. 17.3). There are several clues that can help the clinician to know that the cognitive impairment is secondary to a metabolic disorder and not secondary to a primary cause of dementia.

The first clue is that dementias are progressive, whereas metabolic disorders tend to wax and wane. For example, if the patient with congestive heart failure

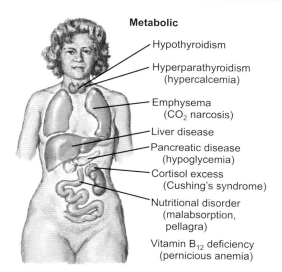

Metabolic

Hypothyroidism

Hyperparathyroidism
(hypercalcemia)

Emphysema
(CO_2 narcosis)

Liver disease

Pancreatic disease
(hypoglycemia)

Cortisol excess
(Cushing's syndrome)

Nutritional disorder
(malabsorption,
pellagra)

Vitamin B_{12} deficiency
(pernicious anemia)

Fig. 17.3 Metabolic disorders can disrupt attention and memory. (Netter illustration from www.netterimages.com. Copyright Elsevier Inc. All rights reserved.)

becomes confused when his heart failure acutely worsens but then is completely back to normal when the heart failure is better, the confusion is unlikely caused by a dementia. A similar scenario can happen with other metabolic disorders such as with liver failure. We have treated a 65-year-old man who has liver disease secondary to chronic alcohol use. When his liver failure was severe (and it was severe enough to require extended hospitalization) he was terribly confused, and even after he left the hospital and his liver function tests returned to just about normal, his cognition was still not what it used to be. This continued cognitive impairment in the setting of near normal liver function tests led his family to worry that he was now developing a dementia on top of everything else. Over a period of months, however, his cognitive function improved rather than worsened, and this was one reason that we knew that the patient was still recovering from his liver failure, and was not developing a dementia.

The second clue that cognitive impairment is a result of a metabolic disorder is that the impairment in cognition is virtually always poor attention. Patients with a metabolic disorder show extreme difficulties in paying attention, both on formal cognitive testing and in observing them at the bedside or in the clinic. Simple tasks, such as counting backward from 20 to 1, reciting the months of the year backward, or spelling the word "WORLD" backward, may be quite difficult for these patients. Memory problems are prominent, but these memory problems are secondary to poor attention. The ability to learn new information is severely impaired during the time when the patient is confused with poor attention, often leading to the patient having no memory of the time that they were confused.

The last thing to note here is that a patient may have an incipient dementia that is made apparent by a metabolic disorder—the so-called "unmasking effect." For example, a 74-year-old patient with no clinical complaints of memory loss by either herself or her family may have a small amount of Alzheimer's pathology in the brain. Under normal circumstances this pathology is "silent," that is, it produces no clinical signs or symptoms. If this patient develops hypercalcemia, however, she may show signs of inattention and memory loss that are due both to the hypercalcemia and to the small amount of Alzheimer's pathology in the brain. Thus her cognitive dysfunction may be worse than that of another 74-year-old with hypercalcemia but without the Alzheimer's pathology. When the hypercalcemia is successfully treated, her cognition returns to normal. How do we know that she has underlying Alzheimer's pathology? We know that she has underlying Alzheimer's pathology if several months or years later she develops the signs and symptoms of Alzheimer's disease when she does not have hypercalcemia or another metabolic disorder.

DIABETES

Diabetes can cause memory loss and other cognitive problems in several different ways. The two most common and concerning are from cerebrovascular disease and hypoglycemia. Along with hypertension, increased cholesterol, and smoking, diabetes predisposes the patient to cerebrovascular disease. These effects are discussed in Chapter 7. Hypoglycemia can also damage the brain. A variety of cognitive, behavioral, and personality changes can be seen (Kössler et al., 2020). Although the specific pathophysiology has not been worked out, hypoglycemia damages both gray and white matter, meaning that both neurons and myelinated axons and dendrites suffer injury (Ma et al., 2009). In our experience there is the not-surprising correlation between how tightly the glucose is trying to be maintained and how frequently episodes of hypoglycemia and subsequent cognitive impairment occur. We would therefore recommend that control of glucose not be so tight such that hypoglycemic episodes are frequent. Tight control is of course particularly dangerous when the patient is not aware of his or her hypoglycemia.

ALCOHOL ABUSE AND ALCOHOLIC KORSAKOFF'S SYNDROME

About half of the 18 million problem drinkers in the U.S. develop cognitive deficits (Oscar-Berman & Marinkovic, 2007) (Fig. 17.4). Most of these individuals develop mild neuropsychological difficulties which improve within a year of abstinence. Approximately two million alcoholics, however, develop lifelong disabling conditions that require custodial care. Factors that contribute to alcohol's effect on the brain include older age, comorbid health conditions, and positive family history.

The brain structures most vulnerable to dysfunction and damage in alcoholism include the frontal lobes, limbic system, and cerebellum. Other structures showing either atrophy or reduced blood flow on MRI include the other regions of the cerebral cortex, corpus callosum, hippocampus, and the amygdala. Additional structures damaged in alcoholic Korsakoff's syndrome are discussed below.

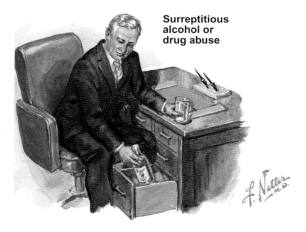

Surreptitious alcohol or drug abuse

Fig. 17.4 Half of problem drinkers develop cognitive deficits. (Netter illustration from www.netterimages. com. Copyright Elsevier Inc. All rights reserved.)

Alcohol's acute effects on the brain include both stimulating effects in low doses and depressant effects in higher doses. Neuropsychologically there is a reduction in working memory, planning, other executive functions, visuospatial ability, and interhemispheric processing speed. Attention and vigilance can be reduced at blood alcohol levels as low as 0.02% to 0.03%, much lower than legal intoxication levels. Regarding behavior, alcohol intoxication increases the likelihood of aggressive behaviors secondary to impulsivity, disinhibition, social or sexual inappropriateness, and impairments in decision-making and executive function. Alcoholics frequently make poor decisions, including decisions regarding their alcohol consumption. Changes in emotion and personality are also seen, including a diminished ability to recognize emotional facial expressions and emotional spoken prosody (tone of voice). Personality traits are often described in terms of "disinhibition," impulsivity, aggression, and a lack of concern for the consequences of inappropriate behaviors. On the neurological examination the most common problems are with gait and balance, typically associated with cerebellar dysfunction. (Cerebellar function is what is typically evaluated in field sobriety tests.)

Common comorbid medical conditions that, in combination with alcoholism, are most likely to result in greater cognitive dysfunction include head injury, liver disease, cardiovascular disease, fetal alcohol syndrome, and malnutrition leading to thiamine (vitamin B1) deficiency. Frequent comorbid psychiatric conditions that can worsen cognition include depression, schizophrenia, and other drug use.

Neurobehavioral functioning can improve within 3 to 4 weeks of abstinence, accompanied by recovery of metabolic functions and partial reversal of brain shrinkage in some patients. Frontal lobe blood flow returns to normal after approximately four years. Most neurocognitive deficits resolve within seven years, with the exception of visuospatial processing deficits, which may not recover.

Patients with alcohol-induced persisting amnestic disorder, more commonly known as the alcoholic Korsakoff's syndrome, show severe anterograde amnesia (inability to remember new information) as well as some retrograde amnesia (loss of previously acquired information). When severe, these patients are permanently unable to remember new information for more than the time the information is being kept in mind—typically just a few seconds. Patients with Korsakoff's syndrome live in the past, and generally retain many older memories formed before the onset of their alcohol-related brain damage. The damaged areas of the brain include the mamillary bodies, basal forebrain, hippocampus, fornix, and medial and anterior nuclei of the thalamus. Although damage to the mamillary bodies is commonly thought to be the cause of the memory deficit in this syndrome, at least one study suggests that it is actually damage to the anterior nucleus of the thalamus that is most closely correlated with the memory deficit (Harding et al., 2000). In addition to memory deficits, patients with Korsakoff's syndrome are abnormally sensitive to proactive interference; have restricted attention; retarded perceptual processing abilities; are impaired on tests of fluency, executive function, and cognitive flexibility; and show perseverative responding and neuropsychiatric symptoms (Moerman-van den Brink et al., 2020). They are also ataxic.

The cerebellum in particular deserves mention. Alcoholism is associated with marked cerebellar atrophy, particularly of the cerebellar vermis. The cerebellum is now understood to be important for normal cognitive and behavioral function (Argyropoulos et al., 2020), particularly executive function including cognitive flexibility, allocation of attentional resources, set shifting ability, inhibition of perseverative errors, abstraction, planning, and inhibition of irrelevant information. Thus damage to the cerebellum may also be responsible for some of the cognitive and behavioral impairment seen in patients with alcoholism.

Most patients with alcoholism complain of memory deficits. If their alcoholism is mainly affecting frontal/executive function, then the memory deficit will be of a "frontal" variety; that is, difficulty learning new information and freely recalling it, but if enough effort is used, new information can be learned and retrieved. If their alcoholism has led to Korsakoff's syndrome, then their memory deficit will be similar to that of a patient with Alzheimer's disease or other hippocampal injury; that is, new information may not be able to be learned, regardless of the effort employed. It is sometimes difficult to distinguish patients with alcoholism and Alzheimer's disease from patients with alcoholism and Korsakoff's syndrome, particularly at a single visit. Both will have frontal executive and episodic memory dysfunction. Over time, however, things become clearer. As long as the patient abstains from drinking, over time the patient with Korsakoff's syndrome will be stable, whereas the patient with Alzheimer's disease will deteriorate.

LYME DISEASE

Lyme neuroborreliosis, Lyme disease affecting the central nervous system, is an uncommon but highly treatable cause of memory problems. The memory problems are typically secondary to difficulties with focusing and sustaining attention, leading to difficulties in encoding (learning).

Lyme disease should be considered in those who live in an area endemic for Lyme who are at risk for deer tick exposure by, for example, taking walks in the woods. Exposure to Lyme disease can be determined from a positive serum immunoglobin (Ig)G. A positive serum IgM indicates active infection. Traditionally, a positive IgA in the cerebral spinal fluid confirms the diagnosis of Lyme neuroborreliosis, although polymerase chain reaction of specific Lyme DNA sequences in the cerebrospinal fluid may be more sensitive and specific (Stanek & Strle, 2009).

Lastly, one review suggests that 28% of patients with treated Lyme neuroborreliosis show some residual symptoms including cognitive disturbances, headache, and fatigue (Dersch et al., 2016).

SUBDURAL AND EPIDURAL HEMATOMAS

Subdural and epidural hematomas may cause a number of symptoms, including drowsiness, inattention, hemiparesis, or seizures, depending upon the size, age, and composition of the fluid collections. Subdural hematomas are when blood accumulates between the brain and the dura, lining the sulci and gyri of the brain with blood. Epidural hematomas are between the dura and the skull, and often appear in the shape of a lens (Fig. 17.5). As the brain atrophies or shrinks with normal aging or with a neurodegenerative disease (such as Alzheimer's disease), the bridging veins between the dura and the brain become relatively longer. The dura may also start to pull away from the skull. Thus the effect of the brain shrinking makes it much more likely that even a minor fall involving the head can lead to a subdural or epidural hematoma. These hematomas are even more likely in some dementias—such as progressive supranuclear palsy (see Chapter 12)—which predispose the patient to falls. In Alzheimer's disease and other dementias with

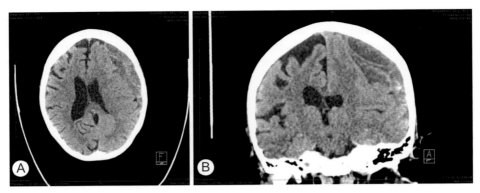

Fig. 17.5 Axial **(A)** and coronal **(B)** views of a large, multilayered, epidural hematoma in a patient with Alzheimer's disease. Note the atrophy apparent in the right hemisphere (left side of image) and the compression from the hematoma, pushing the entire brain to the right. This patient did not recall the fall that led to the hematoma.

prominent memory loss, there is also the problem that the patient may fall but not remember to tell anyone. We have often seen patients who present with bruises to the face and cannot tell their caregivers or doctors how they came about.

VITAMIN B12 DEFICIENCY

Vitamin B12 deficiency should always be looked for when a patient presents with memory loss, because it is generally reversible with treatment. Many cognitive and neuropsychiatric symptoms have been observed in patients who do not have a megaloblastic anemia, including memory loss, psychosis including hallucinations and delusions, fatigue, irritability, depression, and personality changes.

Vitamin B12 deficiency should be suspected when the patient is vegetarian (particularly vegan), and in older adults because inability to absorb B12 owing to atrophic gastritis is common in the elderly. Some medications (e.g., metformin) can also interfere with B12 dietary absorption, as can a number of intestinal infections.

Diagnosis of B12 deficiency can be performed in a number of ways. We typically screen patients for B12 deficiency with a serum B12 level, looking for a value of at least 400 ng/mL, regardless of the stated normal range. However, if the suspicion is strong and the B12 level is low normal we will follow up with serum levels of methylmalonic acid, which is more sensitive.

Treatment is, of course, supplementation with vitamin B12, either orally (if the result of a dietary deficiency such as a vegan diet) or parenterally (if caused by poor absorption such as in atrophy gastritis). There are also nasal formulations available. It is important to monitor serum B12 and/or methylmalonic acid to assure that levels are returning to normal. Cognition should return to normal with treatment.

SEIZURES

Seizures are an uncommon cause of memory problems but must be considered both because they are a treatable disorder and because they can lead to disability and death if they were to occur, for example, while driving a car. Because generalized tonic–clonic seizures are rarely a secret, undiagnosed seizures that cause memory problems are typically focal impaired awareness seizures (previously called partial complex seizures)—focal seizures that interfere with awareness without generalizing.

Sometimes the amnesia caused by the seizure can be profound, such as in the case of transient epileptic amnesia, in which patients have an inability to form any new memories for several hours. More commonly, focal impaired awareness seizures intermittently impair consciousness, causing patients to have difficulty focusing their attention such that their encoding (learning) is intermittently reduced. This intermittent deficit in encoding can lead to intermittent problems with memory that may sound quite similar to those of a patient with amnestic mild cognitive impairment or even mild Alzheimer's disease.

Focal impaired awareness seizures should be suspected in patients of any age in whom there is a history of "episodes" of memory loss that may be quite profound in the setting of otherwise good memory and normal cognitive testing. These seizures should also be considered in patients younger than 65 years of age. Diagnosis can sometimes be made by history alone if a focal impaired awareness seizure is observed. If the seizures are frequent enough, the diagnosis can be confirmed by ambulatory electroencephalogram (EEG) monitoring. Epileptiform activity on the routine EEG can also suggest the diagnosis.

HUMAN IMMUNODEFICIENCY VIRUS–ASSOCIATED NEUROCOGNITIVE DISORDER

Human immunodeficiency virus (HIV), either alone or with concomitant opportunistic infections, can cause cognitive impairment and dementia. Cognitive impairment frequently observed includes slowing of psychomotor speed, information processing, and executive function. Memory deficits are present because of an impaired frontal lobe "file clerk," that is, they are secondary to poor encoding and retrieval (see Appendix C for more on the filing analogy of memory). Apathy is also common. These impairments are thought to be related to the finding that HIV has been found in subcortical and deep gray matter structures such as caudate and nucleus accumbens. Extrapyramidal/parkinsonian motor features are also observed and may increase with age.

There are two main scenarios in which considering HIV-associated neurocognitive disorder arises. The first is in the patient with known HIV. There is a debate in the literature about whether or not to screen for cognitive impairment in these patients. We believe that it is important to do so, because—owing to apathy and loss of insight—symptom reporting is unreliable. We recommend the Montreal Cognitive Assessment (MoCA) as a screening test because it is sensitive to executive dysfunction. More detailed neuropsychological testing may be even more sensitive (Costaggiu et al., 2020). The second scenario is when searching for a cause of cognitive impairment in a patient who is not known to have HIV disease. Because HIV is treatable, it is an important disease to consider when evaluating a patient with apathy, slow processing speed, and executive dysfunction, with or without extrapyramidal motor features. When evaluating such a patient in our clinics we probe for behaviors that have been associated with HIV risk factors and, if present, discuss possible HIV testing with the patient.

BRAIN SAGGING SYNDROME

Spontaneous intracranial hypotension causing brain sagging syndrome is a rare but treatable cause of progressive cognitive decline that can mimic several dementias. Although it most commonly presents as behavioral variant frontotemporal dementia, we have seen amnestic presentations mimicking Alzheimer's disease as well (Vives-Rodriguez et al., 2020). MRI findings include a sagging of the brain with flattening of the pons and cerebellar tonsillar herniation (Fig. 17.6A). It is important to look for, as it may be treatable with epidural blood patch procedures, resulting in radiographic and cognitive improvement (see Fig. 17.6B) (Vives-Rodriguez et al., 2020).

HASHIMOTO'S ENCEPHALOPATHY (STEROID-RESPONSIVE ENCEPHALOPATHY ASSOCIATED WITH AUTOIMMUNE THYROIDITIS)

Hashimoto's encephalopathy, also termed steroid-responsive encephalopathy associated with autoimmune thyroiditis (SREAT), is a rare but treatable autoimmune disorder associated with chronic lymphocytic Hashimoto's thyroiditis (Geschwind, 2016). It often begins with psychiatric symptoms such as depression, personality changes, or psychosis, and then progresses with cognitive decline and one or more of a variety of signs and symptoms including myoclonus, ataxia, pyramidal and extrapyramidal signs, stroke-like episodes, altered levels of consciousness, confusion, and seizures. Because it produces a rapidly progressing dementia it is most commonly mistaken for Creutzfeldt–Jakob disease (see Chapter 16). Seizures, hallucinations, and delusions are common. Women represent 85% of patients with Hashimoto's encephalitis. The course tends to be fluctuating. Patients with Hashimoto's encephalitis can be euthyroid, hypothyroid, or hyperthyroid, although the diagnosis cannot be made until the patient is euthyroid. Elevated levels of either antithyroglobulin or antithyroperoxidase in the appropriate clinical context suggest the diagnosis. EEG is nonspecific and can be confused

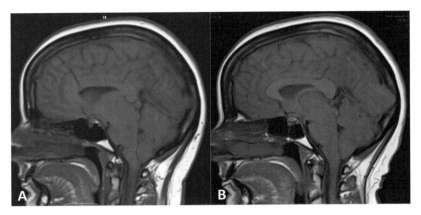

Fig. 17.6 Brain sagging syndrome. Sagittal T1-weighted MRI views pre- **(A)** and post- **(B)** epidural blood patch procedures. Note the downward displacement of brainstem and cerebellar tonsils, flatting of the pons, and narrowing of the quadrigeminal plate, suprasellar, and basilar cisterns **(A)**, all improved after the blood patch procedures **(B)**.

with Creutzfeldt–Jakob disease, as can the cerebrospinal fluid examination because both show increased protein. MRI often shows increased T2-weighted signal in the subcortical mesial temporal white matter, which may resolve after treatment.

The etiology of Hashimoto's encephalitis is not clear, but it is thought to be as a result of the presence of a shared antigen in the brain and the thyroid. More than 90% of patients respond well to immunosuppression. The typical treatment is with high-dose steroids followed by a long, slow taper. Some patients may have persistent symptoms or a fluctuating course. Plasmapheresis has also been used.

REFERENCES

Argyropoulos, G. P. D., van Dun, K., Adamaszek, M., et al. (2020). The cerebellar cognitive affective/Schmahmann syndrome: A task force paper. *Cerebellum (London, England), 19*(1), 102–125.

Bennett, S., & Thomas, A. J. (2014). Depression and dementia: Cause, consequence or coincidence? *Maturitas, 79*(2), 184–190.

Bojar, I., Gujski, M., Raczkiewicz, D., et al. (2013). Cognitive functions, apolipoprotein E genotype and hormonal replacement therapy of postmenopausal women. *Neuro Endocrinology Letters, 34*, 635–642.

Coker, L. H., Espeland, M. A., Rapp, S. R., et al. (2010). Postmenopausal hormone therapy and cognitive outcomes: The Women's Health Initiative Memory Study (WHIMS). *The Journal of Steroid Biochemistry and Molecular Biology, 118*, 304–310.

Costaggiu, D., Pinna, E., Serchisu, L., et al. (2020). The Repeatable Battery for the Assessment of Neuropsychological Status as a screening strategy for HIV-associated neurocognitive disorders. *AIDS Care, 17*, 1–7.

Craig, M. C., Maki, P. M., & Murphy, D. G. (2005). The Women's Health Initiative Memory Study: Findings and implications for treatment. *Lancet Neurology, 4*, 190–194.

Cummings, J. L., Ross, W., Absher, J., et al. (1995). Depressive symptoms in Alzheimer disease: Assessment and determinants. *Alzheimer Disease and Associated Disorders, 9*, 87–93.

Dersch, R., Sommer, H., Rauer, S., et al. (2016). Prevalence and spectrum of residual symptoms in Lyme neuroborreliosis after pharmacological treatment: A systematic review. *Journal of Neurology, 263*(1), 17–24.

Gava, G., Orsili, I., Alvisi, S., et al. (2019). Cognition, mood and sleep in menopausal transition: The role of menopause hormone therapy. *Medicina (Kaunas, Lithuania), 55*(10), 668.

Geschwind. M. D. (2016). Rapidly progressive dementia. *Continuum (Minneapolis, Minn.), 22*(2 Dementia), 510–537.

Harding, A., Halliday, G., Caine, D., et al. (2000). Degeneration of anterior thalamic nuclei differentiates alcoholics with amnesia. *Brain, 123*, 141–154.

Henderson. V. W. (2009). Aging, estrogens, and episodic memory in women. *Cognitive and Behavioral Neurology: Official Journal of the Society for Behavioral and Cognitive Neurology, 22*, 205–214.

Hennies, N., Lambon, R. M. A., Kempkes, M., et al. (2016). Sleep spindle density predicts the effect of prior knowledge on memory consolidation. *The Journal of Neuroscience, 36*(13), 3799–3810.

Kössler, T., Weber, K. S., Wölwer, W., et al. (2020). Associations between cognitive performance and Mediterranean dietary pattern in patients with type 1 or type 2 diabetes mellitus. *Nutrition & Diabetes, 10*(1), 10.

Kuring, J. K., Mathias, J. L., & Ward, L. (2018). Prevalence of depression, anxiety and PTSD in people with dementia: A systematic review and meta-analysis. *Neuropsychology Review, 28*(4), 393–416.

Ma, J. H., Kim, Y. J., Yoo, W. J., et al. (2009). MR imaging of hypoglycemic encephalopathy: Lesion distribution and prognosis prediction by diffusion-weighted imaging. *Neuroradiology, 51*, 641–649.

Moerman-van den Brink, W. G., van Aken, L., Verschuur, E. M. L., et al. (2020). The relationship between executive dysfunction and neuropsychiatric symptoms in patients with Korsakoff's syndrome. *The Clinical Neuropsychologist, 34*(4), 740–754.

Oscar-Berman, M., & Marinkovic, K. (2007). Alcohol: Effects on neurobehavioral functions and the brain. *Neuropsychology Review, 17*, 239–257.

Stanek, G., & Strle, F. (2009). Lyme borreliosis: A European perspective on diagnosis and clinical management. *Current Opinion in Infectious Diseases, 22*, 450–454.

Tractenberg, R. E., Weiner, M. F., Patterson, M. B., et al. (2003). Comorbidity of psychopathological domains in community-dwelling persons with Alzheimer's disease. *Journal of Geriatric Psychiatry and Neurology, 16*, 94–99.

Van der Mussele, S., Fransen, E., Struyfs, H., et al. (2014). Depression in mild cognitive impairment is associated with progression to Alzheimer's disease: A longitudinal study. *Journal of Alzheimer's disease: JAD, 42*, 1239–1250.

Vives-Rodriguez, A., Turk, K. W., Vassey, E. A., et al. (2020). Reversible amnestic cognitive impairment in a patient with brain sagging syndrome. *Neurology: Clinical Practice,* May 2020. doi:10.1212/CPJ.0000000000000860.

18

Goals for the Treatment of Memory Loss, Alzheimer's Disease, and Dementia

---

QUICK START: GOALS FOR THE TREATMENT OF MEMORY LOSS, ALZHEIMER'S DISEASE, AND DEMENTIA

- Treatment of Alzheimer's disease and other causes of memory loss and dementia is best carried out in a partnership between patient, caregiver, and clinician.
- Current FDA approved treatments can help improve or maintain the patient's cognitive and functional status by "turning back the clock" on memory loss.
- New, disease-modifying treatments are being developed and may be available soon.

- Families and other caregivers are helped by treatments that improve the behavioral and psychological symptoms of dementia.
- Nonpharmacological strategies can also help compensate for memory loss.

In our experience, treatment of Alzheimer's disease and other causes of memory loss and dementia is best carried out in a partnership between the patient, caregiver(s), and clinician. As with most diseases, when the diagnosis of Alzheimer's disease is made, the first question that is asked is: "What can be done?" As we explain to our patients and families, there are many aspects to treatment ranging from counseling and education to medication that, when skillfully combined, lead to the best outcomes.

TALKING ABOUT TREATMENTS FOR ALZHEIMER'S DISEASE

Patients for whom we prescribe a cholinesterase inhibitor, memantine, or a combination of the two often ask how these medications work and what else can be done.

We typically have a discussion with these patients and their families that attempts to incorporate the following points.

- Alzheimer's disease is a brain disease. In the most basic sense, brain cells are dying. As you lose brain cells, the abilities to which these cells contribute are also lost. For example, early in the course of the disease individuals with Alzheimer's disease lose cells in a brain structure called the hippocampus. The hippocampus is critical to the formation of new memories and this is why one of the first signs of Alzheimer's disease is difficulty remembering new information. (We sometimes show a photograph or a model of the brain with the hippocampus [such as in Figs. 4.6 and 4.12] and we generally show the patient their computed tomography [CT] or magnetic resonance imaging [MRI] scan and indicate the hippocampus and other regions of atrophy to show where brain cells have been lost.)

- Unlike many other organs in the body, brain cells do not typically regenerate, so, once a brain cell is lost, it is gone forever.
- As more brain cells die, the disease progresses and more abilities are lost.
- The goal is to treat with medications that will help the remaining brain cells—even those that may be diseased—function more efficiently. This improved efficiency can help to compensate for the ongoing loss of brain cells.
- The two most commonly used types of medication to accomplish this goal are cholinesterase inhibitors and memantine.
- These medications do not stop the death of brain cells or even slow it down, but they do help to improve the symptoms of the disease. (We often show or draw them a figure similar to Fig. 18.1 to help them understand what symptomatic benefit means.)
- We often mention that these treatments can "turn back the clock" on the patient's memory to where it was 6 or 12 months ago, but they cannot stop the clock from ticking down nor slow its rate.
- Cholinesterase inhibitors help brain cells that use the neurotransmitter acetylcholine to function more efficiently.
- Memantine helps brain cells that use the neurotransmitters glutamate and dopamine to function more efficiently.
- Acetylcholine, glutamate, and dopamine are all important in human memory.

Following this discussion, patients and families typically grasp the notion that the disease is progressive and that by using these approved medications we are attempting to treat the symptoms of the disease such as memory deficits, but we are not treating the underlying cause, that is, the death of neurons. If at this point they ask if there is anything else that might be done, we discuss the opportunity to participate in clinical trials. Because Alzheimer's is a fatal disease, as in the field of oncology, we believe that the best care allows patients to participate in clinical trials of novel medications if they so choose.

As described in more detail in Chapters 19 and 20, most of our patients with Alzheimer's disease are on a cholinesterase inhibitor and some are also on memantine extended release. Only occasionally do we prescribe Namzaric, which combines memantine extended release at various doses plus donepezil 10 mg (Calhoun et al., 2018). We find it easier to titrate up each pill separately and sometimes patients are on 5 or 15 mg of donepezil. It is also generally less expensive for patients to take generic memantine and generic donepezil than brandname Namzaric. However, for some patients who are living alone, the single, once-a-day pill Namzaric may be easier for them to manage.

STRATEGIES TO TREAT THE SYMPTOMS OF ALZHEIMER'S DISEASE

In the following chapters we discuss several different strategies to treat Alzheimer's disease. In Chapters 19 and 20 we discuss the cholinesterase inhibitors and memantine, respectively. In Chapter 21 whether vitamins, herbs, supplements, and antiinflammatory medications are helpful is discussed. Chapter 22 presents some nonpharmacological strategies to help compensate for memory loss including diet and exercise. Finally, in Chapter 23 some of the possible future treatments for Alzheimer's disease are explored.

TREATING COGNITION AND TREATING BEHAVIOR

Patient JH is a 73-year-old retired high school music teacher who has been having memory and related problems for about a year. He recognizes his memory problems and is anxious to be treated. He lives with his wife and has two children who live nearby. He seems to be in generally good spirits with no symptoms of anxiety or depression. There is no sign of agitation. He sleeps well

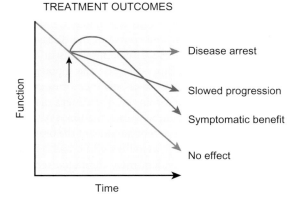

Fig. 18.1 Possible treatment outcomes.

and his appetite and energy level are unchanged. There are no psychiatric symptoms such as hallucinations, delusions, or thought disorder. His primary deficit is in recent memory; he forgets conversations by the next day and cannot remember to take his medications. He also has some recent word-finding problems. We diagnosed him with Alzheimer's disease dementia and then had a discussion with the patient, his wife, and his daughter regarding treatments.

Patient EB is an 84-year-old woman who is living with her two nieces. She moved to the United States at age 22, never married, and worked in the fashion industry in New York, retiring at age 65 years. She has memory problems (denies having conversations which she had and constantly repeats questions), problems with executive functioning (she has great difficulty managing her finances and has inappropriately given away money), and visuospatial functioning (she can become lost walking in her neighborhood). She also entirely denies any cognitive deficits and does not understand why she needs to live with her nieces. She is agitated and this agitation is expressed by constantly berating her nieces, denying her problems, and attempting to wander in the neighborhood. Her nieces are extremely frustrated in attempting to care for her. We diagnosed her with Alzheimer's disease dementia and then had a discussion with the patient and her nieces regarding treatments.

Although both of these patients have the same diagnosis, it is clear that they each present with different treatment needs. Both patients are experiencing cognitive problems, the hallmark of Alzheimer's disease, that require treatment. But patient EB also has what has come to be known as the behavioral and psychological symptoms of dementia (BPSD) (Finkel, 2001, 2002). These behavioral and psychiatric symptoms can manifest in a variety of ways, including hallucinations, delusions, depression, anxiety, and agitation (which can also be expressed in a variety of ways; see Chapter 24). Although it does not occur in all cases of dementia, by some estimates 50% to 90% of Alzheimer's disease patients will experience one or more behavioral and psychiatric symptoms during the course of the disease. Some symptoms, such as depression, occur relatively early in the disease, whereas other symptoms, such as agitation and delusions, tend to occur later in the disease. Whenever they occur, in many cases these behavioral and psychiatric symptoms are more distressing to the family and patient than the cognitive problems and as such demand treatment. In some cases, behavioral and psychiatric symptoms can be treated with behavioral techniques, but often medication is necessary. We will consider diagnosing and treating these symptoms in more detail in Section IV: *Behavioral and Psychological Symptoms of Dementia*. For now, we simply want to acknowledge the presence of this important aspect of Alzheimer's disease treatment. In this section we will focus on treating the cognitive aspect of the disease.

REFERENCES

Calhoun, A., King, C., Khoury, R., et al. (2018). An evaluation of memantine ER + donepezil for the treatment of Alzheimer's disease. *Expert Opinion of Pharmacotherapy*, 19(15), 1711–1717.

Finkel, S. I. (2001). Behavioral and psychological symptoms of dementia: A current focus for clinicians, researchers, and caregivers. *Journal of Clinical Psychiatry*, 62(Suppl. 21), 3–6.

Finkel, S. I. (2002). Behavioral and psychological symptoms of dementia. Assisting the caregiver and managing the patient. *Geriatrics*, 57, 44–46.

19

Cholinesterase Inhibitors

QUICK START: CHOLINESTERASE INHIBITORS	
Mechanism of action and cognitive benefit	• Cholinesterase inhibitors increase the concentration of acetylcholine at the synapse and improve memory, attention, mood, and behavior. • Cholinesterase inhibitors are efficacious and well tolerated.

Indications and recommendations	• For Alzheimer's disease dementia in mild, moderate, and severe stages, we recommend using one of the following once-a-day cholinesterase inhibitor formulations:
	  • Donepezil (generic and Aricept) pill or oral dissolving tablet
	  • Galantamine (generic) extended-release (ER) pill
	  • Rivastigmine (generic and Exelon) patch

Common side effects	• Some common and important side effects are (listed in approximate order of prevalence):
	  • Gastrointestinal: loose stools, loss of appetite, nausea, vomiting, weight loss
	  • Vivid dreams at night
	  • Rhinorrhea
	  • Salivation
	  • Muscle cramps
	  • Bradycardia
	• Cholinesterase inhibitors should not be used in patients with peptic ulcer disease, several other conditions, and certain medications (see text).
	• To evaluate for risk of heart block we recommend obtaining an electrocardiogram (ECG) in all patients started on cholinesterase inhibitors.

Judging efficacy	• It is important to set appropriate expectations as to the magnitude of the average improvement observed with cholinesterase inhibitors: • Most patients improve equivalent to "turning the clock back" 6 to 12 months. • To determine whether the cholinesterase inhibitor is working, ask the patient, ask the family, and evaluate the patient's cognition and function 2 to 3 months after starting the medication.

Off-label uses	• We also recommend a trial of cholinesterase inhibitors in the following disorders:
	  • Mild cognitive impairment due to Alzheimer's disease
	  • Dementia with Lewy bodies (Parkinson's disease dementia) (U.S. Food and Drug Administration approved for rivastigmine [Exelon], off-label for other cholinesterase inhibitors)
	  • Vascular dementia

CHOLINESTERASE INHIBITORS IN ALZHEIMER'S DISEASE

There are currently four cholinesterase inhibitors approved by the U.S. Food and Drug Administration (FDA) for the treatment of Alzheimer's disease dementia (Table 19.1): tacrine (Cognex, no longer marketed), donepezil (generic and Aricept), rivastigmine (generic and Exelon), and galantamine (generic, formerly marketed as Razadyne and Reminyl) (Yiannopoulou & Papageorgiou, 2020). These drugs all work in essentially the same way: they bind to and reversibly inhibit acetylcholinesterase, the enzyme responsible for metabolizing acetylcholine in the synapse (Fig. 19.1). By doing this they increase the level of acetylcholine in the synapse. By increasing the level of acetylcholine in the synapse, the cholinesterase inhibitors are hypothesized to improve cognition. Although no one understands exactly how that happens, one hypothesis is as follows. In most regions of the brain, any individual neuron will receive input from tens or hundreds of other neurons. Because in Alzheimer's disease neurons—particularly cholinergic neurons—are dying, there are fewer cholinergic neurons from which to receive input. The idea is that if the acetylcholine from the remaining cholinergic neurons can bind to the synaptic receptor more times before the acetylcholine is broken down, these remaining neurons will be able to compensate for those neurons which are damaged or dead. There are two basic decisions that a clinician must make regarding the cholinesterase inhibitors:

1. Should I prescribe a cholinesterase inhibitor for my patient with Alzheimer's disease or other dementia?
2. If so, which one should I prescribe?

SHOULD I PRESCRIBE A CHOLINESTERASE INHIBITOR?

As with any medication, the decision to prescribe or not to prescribe is made on an individual basis for each patient and is based on a risk/benefit analysis. Let us consider the pros and cons of this class of medication.

Cholinesterase Inhibitors Are Well Tolerated

In our experience, supported by published clinical trials, cholinesterase inhibitors are tolerated by more than 90% of patients. The most common side effects, occurring in about 10% of patients, are gastrointestinal in nature including loss of appetite, upset stomach, mild nausea, and loose stools. These side effects are the result of muscarinic cholinergic receptors in the gut. In the majority of cases, these gastrointestinal side effects subside in a few days and are not of any notable distress to the patients. In a small percentage of cases, the gastrointestinal side effects are more serious and include nausea and vomiting or loose stools. In these cases, the patient should either stop taking the medication or reduce the dose. The gastrointestinal side effects will then fully resolve within a few days. It is next worth trying at least one other cholinesterase inhibitor, as some patients experience more side effects with one medication than with another. Lastly it is worth trying the rivastigmine (Exelon) patch, as some patients who cannot tolerate oral cholinesterase inhibitors do fine on the 4.6 or 9.5 mg/24 h dose of the patch. Some clinicians may try to manage these side effects with antiemetic agents, but we have not found this to be a particularly helpful strategy (Table 19.2). In general, we suggest that patients take the medication in the evening so that, if they experience mild gastrointestinal side effects during the peak concentrations (these generally occur within 2–6 hours after taking cholinesterase inhibitors), they can sleep through them.

A second common side effect is vivid dreams. These dreams are not nightmares; they are the dreams the patient normally has, just more vivid. These are brought about by the role of brainstem cholinergic systems in producing rapid-eye movement (REM) sleep (dream sleep). Vivid dreams are generally characterized by our patients as being extremely realistic and lifelike. In some instances, patients find these disturbing; in other cases, they are neutral about them; and occasionally, they even find them enjoyable. In cases where patients find these unpleasant, vivid dreams can usually be minimized or eliminated by moving the dosing of the medication to earlier in the day. This will cause the peak concentration of the medication to be during waking hours and the troughs at night.

Other less common side effects reported in the clinical trials of cholinesterase inhibitors are dizziness, insomnia, and headache. Other side effects of note in our clinical experience (and also reported in controlled studies) are rhinorrhea (runny nose), increased salivation, muscle cramping, fasciculations, rash, and rarely seizures or a slowing of the heart rate (one of our

Drug	Mechanism of Action	Half-Life Metabolism/ Elimination	Dosing (Therapeutic Doses in Italics)	Common Side Effects	Comment	FDA Approved	Demonstrated Efficacy
Donepezil (generic and Aricept)	Inhibits acetylcholinesterase	70–80 h liver; CYP450; 2D6; 3A4/urine and feces	Once daily • *5 mg QD* *4 weeks* • *10 mg QD* *3 months* • *23 mg QD* (for moderate to severe patients; see text before prescribing)	Nausea, vomiting, anorexia, diarrhea	Generally well tolerated. Also comes in same strength oral dissolving tablet	Alzheimer's disease. 5 mg QD: mild to moderate; 10 mg QD: mild, moderate, and severe; 23 mg QD: moderate to severe	Cognition (memory, attention), mood, behavior
Rivastigmine (generic and Exelon) capsule	Inhibits acetylcholinesterase (also inhibits butylcholinesterase)	2 h plasma; CYP450/urine 97%, feces 0.4%	Twice daily • *1.5 mg BID* *4 weeks* • *3 mg BID* *4 weeks* • *4.5–6 mg BID*	Nausea, vomiting, anorexia, diarrhea; side effects more frequent than with others	Side effects less if taken with food and titrated slowly	Mild, moderate Alzheimer's disease	Cognition (memory, attention), mood, behavior
Rivastigmine (generic and Exelon) patch	Inhibits acetylcholinesterase (also inhibits butylcholinesterase)	2 h but in continuous release patch plasma; CYP450/urine 97%, feces 0.4%	Once daily • *4.6 mg/24 h QD patch 4 weeks* • *9.5 mg/24 h QD patch* • *13.3 mg/24 h QD patch*	Nausea, vomiting, anorexia, diarrhea; these side effects equal to or less than others; also rash/skin irritation	Well tolerated. Patch should be removed slowly and carefully to reduce skin irritation	Mild, moderate, and severe Alzheimer's disease and mild, moderate Parkinson's disease dementia	Cognition (memory, attention), mood, behavior
Galantamine (generic, formerly Razadyne and Reminyl)	Inhibits acetylcholinesterase (also has allosteric nicotinic modulation)	5–7 h liver partially; CYP450; 2D6; 3A4/urine 95%, feces 5%	Twice daily • *4 mg BID* *4 weeks* • *8 mg BID* *4 weeks* • *12 mg BID*	Nausea, vomiting, anorexia, diarrhea; 12 mg dose side effects more frequent	12 mg dose highly efficacious; side effects less if taken with food	Mild, moderate Alzheimer's disease	Cognition (memory, attention), mood, behavior

(Continued)

Drug	Mechanism of Action	Half-Life Metabolism/ Elimination	Dosing (Therapeutic Doses in Italics)	Common Side Effects	Comment	FDA Approved	Demonstrated Efficacy
Galantamine (ER) (generic, formerly Razadyne and Reminyl)	Inhibits acetylcholinesterase (also has allosteric nicotinic modulation)	5–7 h, released immediately and 12 h later (metabolism/ elimination as galantamine)	Once daily • 8 mg QD 4 weeks • *16 mg QD* 4 weeks • *24 mg QD*	Nausea, vomiting, anorexia, diarrhea 24 mg dose side effects more frequent	24 mg dose highly efficacious; side effects less if taken with food	Mild, moderate Alzheimer's disease	Cognition (memory, attention), mood, behavior
Memantine (generic)	Glutamate antagonist (also dopamine agonist)	60–80 h liver minimally; CYP450/urine	Twice daily • 5 mg QAM 1 week • 5 mg BID 1 week • 10 mg QAM, 5 mg QPM 1 week • *10 mg BID*	Confusion, drowsiness	Can be taken with acetylcho-linesterase inhibitors	Moderate, severe Alzheimer's disease	Cognition (attention, alertness), mood, behavior
Memantine XR (Namenda XR)	Glutamate antagonist (also dopamine agonist)	60–80 h liver minimally; CYP450/urine	Once daily • 7 mg QAM 1 week • 14 mg QAM 1 week • 21 mg QAM 1 week • *28 mg QAM*	Confusion, drowsiness	Can be taken with acetylcho-linesterase inhibitors. Capsule can be opened and sprinkled on food.	Moderate, severe Alzheimer's disease	Cognition (attention, alertness), mood, behavior

Normal cholinergic synapse

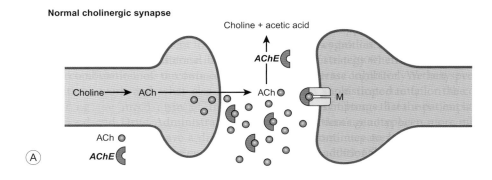

Cholinergic synapse – Alzheimer's disease

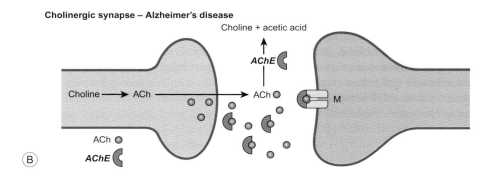

Cholinergic synapse – Alzheimer's disease
AChE inhibitor

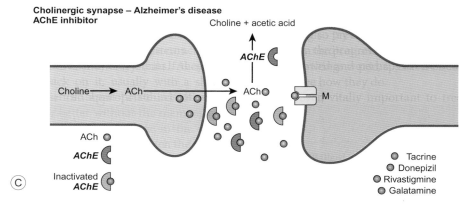

Fig. 19.1 Cholinesterase inhibitor mechanism of action. **(A)** Normal cholinergic synapse with muscarinic receptor *(M)*. Note the large number of acetylcholine *(ACh)* molecules. Acetylcholinesterase *(AChE)* breaks down acetylcholine into choline and acetic acid. **(B)** Cholinergic synapse in Alzheimer's disease. Because the neurons that produce acetylcholine in the nucleus basalis of Mynert are being damaged and destroyed by Alzheimer's disease pathology, there are many fewer molecules of acetylcholine available. **(C)** The cholinesterase inhibitors tacrine, donepezil, rivastigmine, and galantamine reversibly inhibit acetylcholinesterase such that more molecules of acetylcholine are available in the synapse.

TABLE 19.2   Selected Side Effects of Cholinesterase Inhibitors and Possible Management Techniques

Side Effect	Possible Management Technique
Loss of appetite	Take at night or reduce dose
Nausea	Take at night or reduce dose
Vomiting	Reduce dose
Diarrhea/loose stools	Can try over-the-counter loperamide, once or twice a week to reduce bowel movements to 1 or 2 per day. Or reduce dose
Vivid dreams	Take in the morning. Or reduce dose. Or switch to immediate-release galantamine given only in the morning
Dizziness	Depends upon the cause; investigate swiftly whether this could be a sign of bradycardia (slowing of the heart rate)
Dehydration	Determine cause, increase hydration, and/or reduce dose
Insomnia	Take in the morning or reduce dose
Headache	Reduce dose
Rhinorrhea (runny nose)	Can try ipratropium nasal spray 0.06% as needed for social occasions. Or reduce dose
Salivation	Can try ipratropium nasal spray 0.06% in the mouth as needed for social occasions. Or reduce dose
Muscle cramps	Increase water intake, increase electrolyte intake including eating bananas (for potassium) and taking over-the-counter magnesium oxide, or reduce dose
Fasciculations	Reduce dose
Rash	Discontinue immediately. Can later try another cholinesterase inhibitor
Bradycardia (slowing of the heart rate)	Discontinue immediately, and immediately initiate an inpatient cardiac evaluation including continuous cardiac monitor
Seizure	If single brief seizure, reduce dose and initiate seizure evaluation. If multiple or prolonged, discontinue immediately and initiate seizure evaluation

Note: This table contains some of the common and/or serious side effects that our patients have experienced and some strategies that we have found to be successful in dealing with these side effects. It is not meant to be an exhaustive list nor a substitute for clinical judgment. When in doubt regarding a serious side effect, discontinue the cholinesterase inhibitor and fully evaluate the patient.

patients developed syncope and ultimately required a pacemaker). Because of this latter symptom of bradycardia that could be related to heart block, we recommend obtaining an electrocardiogram (ECG) on all patients prescribed cholinesterase inhibitors after they have been on the highest dose of the drug for several weeks, in addition to cautioning patients about the signs and symptoms of bradycardia. We recommend caution in prescribing cholinesterase inhibitors when patients have any of the conditions in Box 19.1. Cholinesterase inhibitors may interact with many other medications. Although in our experience few of these interactions are clinically important, it is important to be aware of them. The most important interactions are related to the characteristics found in Box 19.2. Please consult an up-to-date reference, website, or application when evaluating potential drug interactions in your patient.

Cholinesterase Inhibitors Are Efficacious

Comprehensive reviews of the efficacy of cholinesterase inhibitors generally conclude that the drugs have modest benefits in some, but not all, patients. For example, one comprehensive review carried out by the Cochrane Database of Systematic Reviews (Birks & Harvey,

---

BOX 19.1   Serious Reactions and Conditions That Either Contraindicate or Require Caution When Prescribing Cholinesterase Inhibitors

- Hypersensitivity to the specific drug or class of medications
- Hypersensitivity to cholinergic medications such as succinylcholine
- Syncope/cardiac conduction disorders/sick sinus syndrome/bradycardia—can cause or worsen bradycardia or heart block
  - Check an electrocardiogram in patients prescribed cholinesterase inhibitors
- Seizures and seizure disorders—can lower seizure threshold
- Asthma and chronic obstructive pulmonary disease—can increase secretions and/or cause bronchospasm
- Gastrointestinal bleeding and/or peptic ulcer disease—can worsen peptic ulcer disease
- Concomitant use of nonsteroidal antiinflammatory drugs—can increase risk of peptic ulcer disease
- Urinary obstruction—can worsen bladder obstruction
- Hepatic impairment—can raise cholinesterase inhibitor levels
- Renal impairment—can raise cholinesterase inhibitor levels (particularly for galantamine)
- Anesthesia or surgery—can interact with anesthetic agents and/or paralytics
- Weight <55 kg (121 lbs)—may need a lower than standard dose

Note: This box contains some of the more serious side effects, cautions, and contraindications of the cholinesterase inhibitors that have been reported. It is not meant to be an exhaustive list nor a substitute for clinical judgment. When in doubt regarding a serious side effect, discontinue the cholinesterase inhibitor and fully evaluate the patient. When in doubt regarding whether to start a medication, consult expert colleagues or do not start the cholinesterase inhibitor.
Modified from online.epocrates.com, donepezil, galantamine, and Exelon, accessed September 13, 2014.

BOX 19.2   Cholinesterase Inhibitors Interaction Characteristics

- CYP2D6 substrate
- CYP3A4 substrate
- Bradycardia
- Cholinergic effects
- Lowers seizure threshold

Modified from online.epocrates.com, donepezil, galantamine, and Exelon, accessed September 13, 2014.

This conclusion is certainly consistent with our clinical experience using these drugs in thousands of patients. We have found that in most, but not all, of our patients there is benefit in terms of both cognitive function and daily activities. When we talk to the caregivers, their most common description of the patient taking these medications is that not only do these medications improve memory but also that the patient is "more with it." By this description they mean that the patient is more engaged in family activities, more likely to participate in day-to-day activities in the home such as setting the table or walking the dog, and more likely to engage in conversation in social situations. How much improvement should we and caregivers expect to see? Both studies (for review see Cummings, 2004) and our experience suggest that for the majority of patients the response to cholinesterase inhibitors is equivalent to "turning back the clock" on their disease by 6 to 12 months. In other words, we expect that their memory and general level of functioning will return to where they were 6 to 12 months ago (see Fig. 18.1). For these reasons as well as the data from well-done research studies, we generally recommend a trial on one of these drugs to our patients with Alzheimer's disease.

Thus it is clear from the preceding discussion that cholinesterase inhibitors are safe and effective in the majority of patients. But how do we know if a cholinesterase inhibitor is working in an individual patient?

IS THE MEDICATION WORKING?

One of the thorniest problems facing the practicing clinician who treats patients with Alzheimer's disease is how to judge the benefit (or lack thereof) of an antidementia drug in an individual patient. In our clinical research setting, each patient undergoes a comprehensive cognitive evaluation during most visits. These visits

2018) concluded that, in patients with mild, moderate, or severe dementia due to Alzheimer's disease, those treated with cholinesterase inhibitors showed benefit in cognitive function, activities of daily living, and clinician-rated global clinical state. Additionally, clinicians who were blinded to the results of these objective cognitive tests judged patients on cholinesterase inhibitors to be doing better than patients on placebo.

can take between 1 and 1.5 hours. By using the data from these evaluations in conjunction with interviewing the patients and caregivers we can make highly reliable judgments regarding the efficacy of the treatment. But we certainly recognize that this type of evaluation is not feasible in the context of a busy primary care or even specialty practice. The challenge then becomes to find techniques to judge the efficacy of treatment that work day-to-day in a busy practice setting.

In addition to speaking with the patient and family, we would recommend two general strategies for evaluating the effects on cognition of antidementia compounds. The first is to use a brief objective measure of cognition. The second is to use a global measure of overall functioning of the patient. As the reader may recognize, these strategies are similar to criteria used to measure drug benefit in clinical trials of antidementia compounds.

In terms of visit frequency, we generally see the patient 2 to 3 months after starting a cholinesterase inhibitor and then every six months thereafter.

Measuring Cognition

As discussed in Chapter 2 and in Appendix A, there are numerous brief measures of cognition that can be used to assess the efficacy of cholinesterase inhibitors. Probably the two that are most commonly used are the Mini-Mental State Examination (MMSE) (Folstein, Folstein, & McHugh, 1975) and the Montreal Cognitive Assessment (MoCA) (www.mocatest.org) test. Each of these can be administered in about 10 minutes by office staff. In general, after successful treatment with cholinesterase inhibitors patients tend to improve two or three points on the MMSE and the MoCA.

Measuring General Functioning

In contrast to measures of cognition, there are few measures of general functioning that are appropriate for the practicing clinician. Rather than using a specific instrument, we tend to use a structured interview that generally asks about three areas: cognition, mood and behavior, and function. The interview is typically carried out in about 10 minutes, with the patient and caregiver either together or separately (Table 19.3). At the end of the interview, we attempt to arrive at a judgment as to whether the patient shows:
- Marked improvement
- Moderate improvement

- Mild improvement
- Unchanged
- Mild worsening
- Moderate worsening
- Marked worsening.

Box 19.3 provides some guidelines that we find helpful in determining whether a particular patient is functioning better or worse. We often find it helpful to compare the results of the current interview with the interview we conducted when we initially evaluated the patient to determine how things have changed. If our judgment is that the patient is unchanged or improved in the initial follow-up visit, we take this as evidence that the drug is having benefit—especially when this judgment is supported by the results of a brief cognitive test. (Remember that the expectation is that over a six-month period the patient will decline.) If the patient is only mildly worse, we also typically extend treatment for another six months. For patients who are moderately or markedly worse, we question whether the medication is working, and we would often try another cholinesterase inhibitor.

Sudden Changes

A word of caution when the patient is moderately or significantly worse. If there are sudden and rapid changes we consider the possibility of a medical or psychiatric condition that may affect cognition. The most common medical conditions include a urinary tract infection or pneumonia, either one of which can have dramatic deleterious effects on cognition in our experience. Strokes and other more serious conditions can, of course, also occur. The most common psychiatric conditions, especially early in the disease when the patient maintains insight, are depression and anxiety. In these cases, treating the medical or psychiatric condition will often improve cognition.

WHICH CHOLINESTERASE INHIBITOR SHOULD I PRESCRIBE?

There are currently three FDA-approved cholinesterase inhibitors available. How should a clinician choose? In general, this decision can be made based on four factors: efficacy, safety and tolerability, convenience for the patient/caregiver, and cost. Sample instructions that we give to the patient and family can be found in Box 19.4.

TABLE 19.3   Brief Clinical Interview for Follow-Up Visits

Instructions: Note changes in any of the following cognitive areas. If there are changes, you may find it helpful to briefly note the nature of the changes (i.e., what area has improved or worsened)

	Yes (A Change) (Better or Worse?)	No (No Change)	N/S (Not Sure)
Forgetting information over short periods of time			
Repeating stories or questions about events of the day			
Difficulty handling financial matters (e.g., problems with checkbook or paying bills)			
Problems with judgment (e.g., poor financial decisions, difficulty making decisions)			
Confusion about the correct day, date, month, or year			
Seeming bewildered or confused in a familiar setting			
Difficulty learning something new (e.g., learning to use a new appliance, gadget, or computer program)			
Social withdrawal (e.g., participating less in conversations)			
Loss of interest in usual activities (e.g., hobbies)			
Difficulty with everyday activities (e.g., self-care or dressing, household tasks, finding one's way around, using appliances such as telephone or television)			

BOX 19.3   Criteria for Improvement or Worsening of General Function

- **Mild improvement:** A noticeable improvement in the patient's functioning, social interactions, or mental clarity in any aspect of performance, capabilities, tendencies, or tolerances. The change should be noticeable enough to make a difference in some aspect of day-to-day function and behavior even if it does not result in any greater independence for the patient.
- **Moderate improvement:** Similarly defined but with the additional requirement that some measure of functional independence—social, instrumental, cognitive—has been regained.
- **Marked improvement:** Carries the additional requirement that a major activity in the patient's daily routine or in mental status has been regained, in addition to regaining some measure of functional independence.

- **Mild worsening:** A noticeable decline in patient's functioning, social interactions, or mental clarity in any aspect of performance, capabilities, tendencies, or tolerances. The change should be noticeable enough to make a difference in some aspect of day-to-day function and behavior even if it does not result in any greater dependence on the part of the patient.
- **Moderate worsening:** Similarly defined but with the additional requirement that, on some measure, functional dependence has emerged.
- **Marked worsening:** Carries the additional requirement that a major activity in the patient's daily activity or mental status has been lost, in addition to loss of functional independence on some measure.

Efficacy and Tolerability

Was Joe Louis a better boxer than Mohammed Ali? Were the 1927 Yankees better than the 1998 Yankees? These questions can lead to interesting and sometimes contentious conversation in the local sports bar and they are the stuff that computer simulations are made of. But no amount of debate, discussion, or contention, and no computer program can answer these questions. There is only one way to solve the debate: the 1927 Yankees would have to play the 1998 team on the same

BOX 19.4 Example of Cholinesterase Inhibitor Instructions Given to Patients and Families

Instructions for Donepezil

- You have been started on a new medication today, called donepezil. You should begin taking a 5 mg tablet once daily. After one month, you should increase to 10 mg once daily.
- You can take it any time of day.
- This medicine works by increasing the concentration of a substance in the brain called acetylcholine, which is involved in memory, attention, mood, and behavior.
- **Possible side effects:** This medicine is well tolerated by the majority of patients. But like all medications, there are potential side effects. Some of the most common are reviewed here. Please contact us with any problems.
  - About 1 in 10 patients experience a loss of appetite, loose stools or an increased infrequency of bowel movements, or nausea. Rarely, there can be vomiting. If you experience these side effects, try taking the medication before bed.
  - About 1 in 15 patients experience vivid dreams. If you experience this side effect, try taking the medication in the morning.
  - About 1 in 100 patients experience an increase in saliva, runny nose, or muscle cramps.
  - About 1 in 1000 patients experience slowing of the heart, which can cause one to feel faint, or to faint.
- After you have been on the 10 mg dose for 1 month, you should have an electrocardiogram (ECG) performed by your primary care provider.
- **Follow-up:** Please schedule a follow-up in 2–3 months so we can see how you are doing on the medicine.

field (artificial turf or grass), with the same baseball (live vs. dead ball era), in the same weather, with the same fans. In short, we would need to have "head-to-head" competition.

Is rivastigmine (Exelon) better than galantamine? Is galantamine better than donepezil (Aricept)? There are dozens of studies on each of these drugs individually reporting efficacy and safety. And while it is tempting to compare the percentage of patients who experience side effects on each drug or the number of points that each drug differs from placebo in each trial, these are entirely inappropriate comparisons. Although on the surface the studies appear to have similar patients, designs, and outcome measures, the only way to answer this question (as in the sports analogy) is to conduct a head-to-head comparison. That is, test multiple cholinesterase inhibitors in the same study with the same group of patients, the same experimental design, and the same outcome measures.

The results of the head-to-head studies do not yield any clear choice. To date there have been relatively few head-to-head trials comparing the effects of different cholinesterase inhibitors. The data from the majority of these trials are difficult to interpret because they were conducted using an "open-label design," that is, the patients knew what drugs they were taking (Bullock et al., 2005; Jones et al., 2004; Wilcock et al., 2003; Wilkinson et al., 2002).

In our experience, donepezil (Aricept) at doses of 5 and 10 mg is equally efficacious and well tolerated as galantamine ER (extended release) at doses of 8 and 16 mg. Galantamine ER at the 24 mg dose is probably equivalent to 15 mg (a nonstandard dose) of donepezil (Aricept); in each case the efficacy is greater than the lower dose but so are the side effects. Our clinical experience suggests that the rivastigmine (Exelon) capsule may have somewhat more side effects than either galantamine ER or donepezil (Aricept) at therapeutic doses, consistent with one of the open-label trials (Wilkinson et al., 2002). However, our experience is also that the rivastigmine (Exelon) patch is both efficacious and may have the least gastrointestinal side effects of any cholinesterase inhibitor formulation at the 4.6 and 9.5 mg/24 h doses.

In brief, there is no reason to believe that one cholinesterase inhibitor is more or less effective than any other.

Convenience

Besides efficacy and tolerability, a third factor that can lead to favoring one cholinesterase inhibitor over another is convenience (Table 19.1). Two primary factors seem important: (1) how frequently is the drug taken and (2) how complex is the titration scheme.

Remembering to take medications is challenging for everyone. It is especially challenging for patients with memory problems. Because of this, medications that are taken less frequently may be desirable.

WHAT IS THE BEST DOSE?

In general, the higher the dose of a cholinesterase inhibitor the greater the efficacy but also the greater the likelihood of side effects. Most studies of cholinesterase inhibitors have found that higher doses are more efficacious than lower doses. But higher doses are more likely to produce side effects, typically loss of appetite, nausea, vomiting, and loose stools as discussed. So the prescribing clinician will generally attempt to achieve a balance of using the highest dose without producing side effects.

Each of the three cholinesterase inhibitors mentioned provides instructions in the labeling to guide the clinician through a tested titration scheme (Table 19.1). Our experience suggests that these titration schemes work for most patients who can achieve the highest dose in the absence of side effects. In some cases, however, an even more gradual titration scheme may help some patients achieve the highest recommended dose.

For example, the common titration scheme for donepezil (Aricept) is that the patient begins with a dose of 5 mg once per day, taken in the evening. This dose continues for one month and, if it is well tolerated, the dose is increased to 10 mg, the highest recommended dose for mildly affected patients. In some cases, the patient tolerates the 5 mg dose with no side effects, but when the dose is increased to 10 mg he or she may experience gastrointestinal distress or other side effects. In these cases, we immediately return the patient to the 5 mg dose until the side effects resolve. We may then attempt a slower titration schedule. For example, we may have them alternate 5 and 10 mg doses (5 mg every other day with 10 mg on the alternate days) for several weeks before increasing to 10 mg daily. In some patients we have found that this will help them tolerate the higher dose. For some patients 5 mg in the morning and 5 mg in the evening is easier than 10 mg all at once. And although not quite as good as 10 mg/day, 5 mg daily is a perfectly acceptable dose. Note that some clinicians (including us) have used donepezil off-label in a 15 mg dose. Again, the logic is that, for those who can tolerate the dose, more is better. A 23 mg dose of donepezil is also available for patients with moderate to severe Alzheimer's disease. Patients can be tried on this higher dose after being on the 10 mg dose for three months. Our experience is that although there may be greater efficacy, few patients can tolerate it, and we rarely use the 23 mg

dosage. Note that transdermal donepezil administration is being developed (Bashyal et al., 2020), and a once-a-week donepezil patch may soon be approved by the FDA (https://www.nia.nih.gov/alzheimers/clinical-trials/donepezil-transdermal-patch).

For galantamine we would generally recommend the extended release (galantamine ER) formulation as it is both once-a-day and it is also better tolerated than the older, immediate release, galantamine. Both 16 mg and 24 mg are good therapeutic doses. The 24 mg dose may have somewhat greater efficacy but also somewhat more frequent side effects compared with the 16 mg dose. As mentioned above, in our experience 16 mg of galantamine ER is roughly equivalent to 10 mg of donepezil (Aricept), and 24 mg of galantamine ER is roughly equivalent to 15 mg of donepezil (Aricept).

For rivastigmine (Exelon) we would always recommend the patch as it is both once-a-day and also better tolerated than the capsules. Studies have shown that 9.5 mg/24 h is a good therapeutic dose; we have also found that a lower dose of 4.6 mg/24 h is the best dose for some patients who are particularly sensitive to cholinesterase inhibitors. The patch has one particular side effect which is related to its being a patch: there can be skin irritation when it is removed. Although there is some debate regarding the exact cause of this irritation, in our experience it is at least in part local irritation related to how the patch is pulled off. The patch should be pulled off slowly. It should not be pulled off quickly like a Band-Aid. The patch sticks on very tight. The strong adhesive has the advantage of allowing the patient to swim and shower with it—without it falling off. But it has the disadvantage that it must be carefully taken off, usually slowly by the caregiver using two hands, one to lift up the patch, and one to hold down the skin. Additional instructions can be found on the comprehensive package insert.

WHEN SHOULD THE MEDICATIONS BE TAKEN?

Donepezil (generic and Aricept) is taken once a day. In general, we start patients taking the drug in the evening. The rationale is that, if they experience mild gastrointestinal side effects, they will sleep through them. But another common side effect of donepezil (Aricept) is vivid dreams. These are not nightmares and most cases are not disturbing to patients—some patients even enjoy these dreams—but in some cases patients do complain of these dreams. In these cases we recommend that the patients take the medication in the morning and this usually alleviates the vivid dreams. For galantamine ER we usually start patients taking the drug in the morning and then switch to evening if needed to help reduce gastrointestinal side effects. We would note that we occasionally use a single morning dose of immediate release galantamine for those patients who have severe problems with vivid dreams at night; because of its short half-life, the morning dose of immediate release galantamine is mostly gone by bedtime. For the rivastigmine (Exelon) patch the medication is delivered continuously, such that the time of day the new patch is applied does not matter.

DOES IT HELP TO SWITCH MEDICATIONS?

One question that often comes up is whether switching from one cholinesterase inhibitor to another might be beneficial in terms of either efficacy or side effects. Although the medications all work in the same way so that in theory there is no reason why a patient should show greater benefits or side effects on one medication than another, in practice there is some variability of response, both real and perceived. If shortly after starting one cholinesterase inhibitor there is not only no improvement but also no stabilization (or there is a decline), and/or there are notable side effects, we may try another cholinesterase inhibitor. Everyone is different, and some patients do better with one medication than another. Note, however, that in our clinic switching is uncommon and we will end up doing this in fewer than one in 25 patients.

In a different scenario, sometimes after a patient has been on a cholinesterase inhibitor for a time, either the patient or the family will ask whether switching to another cholinesterase inhibitor might provide him or her with more benefit. As long as the patient had a good response initially, we would recommend that he or she continue the current medication as it is unlikely that the patient will benefit more from one cholinesterase inhibitor than another, and the new medication may not work as well as the original. We may try increasing the dose of the cholinesterase inhibitor.

HOW DO I DISCUSS WITH THE PATIENT WHETHER THE CHOLINESTERASE INHIBITOR IS WORKING?

Determining whether an antihypertensive medication is efficacious is a straightforward process: you measure blood pressure and ask about side effects. Determining whether an antidementia compound is working is more complex for several reasons, as follows.

- As discussed, we do not have a "blood pressure cuff" for cognition. There is no single, readily used measure that is appropriate in day-to-day practice that gives an accurate measure of changes in cognition.
- The patient may be benefiting from the antidementia medication even if there is no apparent symptomatic improvement. About half of our patients and their families report improved cognition with the use of cholinesterase inhibitors. But the other half report no change. No change, however, may actually be a benefit in a progressive degenerative disease such as Alzheimer's. Any drug that can "turn the clock back" on this decline is beneficial. But conveying this information to patients and their families can be challenging.

When we treat patients with cholinesterase inhibitors, we try first to explain (1) what is happening in their brain, (2) how these drugs affect the ongoing process in their brain, (3) what they can expect from these drugs, and (4) how we will measure this. We often draw a graph similar to Figure 18.1 showing the "no treatment" and "symptomatic benefit" lines so that they know what to expect in the future. The conversation might proceed as follows:

Mrs. Jones, as we have discussed, the cause of your memory and related problems is Alzheimer's disease. Alzheimer's is a brain disease. What is happening in your brain is that brain cells called neurons are slowly dying. Unlike cells in other parts of your body, brain cells do not regenerate. Once they die they are lost forever. Although the drug that you will be taking will not prevent these brain cells from dying, it can help with the symptoms of your disease—your thinking and memory—by allowing the remaining brain cells to function more efficiently. By doing this we hope that we can turn the clock back on your brain disorder. If the medication is working we will expect that your thinking and memory will return to how they were about 6 to 12 months ago. So, we would not expect any huge changes, but we do hope to see small but noticeable and important changes. We will see you back in 2 to 3 months to get a sense as to how you are doing and whether the medication is working. Even if you do not notice any changes, the medication may still be working. We will talk with you and your family and we will also give you tests of memory, much like the ones you have already done in this clinic. We will decide together at that time whether to continue the medication or try another. After that we will see you about every 6 months. Many of our patients ask if we can stop the decline of Alzheimer's disease. With the medications currently available we cannot. Although we can turn the clock back on your memory loss, we cannot stop the clock from ticking down; we cannot stop decline that occurs over time. However, the vast majority of people do benefit from this medication, and there are new medications being developed every day, many of which do have the potential to slow down or halt this disease.

We have found that, when we establish appropriate expectations at the beginning of the medication trial, patients are more likely to remain on medication for a long enough period of time to determine if it is indeed providing benefit. As discussed, using Table 19.3 and Box 19.3 for measuring the general functional outcome can be useful, along with talking with the patient, talking with family or other caregivers, and (if possible) repeating a brief cognitive test.

CHOLINESTERASE INHIBITORS IN LATE-STAGE DISEASE

Donepezil (generic and Aricept) is FDA approved to treat severe Alzheimer's disease, and in our experience all of the cholinesterase inhibitors can be helpful to preserve function and delay nursing home placement in late-stage disease (Howard et al., 2015). For this reason, we would always continue the patient's cholinesterase inhibitor into the severe stage of Alzheimer's disease dementia (supported by Howard et al., 2012). We

recommend discontinuing the cholinesterase inhibitor when the patient is no longer able to enjoy any aspect of life and the goal of treatment changes to that of trying to help the patient die with comfort and dignity. Typically, this occurs after the patient has been living in a nursing home for a number of years, can no longer feed him- or herself, and no longer takes any pleasure in visits with family members. Within two weeks of discontinuing the cholinesterase inhibitor the patient generally shows a fairly dramatic decline in function (equivalent to about a 6- to 12-month decline), which generally hastens death.

We also recommend starting a cholinesterase inhibitor in the severe stage of the disease as long as there is function that one wishes to preserve. The one difference in starting a cholinesterase inhibitor at this stage of Alzheimer's disease is that we do not expect to see benefit or even stabilization. All the studies of patients with severe Alzheimer's disease have consistently shown less decline, rather than improvement or stabilization, with cholinesterase inhibitors compared with control.

HUPERZINE A

Huperzine A is a cholinesterase inhibitor that is derived from the Chinese folk medicine *Huperzia serrata* (Qian & Ke, 2014). It is licensed in China as a treatment for Alzheimer's disease and is available in the U.S. as a nutraceutical (not regulated by the FDA). There is reasonably good evidence that shows huperzine A is effective in Alzheimer's disease and perhaps vascular dementia as well (Xing et al., 2014). The usual starting dose is 100 micrograms twice a day, increasing after one month to 200 micrograms twice a day—the dose used most often in clinical trials of the compound. Our experience is that it does indeed work similarly to other cholinesterase inhibitors but is less potent, perhaps equivalent to 2.5 or 5 mg of donepezil. The other issue with all nutraceuticals is that there are no real standards or quality controls. We therefore use huperzine A infrequently. We typically suggest it when patients refuse standard medications and want to use only natural, herbal remedies. If patients are going to purchase it we recommend they do so at a large national pharmacy chain, with the presumption that the pharmacy will make sure that the drug is relatively pure and the dose is accurate.

CHOLINESTERASE INHIBITORS IN OTHER DISORDERS

Should cholinesterase inhibitors be used in disorders other than Alzheimer's disease? Other causes of dementia? Other memory disorders? There are a number of studies that have examined the use of cholinesterase inhibitors in disorders other than Alzheimer's disease, and we have had experience using cholinesterase inhibitors in these plus a few additional disorders (Box 19.5). As discussed in the relevant chapters, there are a number of well-conducted randomized double-blind placebo-controlled trials examining the use of cholinesterase inhibitors in mild cognitive impairment due to Alzheimer's disease (e.g., Petersen et al., 2005), vascular dementia (e.g., Moretti et al., 2003), and Parkinson's disease dementia (dementia with Lewy bodies) (e.g., McKeith et al., 2000). The majority of these studies have found benefit with cholinesterase inhibitors. Further, the FDA has approved the rivastigmine (Exelon) patch for Parkinson's disease dementia. Our clinical experience in all of these disorders is similar: we believe that cholinesterase inhibitors are of benefit, with patients showing improvement of the same order of magnitude as patients with Alzheimer's disease experience. Therefore we generally recommend or prescribe cholinesterase inhibitors for patients with mild cognitive impairment due to Alzheimer's disease, vascular dementia, and Parkinson's disease dementia (dementia with Lewy bodies), just as we would for Alzheimer's disease.

There are a few additional disorders that we have also had positive experience with using cholinesterase inhibitors and/or there are suggestive studies (though not necessarily randomized, double-blind, and placebo-controlled). There are a number of studies that have examined either multiple sclerosis (Christodoulou et al., 2006) or traumatic brain injury (Kim et al., 2009), almost all of which found that cholinesterase inhibitors showed benefit. Our experience is similar: patients with multiple sclerosis and traumatic brain injury generally show benefit from cholinesterase inhibitors, particularly if memory and/or attention is one of the major problems for these patients. Although there are few or no studies to support it, we have also found that patients who experience memory problems because of single strokes or tumor resections may also benefit from cholinesterase inhibitors. In general, we find that as a class the cholinesterase inhibitors are medications that can improve memory, regardless of the underlying cause of the memory loss. Therefore if there are patients who experience memory loss from other disorders (e.g., encephalitis), we would be willing to give a trial of a cholinesterase inhibitor to see if it is helpful.

Lastly, there are a few disorders in which we would not recommend cholinesterase inhibitors or we would recommend using extreme caution. Patients with frontotemporal dementias typically do not benefit from cholinesterase inhibitors. There is no biochemical deficit of acetylcholine in frontotemporal dementia, and our experience is that sometimes these patients become further agitated and/or disinhibited when given a cholinesterase inhibitor. Similarly, we would tend to avoid cholinesterase inhibitors in patients with bipolar disorder, or other tendencies toward mania. Please also see Box 19.1 for additional disorders that require caution in the use of cholinesterase inhibitors.

BOX 19.5 Other Disorders to Consider the Use of Cholinesterase Inhibitors

- Mild cognitive impairment (MCI) due to Alzheimer's disease
- Dementia with Lewy bodies
- Vascular dementia
- Multiple sclerosis impairing memory
- Traumatic brain injury impairing memory
- Chronic traumatic encephalopathy impairing memory
- Single strokes impairing memory
- Tumor resection impairing memory

REFERENCES

Bashyal, S., Shin, C. Y., Hyun, S. M., et al. (2020). Preparation, characterization, and in vivo pharmacokinetic evaluation of polyvinyl alcohol and polyvinyl pyrrolidone blended hydrogels for transdermal delivery of donepezil HCl. *Pharmaceutics*, *12*(3), E270.

Birks, J. S., & Harvey, R. J. (2018). Donepezil for dementia due to Alzheimer's disease. *Cochrane Database of Systematic Reviews*, *6*(6), CD001190.

Bullock, R., Touchon, J., Bergman, H., et al. (2005). Rivastigmine and donepezil treatment in moderate to moderately-severe Alzheimer's disease over a 2-year period. *Current Medical Research and Opinion*, *21*, 1317–1327.

Christodoulou, C., Melville, P., Scherl, W. F., et al. (2006). Effects of donepezil on memory and cognition in multiple sclerosis. *Journal of the Neurological Sciences, 245,* 127–136.

Cummings. J. L. (2004). Alzheimer's disease. *The New England Journal of Medicine, 351,* 56–67.

Folstein, M. F., Folstein, S. E., & McHugh, P. R. (1975). A practical method for grading the cognitive state of patients for the clinician. *Journal of Psychiatric Research, 12,* 189–198.

Howard, R., McShane, R., Lindesay, J., et al. (2012). Donepezil and memantine for moderate-to-severe Alzheimer's disease. *The New England Journal of Medicine, 366,* 893–903.

Howard, R., McShane, R., Lindesay, J., et al. (2015). Nursing home placement in the Donepezil and Memantine in Moderate to Severe Alzheimer's Disease (DOMINO-AD) trial: Secondary and post-hoc analyses. *Lancet Neurology, 14*(12), 1171–1181. https://doi.org/10.1016/S1474-4422(15)00258-6.

Jones, R. W., Soininen, H., Hager, K., et al. (2004). A multinational, randomised, 12-week study comparing the effects of donepezil and galantamine in patients with mild to moderate Alzheimer's disease. *International Journal of Geriatric Psychiatry, 19,* 58–67.

Kim, Y. W., Kim, D. Y., Shin, J. C., et al. (2009). The changes of cortical metabolism associated with the clinical response to donepezil therapy in traumatic brain injury. *Clinical Neuropharmacology, 32,* 63–68.

McKeith, I., Del Ser, T., Spano, P., et al. (2000). Efficacy of rivastigmine in dementia with Lewy bodies: A randomised, double-blind, placebo-controlled international study. *Lancet, 356,* 2031–2036.

Moretti, R., Torre, P., Antonello, R. M., et al. (2003). Rivastigmine in subcortical vascular dementia: A randomized, controlled, open 12-month study in 208 patients. *American Journal of Alzheimer's Disease and Other Dementias, 18,* 265–272.

Petersen, R. C., Thomas, R. G., Grundman, M., et al. (2005). Vitamin E and donepezil for the treatment of mild cognitive impairment. *The New England Journal of Medicine, 352,* 2379–2388.

Qian, Z. M., & Ke, Y. (2014). Huperzine A: Is it an effective disease-modifying drug for Alzheimer's disease? *Frontiers in Aging Neuroscience, 6,* 216.

Wilcock, G., Howe, I., Coles, H., et al. (2003). A long-term comparison of galantamine and donepezil in the treatment of Alzheimer's disease. *Drugs & Aging, 20,* 777–789.

Wilkinson, D. G., Passmore, A. P., Bullock, R., et al. (2002). A multinational, randomised, 12-week, comparative study of donepezil and rivastigmine in patients with mild to moderate Alzheimer's disease. *International Journal of Clinical Practice, 56,* 441–446.

Xing, S. H., Zhu, C. X., Zhang, R., et al. (2014). Huperzine A in the treatment of Alzheimer's disease and vascular dementia: A meta-analysis. *Evidence-Based Complementary and Alternative Medicine: eCAM, 2014,* 363985.

Yiannopoulou, K. G., & Papageorgiou, S. G. (2020). Current and future treatments in Alzheimer disease: An update. *Journal of Central Nervous System Disease* 2020;12:1179573520907397.

Memantine

Memantine (Namenda) was approved by the U.S. Food and Drug Administration (FDA) for the treatment of moderate to severe Alzheimer's disease in 2003. In 2014 twice-daily Namenda was discontinued, once-daily Namenda extended-release (XR) was introduced, and sometime later twice-daily memantine became available as generic. Memantine has become the second most widely used drug after donepezil (Aricept) to treat Alzheimer's disease.

MECHANISM OF ACTION

Memantine has an entirely different mechanism of action than the cholinesterase inhibitors. There are, in fact, at least two mechanisms of action for memantine that may be clinically relevant: modulating glutamate and enhancing dopamine transmission.

Modulating Glutamate Transmission

Memantine acts on neurons that use glutamate as a neural transmitter. Glutamate is the most abundant excitatory neural transmitter in the central nervous system, present in about 40% of synapses, and it is critical for learning and memory (Stanley et al., 2017). Numerous preclinical studies conducted in animals have shown that, when glutamate synapses are blocked, new memories cannot be formed (Ryu, Kim, & Lee, 2020). Additionally, there is evidence that the amnesia produced in humans from anoxia (e.g., oxygen deficiency due to cardiac arrest) is the result of the death of glutamatergic neurons.

When glutamate is released from the presynaptic neuron, it crosses the synapse and affects one or a number of different kinds of receptors on the postsynaptic neuron. One of these is the N-methyl-D-aspartic acid (NMDA) receptor. The NMDA receptor appears to be the crucial receptor in the formation of new memories. Memantine acts by regulating the NMDA receptor (Fig. 20.1).

Enhancing Dopamine Transmission

In addition to its effects at the NMDA receptor, there is also much evidence that memantine is a dopamine agonist. It stimulates dopamine receptors in vitro (Peeters, Maloteaux, & Hermans, 2003), increases dopaminergic function in animal models (Takahashi et al., 2018), and patients with Parkinson's disease show improvement in their parkinsonian symptoms (Moreau et al., 2013). Why memantine has this effect is not entirely clear, but it is structurally similar to amantadine (Symmetrel), which is a known dopamine agonist used to treat patients with Parkinson's disease (Fig. 20.2).

WHICH PATIENTS SHOULD TAKE MEMANTINE?

Memantine has been approved in Europe for the treatment of vascular dementia since the 1980s. The initial research using memantine for Alzheimer's disease was begun in the mid-1990s. Unlike the cholinesterase inhibitors, which are FDA approved for patients with mild, moderate, and severe Alzheimer's disease dementia, memantine is FDA approved only for patients in the moderate to severe stages of the disease (about Mini-Mental State Examination [MMSE] score <15 and Montreal Cognitive Assessment [MoCA] score <11). Clinical trials in this stage of disease have shown that the magnitude of the benefit of the drug is smaller than that seen with cholinesterase inhibitors (Knight et al., 2018), although there have been no head-to-head studies. Memantine has also been shown to benefit Alzheimer's disease dementia patients who are residing in nursing homes (Winblad & Poritis, 1999).

EFFICACY OF MEMANTINE

A number of randomized, double-blind studies have demonstrated that, compared with placebo, patients with moderate to severe Alzheimer's disease dementia treated with memantine do better in terms of both objective cognitive tests and clinician ratings (Grossberg et al., 2013; Reisberg et al., 2003; Winblad & Poritis, 1999). Cognitively, memantine mainly improves attention and alertness. Most importantly, all the studies with memantine show improvements in social engagement and function.

What we hear most from families regarding patients in the moderate to severe stage of Alzheimer's disease are statements like, "He's got his spark back!," or "I've got the old Joe back," or "He's more like his old self." Other comments include the patient being more alert, talkative, engaged, outgoing, and "brighter" overall. Sometimes the results from patients in the severe stage of the disease can be quite dramatic.

One of our patients was severely impaired although still able to live at home because she was not incontinent or agitated. She went to daycare 5 days a week, and would mainly spend her time napping in a chair there. We started her on memantine and after about 4 weeks received this phone message that was saved on our voicemail:

I think the medicine is helping her, she seems a little bit more alert, she's talking a little more, and she seems to be happier. I called the daycare and they can tell a difference with her, she's not sleeping as much as she has, and she's doing more joking,

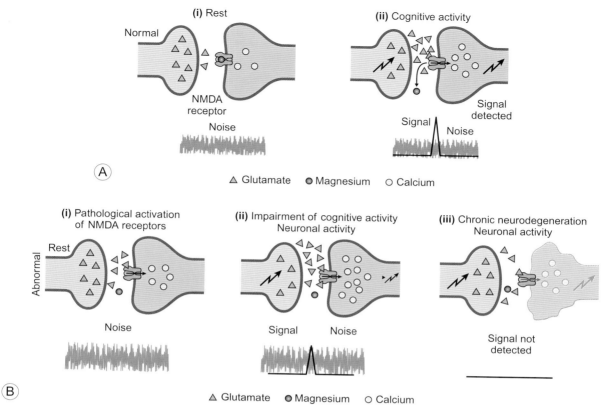

Fig. 20.1 Possible mechanism of action of memantine (Namenda) at the *N*-methyl-D-aspartic *(NMDA)* receptor. **(A)** Normal physiological function of the NMDA receptor. (i) At rest the presynaptic neuron *(left)* is filled with glutamate and a magnesium ion blocks the channel of the NMDA receptor on the postsynaptic neuron *(right)*. Very few glutamate molecules are in the synaptic cleft. (ii) During cognitive activity an action potential *(lightning arrow)* reaches the presynaptic neuron, (1) glutamate is released from the presynaptic neuron, (2) interacts with the NMDA receptor on the postsynaptic neuron, (3) the magnesium ion pops off, (4) calcium enters the cell, and (5) an action potential *(lightning arrow)* is generated in the postsynaptic neuron. If we had an electrode measuring the current of the postsynaptic receptor we would find a low level of noise at rest (i), and enough of a calcium signal to rise up above the level of the noise, triggering an action potential in the postsynaptic neuron (ii). **(B)** Pathological state owing to Alzheimer's disease. (i) Because of Alzheimer's disease, cells are dying, releasing their intracellular stores of glutamate, and thus too much glutamate is in the extracellular fluid. Some of this excess glutamate finds its way into the synaptic cleft and interacts with the NMDA receptor, causing the magnesium ion to pop off and calcium to trickle into the cell—even though no action potential has occurred. This trickle of calcium into the cell causes a high level of noise. (ii) Now when an action potential *(lightning arrow)* reaches the presynaptic neuron *(left)*, again glutamate is released from the presynaptic neuron and interacts with the NMDA receptor of the postsynaptic neuron *(right)*. But this time, because the magnesium ion has already popped off and calcium has been trickling into the cell, the signal cannot be detected above the high level of noise, and an action potential cannot be generated. (iii) Additionally, when calcium chronically trickles into cells it is toxic to them, killing the cells. **(C)** Memantine restores physiological function. (i) The pathological state due to Alzheimer's disease [same as B(i)]. (ii) Despite there being too much glutamate in the extracellular fluid, stimulating the NMDA receptor, memantine sits in the ion channel—like a "super" magnesium ion—stopping calcium from trickling into the cell, and reducing the noise to a normal, low level. (iii) When the action potential *(lightning arrow)* reaches the presynaptic neuron on the left and a large amount of glutamate is released, it again interacts with the NMDA receptor of the postsynaptic neuron. Now the memantine molecule pops off just like the magnesium ion and calcium can enter the cell, propagating the action potential *(lightning arrow)* in the postsynaptic neuron, and physiological function is restored. (From Parsons, C. G., Danysz, W., & Quack, G. (1999). Memantine is a clinically well tolerated *N*-methyl-D-aspartate (NMDA) receptor antagonist: A review of preclinical data. *Neuropharmacology, 38*, 735–767; Parsons, C. G., Stoffler, A., & Danysz, W. (2007). Memantine: An NMDA receptor antagonist that improves memory by restoration of homeostasis in the glutamatergic system: too little activation is bad, too much is even worse. *Neuropharmacology 53*, 699–723.)

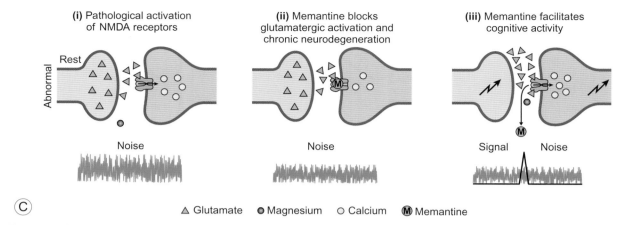

Fig. 20.1 (*Continued*)

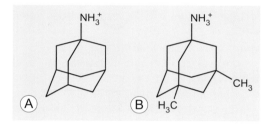

Fig 20.2 Chemical structure of amantadine (Symmetrel [**A**]) and memantine (Namenda [**B**]).

and she seems to be happy. She hasn't had any side effects from what I can see, so maybe it's a good sign …

SAFETY AND TOLERABILITY OF MEMANTINE

In general, memantine is a well-tolerated drug. The most common side effects reported during the clinical trials were headache, constipation, dizziness, agitation, and confusion. None of these, however, occurred significantly more in patients treated with memantine than in those treated with placebo (and agitation was actually numerically less than those treated with placebo).

The most common side effects that we routinely see with memantine (generic and Namenda) are confusion and drowsiness. That confusion and drowsiness are common side effects means that one needs to be careful in prescribing this medication, because confusion and drowsiness are common in any patient with dementia, and it can sometimes be tricky in sorting out when confusion is caused by a medication side effect and when it is simply a part of the dementia (or due to an infection, etc.). However, if you, as the clinician, always evaluate the patient after he or she has been started on the medication as described below, it should be possible to distinguish between these possibilities without too much difficulty.

One potentially interesting aspect of these side effects is that we tend to observe them more in patients with milder disease. As discussed below, we will sometimes prescribe memantine to patients in the mild stage of Alzheimer's disease, and in our experience it is these patients who are most likely to encounter difficulties with confusion and/or drowsiness.

SHOULD I PRESCRIBE GENERIC MEMANTINE OR NAMENDA XR?

Both generic memantine and Namenda XR are effective and well tolerated. The main benefit of Namenda XR is once-a-day dosing. The benefit of generic memantine is cost. Which formulation you prescribe should depend upon factors relevant to the patient and caregiver. Most of our patients are already taking medications twice a day and it is not difficult to add generic memantine to their morning and evening medications. For patients who are only taking medications once a day, however, the convenience and simplicity of the once-daily Namenda XR may be more important than cost—particularly if the patient lives alone. Lastly, the Namenda XR capsule can be opened and the contents sprinkled on food such as applesauce.

TITRATING MEMANTINE

Generic memantine is taken twice daily and is titrated over a four-week period to the maximum dose of 20 mg/day (10 mg, BID); brand-name Namenda XR is also titrated over a four-week period but it is taken once daily with a maximum dose of 28 mg/day (Tables 19.1 and 20.1). Higher doses of memantine are more efficacious and, in the absence of side effects at the lower doses, the goal is to titrate patients to the highest dose. We generally provide patients with one prescription for the titration pack (blister pack) that takes them through the four-week titration and another prescription for either generic memantine 10 mg BID or Namenda XR 28 mg QD with instructions to fill the second prescription if they do not experience side effects during the titration period. In our experience, most patients have no difficulty with the titration. We typically see them back in two to three months to evaluate the medication's benefit and any side effects, with the instructions to call us sooner if they experience dizziness, drowsiness, confusion, or other side effects.

If patients do experience side effects, it is almost always dose related; that is, there is usually a dose in which they were doing well, and we have now exceeded that dose. We encourage patients (with their family's help) to decrease the medication until they reach a dose that provides the desired benefits (improved attention, alertness, etc.) without side effects.

COMBINING MEMANTINE WITH CHOLINESTERASE INHIBITORS

Because memantine and the cholinesterase inhibitors work on different neurotransmitter systems, it is a reasonable hypothesis that combining the two medications would provide more benefit than either alone.

Indeed, a number of studies have shown that adding memantine to cholinesterase inhibitors produces additional benefit. The first of these studies was carried out in 404 patients with moderate to severe Alzheimer's disease (MMSE 5–14) who were stable on donepezil (Aricept) (Tariot et al., 2004). These patients were typically taking donepezil (Aricept) at 10 mg for an average duration of

| TABLE 20.1   Memantine Generic and Namenda XR Titration ||
Generic Memantine	Namenda XR
• Week 1: 5 mg QAM	• Week 1: 7 mg QD
• Week 2: 5 mg BID	• Week 2: 14 mg QD
• Week 3: 10 mg QAM, 5 mg QPM	• Week 3: 21 mg QD
• Week 4: 10 mg BID	• Week 4: 28 mg QD

approximately two years. In this double-blind study, half of the patients were randomized to a group that added memantine (Namenda) to the donepezil (Aricept) and the other half added a placebo. At the end of a 24-week period, patients on the combination therapy were doing significantly better than patients taking Aricept alone. There are also data for patients taking either rivastigmine (Exelon) (Olin et al., 2010) or galantamine (Porsteinsson et al., 2008) along with memantine (Namenda).

Two retrospective studies have looked at the effects of combining memantine and cholinesterase inhibitors over longer periods of time. Lopez et al. (2009) found that time to nursing home placement was delayed by cholinesterase inhibitors alone and that this effect was significantly augmented when memantine (Namenda) was added. Interestingly (and we would argue importantly) there was no change in time to death for either cholinesterase inhibitors alone or in combination with memantine (Lopez et al., 2009). Atri et al. (2008) analyzed a large amount of retrospective data and were able to look at cognitive function and activities of daily living for up to four years, again finding a significant benefit of combination therapy over cholinesterase inhibitors alone in patients with very mild, mild to moderate, and moderate to severe Alzheimer's disease. These latter data are particularly interesting because this benefit was found in patients with very mild Alzheimer's disease, although the largest effects were seen in patients with moderate to severe disease.

In general, we have found that most patients tolerate the combination of a cholinesterase inhibitor and memantine about as well as they tolerate these medications individually. Based on the results of the studies reviewed above and on our clinical experience, we typically start our patients with Alzheimer's disease on a cholinesterase inhibitor, titrating them to their highest tolerated dose. We generally add memantine (generic or

Namenda XR) when patients reach the moderate stage of disease (MMSE <15, MoCA <11), continuing the cholinesterase inhibitor. We then evaluate the patient to make sure that the memantine is providing additional benefit—and not the side effects of drowsiness or confusion.

MEMANTINE IN THE MILD STAGE OF ALZHEIMER'S DISEASE

Whereas the data strongly suggest that memantine is beneficial for the treatment of patients with Alzheimer's disease in the moderate to severe stages of dementia, the data regarding patients in earlier stages of Alzheimer's disease are equivocal, with some studies showing benefit and others not. Similarly, the studies that have been conducted adding memantine to donepezil (Aricept) in mild Alzheimer's disease have not shown any additional benefit over taking donepezil alone. Based on these data, the FDA did not grant an approval of memantine for mild disease.

Nevertheless, some clinicians feel that they have seen patients in earlier disease stages benefit from memantine, and we see many patients with mild Alzheimer's disease who come to our clinic already taking this medication "off-label." The first thing that we do in this situation is to ask the patient and family if they recall any improvement when they started memantine. If there is a clear consensus that the patient became better on it, we leave them on it. In the more common scenario, in which no one is sure if there was any benefit, we take the patient off of memantine for one month, to see if they actually improve. If they are the same or actually improved off of memantine, they stay off it. If they are worse, we put them back on it, usually with a short titration. In our experience, about two-thirds of mild patients are the same or better without the memantine. Note that if we take them off memantine in the mild stage, we may still try it again when they reach the moderate stage of disease.

MEMANTINE IN OTHER DEMENTIAS

Should memantine (generic or Namenda XR) be used in other dementias? Several published studies address this issue. Memantine showed benefit in a large-scale study of patients with vascular dementia (MMSE ranging from 12 to 20) (Orgogozo et al., 2002). Improvements were seen on the MMSE, a cognitive scale (ADAS-cog), as well as a behavioral scale (Nurses' Observational Scale for Geriatric Patients). A somewhat smaller study found that memantine provided benefit in patients with dementia with Lewy bodies and Parkinson's disease dementia (Aarsland et al., 2009). This study found improvement in these patients cognitively in their speed on attentional tasks, and most importantly on the Clinical Global Impression of Change. Treatment in patients with frontotemporal dementia has been more mixed, with benefits found in some patients and studies but not in others (Boxer et al., 2009; Diehl-Schmid et al., 2008; Swanberg, 2007), with the largest and best-controlled trial showing no overall benefit (Boxer et al., 2013).

Our clinical experience parallels these studies. We find that most of our patients with vascular dementia and dementia with Lewy bodies (or Parkinson's disease dementia) benefit from memantine, particularly when they reach the moderate to severe stage of these disorders, or when they are experiencing problems with alertness, attention, or apathy. Our experience in patients with frontotemporal dementias is mixed. Some patients seem to benefit significantly, whereas other patients show no change or a decrement in function. This variability in the response to memantine in frontotemporal dementia may reflect differences in either clinical phenotype or in the underlying pathophysiology.

In short, we will generally try memantine in patients with vascular dementia or dementia with Lewy bodies in the same manner as if they had Alzheimer's disease. In patients with frontotemporal dementias we will sometimes also try memantine, but explain to the family that this medication may or may not be helpful and could make things worse, so that we need to watch them closely to see how they do.

REFERENCES

Aarsland, D., Ballard, C., Walker, Z., et al. (2009). Memantine in patients with Parkinson's disease dementia or dementia with Lewy bodies: A double-blind, placebo-controlled, multicentre trial. *Lancet Neurology, 8*, 613–618.

Atri, A., Shaughnessy, L. W., Locascio, J. J., et al. (2008). Long-term course and effectiveness of combination therapy in Alzheimer disease. *Alzheimer Disease and Associated Disorders, 22*, 209–221.

Boxer, A. L., Knopman, D. S., Kaufer, D. I., et al. (2013). Memantine in patients with frontotemporal lobar degeneration: A multicentre, randomised, double-blind, placebo-controlled trial. *Lancet Neurology, 12*, 149–156.

Boxer, A. L., Lipton, A. M., Womack, K., et al. (2009). An open-label study of memantine treatment in 3 subtypes of frontotemporal lobar degeneration. *Alzheimer Disease and Associated Disorders, 23,* 211–217.

Diehl-Schmid, J., Forstl, H., Perneczky, R., et al. (2008). A 6-month, open-label study of memantine in patients with frontotemporal dementia. *International Journal of Geriatric Psychiatry, 23,* 754–759.

Grossberg, G. T., Manes, F., Allegri, R. F., et al. (2013). The safety, tolerability, and efficacy of once-daily memantine (28 mg): A multinational, randomized, double-blind, placebo-controlled trial in patients with moderate-to-severe Alzheimer's disease taking cholinesterase inhibitors. *CNS Drugs, 27,* 469–478.

Knight, R., Khondoker, M., Magill, N., et al. (2018). A systematic review and meta-analysis of the effectiveness of acetylcholinesterase inhibitors and memantine in treating the cognitive symptoms of dementia. *Dementia and Geriatric Cognitive Disorders, 45*(3–4), 131–151.

Lopez, O. L., Becker, J. T., Wahed, A. S., et al. (2009). Long-term effects of the concomitant use of memantine with cholinesterase inhibition in Alzheimer disease. *Journal of Neurology, Neurosurgery, and Psychiatry, 80,* 600–607.

Moreau, C., Delval, A., Tiffreau, V., et al. (2013). Memantine for axial signs in Parkinson's disease: A randomised, double-blind, placebo-controlled pilot study. *Journal of Neurology, Neurosurgery, and Psychiatry, 84*(5), 552–555.

Olin, J. T., Bhatnagar, V., Reyes, P., et al. (2010). Safety and tolerability of rivastigmine capsule with memantine in patients with probable Alzheimer's disease: A 26-week, open-label, prospective trial (Study ENA713B US32). *International Journal of Geriatric Psychiatry, 25,* 419–426.

Orgogozo, J. M., Rigaud, A. S., Stoffler, A., et al. (2002). Efficacy and safety of memantine in patients with mild to moderate vascular dementia: A randomized, placebo-controlled trial (MMM 300). *Stroke, 33,* 1834–1839.

Parsons, C. G., Danysz, W., & Quack, G. (1999). Memantine is a clinically well tolerated *N*-methyl-D-aspartate (NMDA) receptor antagonist: A review of preclinical data. *Neuropharmacology, 38,* 735–767.

Parsons, C. G., Stoffler, A., & Danysz, W. (2007). Memantine: An NMDA receptor antagonist that improves memory by restoration of homeostasis in the glutamatergic system: Too little activation is bad, too much is even worse. *Neuropharmacology, 53,* 699–723.

Peeters, M., Maloteaux, J. M., & Hermans, E. (2003). Distinct effects of amantadine and memantine on dopaminergic transmission in the rat striatum. *Neuroscience Letters, 343,* 205–209.

Porsteinsson, A. P., Grossberg, G. T., Mintzer, J., et al. (2008). Memantine treatment in patients with mild to moderate Alzheimer's disease already receiving a cholinesterase inhibitor: A randomized, double-blind, placebo-controlled trial. *Current Alzheimer Research, 5,* 83–89.

Reisberg, B., Doody, R., Stoffler, A., et al. (2003). Memantine in moderate-to-severe Alzheimer's disease. *The New England Journal of Medicine, 348,* 1333–1341.

Ryu, H. H., Kim, S. Y., & Lee, Y. S. (2020). Connecting the dots between SHP2 and glutamate receptors. *The Korean Journal of Physiology & Pharmacology: Official Journal of the Korean Physiological Society and the Korean Society of Pharmacology, 24*(2), 129–135.

Stanley, J. A., Burgess, A., Khatib, D., et al. (2017). Functional dynamics of hippocampal glutamate during associative learning assessed with in vivo 1H functional magnetic resonance spectroscopy. *NeuroImage, 153,* 189–197.

Swanberg, M. M. (2007). Memantine for behavioral disturbances in frontotemporal dementia: A case series. *Alzheimer Disease and Associated Disorders, 21,* 164–166.

Takahashi, K., Nakagawasai, O., Nemoto, W., et al. (2018). Memantine ameliorates depressive-like behaviors by regulating hippocampal cell proliferation and neuroprotection in olfactory bulbectomized mice. *Neuropharmacology, 137,* 141–155.

Tariot, P. N., Farlow, M. R., Grossberg, G. T., et al. (2004). Memantine treatment in patients with moderate to severe Alzheimer disease already receiving donepezil: A randomized controlled trial. *The Journal of the American Medical Association, 291,* 317–324.

Winblad, B., & Poritis, N. (1999). Memantine in severe dementia: results of the 9M-Best Study (Benefit and efficacy in severely demented patients during treatment with memantine). *International Journal of Geriatric Psychiatry, 14,* 135–146.

21

Vitamins, Herbs, Supplements, and Antiinflammatories

QUICK START: VITAMINS, HERBS, SUPPLEMENTS, AND ANTIINFLAMMATORIES

- Vitamin D:
  - Increased risk of all-cause dementia and Alzheimer's disease has been observed in those with vitamin D deficiency.
  - We recommend vitamin D supplementation for our patients with vitamin D deficiency.
- Vitamin E:
  - Two studies were positive in patients with Alzheimer's disease, but both had issues and many other studies were negative.
  - We do not recommend vitamin E for our patients.
- B complex vitamins—folic acid, B6, B12:
  - There is much retrospective and theoretical data to suggest that these vitamins would be helpful in Alzheimer's disease.
  - A large 18-month study showed no benefit for patients with Alzheimer's disease.
  - We do not recommend B complex vitamins for our patients unless they have a B vitamin deficiency.
- *Ginkgo biloba*
  - One study was positive in patients with Alzheimer's disease, but many other studies were negative.
  - We do not recommend ginkgo for our patients.

- DHA (phosphatidylcholine docosahexaenoic acid) (fish oil):
  - Large, retrospective studies suggested that DHA may reduce the risk of Alzheimer's disease.
  - A large, multicenter, randomized, placebo-controlled trial showed no benefit.
  - We neither encourage nor discourage taking DHA for our patients.
- Antiinflammatories:
  - Several large retrospective studies suggested that nonsteroidal antiinflammatory drugs (NSAIDs) may help prevent Alzheimer's disease.
  - Several randomized controlled clinical trials for NSAIDs, cyclo-oxygenase (COX)-2 inhibitors, and minocycline showed no benefit related to Alzheimer's disease.
  - NSAIDs, COX-2 inhibitors, and minocycline all have significant side effects and risks associated with them, and we therefore do not recommend them for our patients.
- We do not recommend other over-the-counter supplements (such as Prevagen) for our patients.

Many of our patients and their families ask us about whether they should take any one of the many supplements, herbs, vitamins, or over-the-counter medications they have seen in the supermarkets or on television infomercials. Other patients are already taking some of these additives and wonder if they are doing any good or even whether they are harmful. Because many of these compounds have demonstrated or are purported to have antioxidant effects, and because oxidative stress is thought to be harmful to brain cells, there is a rational basis for hypothesizing that these drugs could slow progression of Alzheimer's disease. We generally explain this rationale to the patient and family, but we also explain to them that, unlike medication approved by the U.S. Food and Drug Administration (FDA), these supplements have not undergone careful evaluation, and, just like prescription medications, vitamins and supplements have possible risks and side effects, and the decision of whether to take them should be made by weighing the relative risks and side effects versus the potential benefits.

VITAMIN D

A study published in September 2014 of over 1500 healthy older adults found that those who had vitamin D deficiency were between 1.7 (mild deficiency) and 2.2 (severe deficiency) times more likely to develop all-cause dementia and Alzheimer's disease (Fig. 21.1) (Littlejohns et al., 2014). Since then, other studies have also found correlations between insufficient levels of vitamin D poor cognitive performance (Amini et al., 2020; Laughlin et al., 2017). However, a prior study found that vitamin D supplementation on healthy older women had no effect on cognition or the development of mild cognitive impairment (MCI) or dementia (Rossom et al., 2012). How do we reconcile these studies? The simple answer is most likely that supplementation of vitamin D is helpful if an individual's levels are low. Vitamin D levels are, in fact, low in many older adults. Moreover, there are other proven benefits of vitamin D in the older adult, such as improving bone health (when combined with calcium), and there are few reported side effects of vitamin D when taken in recommended dosages. We therefore recommend that our older adults with memory problems (whether because of normal aging or disease) either have their vitamin D levels checked or simply take vitamin D supplementation. Because there have been no positive trials in improving cognition or reducing dementia, the exact dose and form of vitamin D to recommend (D2, ergocalciferol vs. D3, cholecalciferol) is unclear at this time. The FDA recommends 400 IU (10 mcg) daily. Many guidelines recommend between 400 and 1000 IU daily, and most experts recommend the D3 (cholecalciferol) form. In our clinic we generally recommend 2000 IU of vitamin D3, or whatever dose is needed to achieve levels between 30 and 50 ng/mL. Note that there are some important and

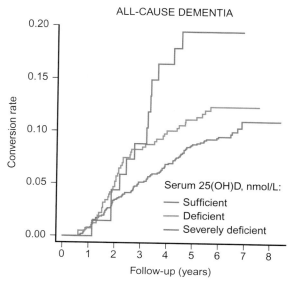

Fig. 21.1 Kaplan-Meier curves for unadjusted rates of all-cause dementia by serum 25-hydroxyvitamin D [25(OH)D] concentrations. (From Littlejohns, T. J., Henley, W. E., Lang, I. A., et al. (2014). Vitamin D and the risk of dementia and Alzheimer disease. *Neurology, 83*, 920–928.)

common drug interactions with vitamin D, including with digoxin, diltiazem, verapamil, thiazide diuretics, and others, so interactions should be checked before recommending vitamin D to your patient.

VITAMIN E

A paper published in the *New England Journal of Medicine* in 1997 reported the results of a 2-year, double-blind, placebo-controlled, randomized trial in 341 patients with mild to moderate Alzheimer's disease receiving either high doses (2000 IU/day) of vitamin E (alpha-tocopherol), selegiline 10 mg/day, both, or placebo. The results showed no statistically significant difference in the outcomes among the four groups. However, after adjustment for unequal baseline Mini-Mental State Examination (MMSE) scores by including MMSE as a covariate, all treatment groups—vitamin E, selegiline, and combined—showed better outcomes than the placebo (Sano et al., 1997). In 2014 the *Journal of the American Medical Association (JAMA)* reported the results of a double-blind, placebo-controlled, randomized trial evaluating 613 patients with mild to moderate Alzheimer's disease treated with vitamin E 2000 IU/day, memantine (Namenda) 20 mg/day, both, or placebo. The authors found that, compared with placebo, there was a slower rate of decline in the vitamin E group, but not in the memantine-alone group nor in the group treated with both vitamin E and memantine (Dysken et al., 2014). A randomized, double-blind, placebo-controlled study that evaluated vitamin E 2000 IU/day versus donepezil (Aricept) 10 mg versus placebo in over 750 patients with mild cognitive impairment over 3 years showed no benefit for vitamin E (Petersen et al., 2005). Another study examined 7540 patients with vitamin E 400 IU/day for 6 years and found no effects on the prevention of Alzheimer's disease (Kryscio et al., 2017).

How are we to best understand these somewhat conflicting data? How do we interpret a study in which there were no effects of treatment until a covariate analysis was performed to correct for unequal baseline, and then all treatments showed effects? What does it mean that another study found benefit for vitamin E alone but not when combined with memantine; does that mean that vitamin E is beneficial but memantine counteracts its beneficial effect? In our view, the data show that vitamin E provides no benefit in patients with mild cognitive impairment, and the data for the use of vitamin E in patients with mild to moderate Alzheimer's disease remain unclear. Vitamin E may increase the risk of cardiac events in individuals with vascular disease or diabetes (Miller et al., 2005), and vitamin E may cause problems with bleeding and/or easy bruising in some individuals (Traber, 2008), including hemorrhagic stroke (Browne et al., 2019).

Based upon the available data, regardless of whether they are cognitively healthy or they have been diagnosed with mild cognitive impairment or Alzheimer's disease, we do not recommend vitamin E supplementation for our patients, and if they are already taking vitamin E solely to prevent or retard Alzheimer's disease, we recommend that they discontinue it.

B COMPLEX VITAMINS: FOLIC ACID, B6, B12

On Valentine's Day in 2002, an article from the Framingham Heart Study was published in the *New England Journal of Medicine* showing that elevated plasma levels of homocysteine were a risk factor for the development of dementia and Alzheimer's disease (Seshadri et al., 2002). Later that year another study was published in the journal *Neurology* suggesting that elevated levels of homocysteine were related to cerebrovascular disease and not the plaques and tangles of Alzheimer's pathology (Miller et al., 2002).

It is well known that deficiencies of folic acid or its cofactors vitamins B6 and B12 can cause an elevation of homocysteine levels (Tinelli et al., 2019). Some studies have found that low levels of these vitamins directly correlate with cognitive decline or brain pathology (Kado et al., 2005; Scott et al., 2004). Studies have also examined whether the combination of vitamins B6, B12, and folic acid could lower the levels of homocysteine in patients with Alzheimer's disease, and found that they could (Aisen, Egelko, et al., 2003). Studies have also examined retrospectively whether individuals who took higher amounts of the vitamins folic acid, B6, or B12 were less likely to develop Alzheimer's disease. One study found that higher levels of folic acid intake (but not B6 or B12) did decrease the risk of later developing Alzheimer's disease (Luchsinger et al., 2008).

So, can we reduce the risk of developing Alzheimer's disease or perhaps slow the progression of the disorder in those already diagnosed? One very small study reported a positive effect of folic acid supplementation in those who had mild Alzheimer's disease (Connelly et al., 2008), but most studies have found no effect. A multicenter study in 409 patients with mild to moderate Alzheimer's disease over 18 months from the Alzheimer's Disease Cooperative Study (ADCS) group found no benefit to supplementation with folic acid, B6, and B12 (Aisen et al., 2008), nor did a meta-analysis of 11 trials with data for over 22,000 individuals (Clarke et al., 2014).

In summary, the data suggest the following. First, there is an association between elevated levels of homocysteine and Alzheimer's disease. Second, there is an association between elevated levels of homocysteine and cerebrovascular disease in patients with Alzheimer's disease. Third, there is also an association between low levels of folic acid and Alzheimer's disease. And fourth, levels of homocysteine were reduced in patients with Alzheimer's disease when they took supplementation with folic acid, B6, and B12. Unfortunately, despite all these promising preliminary data, there is no evidence that supplementation with folic acid, B6, and B12 has a beneficial effect in patients with Alzheimer's disease.

We therefore do not recommend supplementation with the B complex vitamins—folic acid, B6, and B12—for our patients whose vitamin B12 levels are normal. If a patient is deficient in any of these B-complex vitamins, we certainly recommend supplementation to bring the levels back to normal.

GINKGO BILOBA

We see many patients for initial evaluation who are already taking ginkgo. Ginkgo is purported to have antioxidant properties and is also purported to enhance memory. A study of ginkgo in Alzheimer's disease patients published in the *Journal of the American Medical Association* (LeBars et al., 1997) in 1997 was portrayed by the media as showing benefit in patients with Alzheimer's disease. Several more recent studies and meta-analyses have also suggested benefit (see Liu, Ye, & Guo, 2020, for review). More careful scrutiny of these studies, however, reveals that the putative benefit for Alzheimer's disease patients was minimal, and not nearly what is seen with FDA-approved medications. Moreover, there have been other randomized trials that have not shown any benefit in Alzheimer's disease patients. Other studies have shown that there is no effect of ginkgo in reducing the development of Alzheimer's disease or dementia in those with normal cognition or mild cognitive impairment (DeKosky et al., 2008). Additionally, a placebo-controlled, double-blind, randomized trial in healthy elderly also showed no cognitive benefit for ginkgo (Solomon et al., 2002).

Ginkgo is generally a safe drug, but it can have side effects. Most prominent is its anticoagulant effects. This may pose a particular risk when ginkgo is taken in conjunction with aspirin or warfarin, both of which are common in the aging population we treat. Based on the results of these studies we do not recommend *Ginkgo biloba* either as a treatment or as a preventative therapy for Alzheimer's disease.

DHA (FISH OIL)

There has been considerable interest in the potential beneficial effects on cognition and the prevention of Alzheimer's disease by DHA (phosphatidylcholine docosahexaenoic acid), an omega-3 polyunsaturated fatty acid which is found in fish oil.

In one study, researchers followed 899 men and women over a 9-year period who were part of the Framingham Heart Study (Schaefer et al., 2006). During this time, 71 of these participants developed Alzheimer's disease. But people with the highest levels of DHA in their blood had a 39% lower risk of developing Alzheimer's disease. People in this study with the highest DHA levels reported that they ate two to three servings of fish per week, much more than those with lower DHA levels. Fatty fish like mackerel, lake trout, herring, sardines, albacore tuna, and salmon are high in DHA. Based on this study and other results, the ADCS conducted a prospective, randomized trial in 295 patients over 18 months to determine whether DHA can slow the progression of Alzheimer's disease. They found that, compared with those taking placebo, patients with mild to moderate Alzheimer's disease dementia taking 2 g per day of DHA showed no benefit on cognitive tests, overall functioning, or brain volumes (Quinn et al., 2010). Other studies have suggested that DHA may be helpful in patients with mild cognitive impairment (Lee et al., 2013) or normal aging (in APOE ε4-negative individuals; Daiello et al., 2015); unfortunately, these studies are limited because of small sample size and being retrospective, respectively. Meta-analyses have suggested that DHA may be lower in individuals with either Alzheimer's disease or mild cognitive impairment (Hosseini et al., 2020).

We neither recommend nor discourage our patients from taking DHA. We certainly do recommend that they eat several servings of fish per week (see Chapter 22).

ANTIINFLAMMATORIES

A retrospective study from the Baltimore Longitudinal Study of Aging examined 1686 older individuals regarding their risk of Alzheimer's disease in relation to their use of aspirin or other nonsteroidal antiinflammatory drugs (NSAIDs). The results showed that individuals taking NSAIDs for more than 2 years—compared with aspirin or acetaminophen—were much less likely to develop Alzheimer's disease (Rich et al., 1995; Stewart et al., 1997). Other retrospective studies provided similar results (Szekely et al., 2004). The hypothesis put forth to explain this finding was that amyloid plaques could cause local inflammation in the brain, which in turn could injure neurons. In support of this hypothesis, a number of markers of inflammation including activated microglia and astrocytes, complement components, and inflammatory cytokines are associated with Alzheimer's disease (Tuppo & Arias, 2005).

Based upon these retrospective findings of disease prevention, randomized prospective studies have evaluated the use of antiinflammatories to treat patients who were already diagnosed with Alzheimer's disease. The Alzheimer's Disease Cooperative Study (ADCS) conducted a study in which patients were randomized to receive the cyclo-oxygenase (COX)-2 inhibitor rofecoxib (Vioxx), the nonspecific NSAID naproxen (Naprosyn), or a placebo. Patients with mild to moderate disease took daily doses of the assigned drug for 1 year. The results indicated that there was no change in the rate of cognitive decline in those taking rofecoxib (Vioxx) or naproxen (Naprosyn) compared with placebo (Aisen, Schafer, et al., 2003). A recent trial using the tetracycline antibiotic minocycline, which has antiinflammatory properties, both failed to slow decline in mild Alzheimer's disease and caused multiple side effects (Howard et al., 2019). Thus, despite these agents' possible use in the prevention of Alzheimer's disease, they are not helpful in treating the disease once it has already been diagnosed.

In brief, although retrospective studies suggested a benefit of NSAIDs, randomized controlled trials do not (for reviews see Gupta et al., 2015 and Wang et al., 2015). We therefore do not recommend treatment with either NSAIDs or COX-2 inhibitors for our patients with Alzheimer's disease. The controlled trials do not show benefit and the side effects and risks of these medications related to gastrointestinal bleeding and heart disease are well known.

PREVAGEN

As its advertising claims, Prevagen is the best-selling memory supplement on the market. Unfortunately, it is expensive, shows no benefit to any population, and has multiple side effects (Spence et al., 2017). For this reason, its manufacturer has been issued warnings by both the FDA and the Federal Trade Commission for making false and unsubstantiated claims (https://www.ftc.gov/news-events/press-releases/2017/01/ftc-new-york-state-charge-marketers-prevagen-making-deceptive). Needless to say, if our patients are taking Prevagen, we tell them to stop wasting their money.

REFERENCES

Aisen, P. S., Egelko, S., Andrews, H., et al. (2003). A pilot study of vitamins to lower plasma homocysteine levels in Alzheimer disease. *The American Journal of Geriatric Psychiatry, 11*, 246–249.

Aisen, P. S., Schafer, K. A., Grundman, M., et al. (2003). Effects of rofecoxib or naproxen vs placebo on Alzheimer disease progression: A randomized controlled trial. *The Journal of the American Medical Association, 289*, 2819–2826.

Aisen, P. S., Schneider, L. S., Sano, M., et al. (2008). High-dose B vitamin supplementation and cognitive decline in Alzheimer disease: A randomized controlled trial. *The Journal of the American Medical Association, 300*, 1774–1783.

Amini, Y., Saif, N., Greer, C., et al. (2020). The role of nutrition in individualized Alzheimer's risk reduction. *Current Nutrition Reports, 9*, 55–63.

Browne, D., McGuinness, B., Woodside, J. V., McKay, G. J. (2019). Vitamin E and Alzheimer's disease: What do we know so far? *Clinical Interventions in Aging, 14*, 1303–1317.

Clarke, R., Bennett, D., Parish, S., et al. (2014). Effects of homocysteine lowering with B vitamins on cognitive aging: Meta-analysis of 11 trials with cognitive data on 22,000 individuals. *The American Journal of Clinical Nutrition, 100*, 657–666.

Connelly, P. J., Prentice, N. P., Cousland, G., et al. (2008). A randomised double-blind placebo-controlled trial of folic acid supplementation of cholinesterase inhibitors in Alzheimer's disease. *International Journal of Geriatric Psychiatry, 23*, 155–160.

Daiello, L. A., Gongvatanac, A., Dunsigerd, S., et al. (2015). Association of fish oil supplement use with preservation of brain volume and cognitive function. *Alzheimer's & Dementia: The Journal of the Alzheimer's Association, 11*, 226–235.

DeKosky, S. T., Williamson, J. D., Fitzpatrick, A. L., et al. (2008). *Ginkgo biloba* for prevention of dementia: A randomized controlled trial. *The Journal of the American Medical Association, 300*, 2253–2262.

Dysken, M. W., Sano, M., Asthana, S., et al. (2014). Effect of vitamin E and memantine on functional decline in Alzheimer disease: The TEAM-AD VA cooperative randomized trial. *The Journal of the American Medical Association, 311*, 33–44.

Gupta, P. P., Pandey, R. D., Jha, D., et al. (2015). Role of traditional nonsteroidal anti-inflammatory drugs in Alzheimer's disease: A meta-analysis of randomized clinical trials. *American Journal of Alzheimer's Disease and Other Dementias, 30*, 178–182.

Howard, R., Zubko, O., Bradley, R., et al. (2019). Minocycline at 2 different dosages vs placebo for patients with mild Alzheimer disease: A randomized clinical trial [published online ahead of print, 18 Nov 2019]. *JAMA Neurology, 77*(2), 164–174.

Hosseini, M., Poljak, A., Braidy, N., Crawford, J., & Sachdev, P. (2020). Blood fatty acids in Alzheimer's disease and mild cognitive impairment: A meta-analysis and systematic review. *Ageing Research Reviews, 60,* 101043. https://doi.org/10.1016/j.arr.2020.101043.

Kado, D. M., Karlamangla, A. S., Huang, M. H., et al. (2005). Homocysteine versus the vitamins folate, B6, and B12 as predictors of cognitive function and decline in older high-functioning adults: MacArthur Studies of Successful Aging. *The American Journal of Medicine, 118,* 161–167.

Kryscio, R. J., Abner, E. L., Caban-Holt, A., et al. (2017). Association of antioxidant supplement use and dementia in the prevention of Alzheimer's disease by vitamin E and selenium trial (PREADViSE). *JAMA Neurology, 74*(5), 567–573.

Laughlin, G. A., Kritz-Silverstein, D., Bergstrom, J., et al. (2017). Vitamin D insufficiency and cognitive function trajectories in older adults: The Rancho Bernardo Study. *Journal of Alzheimer's Disease: JAD, 58*(3), 871–883.

LeBars, P. L., Katz, M. M., Berman, N., et al. (1997). A placebo-controlled, double-blind, randomized trial of an extract of *Ginkgo biloba* for dementia. North American EGb Study Group. *The Journal of the American Medical Association, 278,* 1327–1332.

Lee, L. K., Shahar, S., Chin, A.-V., et al. (2013). Docosa-hexaenoic acid-concentrated fish oil supplementation in subjects with mild cognitive impairment (MCI): A 12-month randomised, double-blind, placebo-controlled trial. *Psychopharmacology, 225,* 605–612.

Littlejohns, T. J., Henley, W. E., Lang, I. A., et al. (2014). Vitamin D and the risk of dementia and Alzheimer disease. *Neurology, 83,* 920–928.

Liu, H., Ye, M., & Guo, H. (2020). An updated review of randomized clinical trials testing the improvement of cognitive function of *Ginkgo biloba* extract in healthy people and Alzheimer's patients. *Frontiers in Pharmacology, 10,* 1688. https://doi.org/10.3389/fphar.2019.01688. Published 21 Feb 2020.

Luchsinger, J. A., Tang, M. X., Miller, J., et al. (2008). Higher folate intake is related to lower risk of Alzheimer's disease in the elderly. *The Journal of Nutrition, Health & Aging, 12,* 648–650.

Miller, E. R., 3rd, Pastor-Barriuso, R., Dalal, D., et al. (2005). Meta-analysis: High-dosage vitamin E supplementation may increase all-cause mortality. *Annals of Internal Medicine, 142,* 37–46.

Miller, J. W., Green, R., Mungas, D. M., et al. (2002). Homocysteine, vitamin B6, and vascular disease in AD patients. *Neurology, 58,* 1471–1475.

Petersen, R. C., Thomas, R. G., Grundman, M., et al. (2005). Vitamin E and donepezil for the treatment of mild cognitive impairment. *The New England Journal of Medicine, 352,* 2379–2388.

Quinn, J. F., Raman, R., Thomas, R. G., et al. (2010). Docosahexanoic acid and cognitive decline in Alzheimer's disease. *The Journal of the American Medical Association, 304,* 1903–1911.

Rich, J. B., Rasmusson, D. X., Folstein, M. F., et al. (1995). Nonsteroidal anti-inflammatory drugs in Alzheimer's disease. *Neurology, 45,* 51–55.

Rossom, R. C., Espeland, M. A., Manson, J. E., et al. (2012). Calcium and vitamin D supplementation and cognitive impairment in the women's health initiative. *Journal of the American Geriatrics Society, 60,* 2197–2205.

Sano, M., Ernesto, C., Thomas, R. G., et al. (1997). A controlled trial of selegiline, alpha-tocopherol, or both as treatment for Alzheimer's disease. The Alzheimer's Disease Cooperative Study. *The New England Journal of Medicine, 336,* 1216–1222.

Schaefer, E. J., Bongard, V., Beiser, A. S., et al. (2006). Plasma phosphatidylcholine docosahexaenoic acid content and risk of dementia and Alzheimer disease: The Framingham Heart Study. *Archives of Neurology, 63,* 1545–1550.

Scott, T. M., Tucker, K. L., Bhadelia, A., et al. (2004). Homocysteine and B vitamins relate to brain volume and white-matter changes in geriatric patients with psychiatric disorders. *The American Journal of Geriatric Psychiatry, 12,* 631–638.

Seshadri, S., Beiser, A., Selhub, J., et al. (2002). Plasma homocysteine as a risk factor for dementia and Alzheimer's disease. *The New England Journal of Medicine, 346,* 476–483.

Solomon, P. R., Adams, F., Silver, A., et al. (2002). Ginkgo for memory enhancement: A randomized controlled trial. *The Journal of the American Medical Association, 288,* 835–840.

Spence, J., Chintapenta, M., Kwon, H. I., et al. (2017). A brief review of three common supplements used in Alzheimer's disease. *The Consultant Pharmacist: The Journal of the American Society of Consultant Pharmacists, 32*(7), 412–414.

Stewart, W. F., Kawas, C., Corrada, M., et al. (1997). Risk of Alzheimer's disease and duration of NSAID use. *Neurology, 48,* 626–632.

Szekely, C. A., Thorne, J. E., Zandi, P. P., et al. (2004). Nonsteroidal anti-inflammatory drugs for the prevention of Alzheimer's disease: A systematic review. *Neuroepidemiology, 23,* 159–169.

Tinelli, C., Di Pino, A., Ficulle, E., et al. (2019). Hyperhomocysteinemia as a risk factor and potential nutraceutical target for certain pathologies. *Frontiers in Nutrition*, 6, 49.

Traber, M. G. (2008). Vitamin E and K interactions: A 50-year-old problem. *Nutrition Reviews*, 66, 624–629.

Tuppo, E. E., & Arias, H. R. (2005). The role of inflammation in Alzheimer's disease. *The International Journal of Biochemistry & Cell Biology*, 37, 289–305.

Wang, J., Tan, L., Wang, H. F., et al. (2015). Anti-inflammatory drugs and risk of Alzheimer's disease: An updated systematic review and meta-analysis. *Journal of Alzheimer's Disease: JAD*, 44, 385–396.

22

Nonpharmacological Treatment of Memory Loss, Alzheimer's Disease, and Dementia

QUICK START: NONPHARMACOLOGICAL TREATMENT OF MEMORY LOSS, ALZHEIMER'S DISEASE, AND DEMENTIA

- Nonpharmacological treatments to help memory loss can improve function equal to or greater than medication.
- External memory aids such as calendars, lists, and whiteboards can be helpful in keeping patients functional.
- It is important to keep the memory aid in the same place.
- Learning habits (using procedural memory) allow patients with even moderate Alzheimer's disease to improve their function.
- Pictures are easier to remember for patients with Alzheimer's disease.

- Music can be helpful for patients at all stages of Alzheimer's disease.
- Mediterranean-style diets have been shown to reduce the risk of memory loss and Alzheimer's disease, although their value is currently uncertain in those who have already developed dementia.
- Social and cognitively stimulating activities, as found in an enriched environment, have been shown to improve function.
- Aerobic exercise can stimulate the development of new neurons in the hippocampus, improve cognition, and reduce the risk for Alzheimer's disease in addition to its effects on cardiovascular health and mood.

Pharmacological treatment of memory loss, present or future, can only help so much when dealing with Alzheimer's and other diseases affecting memory. Nonpharmacological treatments are invaluable, and can often help daily function as much as, if not more than, medications (Burgener et al., 2009). An entire book could be written on this important subject—and, in fact, we wrote one entitled, *Seven Steps to Managing Your Memory: What's Normal, What's Not, and What to Do About It* (Budson & O'Connor, 2017), which may be helpful for those with mild memory problems. In this chapter we briefly touch on a number of relevant topics.

HELPFUL HABITS

Using a system that can become a habit is critically important when teaching a patient with memory loss new skills. Habits do not depend upon the episodic memory system—the memory system that is affected by Alzheimer's disease and most other disorders of memory. Habits depend upon a different kind of memory, procedural memory. Procedural memory is the type of memory we use when riding a bike, touch typing, playing the violin, and typing with our thumbs on our phone. It is due to procedural memory that, when we are not paying attention to where we are driving, we may make turns toward a familiar location—but not necessarily the one we had intended to go to! Procedural memory is quite well preserved in Alzheimer's disease until quite late in the disease. This preservation of procedural memory allows us to teach the patient with Alzheimer's new functional skills even when their episodic memory is devastated. Teaching by doing is the key to learning with procedural memory. Think again about learning to ride a bike; it is not learning verbally with words. See Appendix C for more on the different types of memory systems in the brain.

Here is an example. The wife of a patient with mild Alzheimer's disease has just bought a new wall calendar that she is keeping all of their appointments on. Although they had not previously used a wall calendar, she is very pleased with her new system, which works very well for her. She reports to us, however, that it is not working for her husband. He is continually asking her what they are doing for the day. Although she has told him a thousand times to go look at the calendar, he never goes on his own; he will go to it, however, after she tells him to. We then explained to her that she needs to actually lead him to the calendar each time he asks what they are doing for the day, so that "his feet can learn where to go." At first it seems like no progress is being made. But over the course of a few weeks of her leading him to the calendar every time he asks, he begins to go to look at the calendar automatically.

EXTERNAL MEMORY AIDS

Almost all of us use external devices to augment our memory. These include traditional simple items, such as a list, calendar, or organizer, as well as electronic devices including smartphones and tablets to store names, addresses, phone numbers, appointments, and other information. Before their illness, most patients with memory problems also used such devices to a greater or lesser extent. Not surprisingly, patients who always depended upon external devices are, in general, able to continue using them early on in the disorder to compensate for their declining memory. Patients who, by contrast, always depended upon their memory to keep themselves organized tend to suffer more swift and severe functional impairment as their memory declines, because they do not automatically reach for external devices to compensate for their impaired memory. As

their illness progresses, however, almost all patients would benefit from additional use of external devices to compensate for their memory problems. What follows are some of the simple ways that a number of our patients have found functional improvement in the face of memory impairment.

Calendar

Knowing the day, date, month, season, and year are important basic components of knowledge that most of us take for granted. Such knowledge is important insofar as we have appointments, meetings, lunch dates, or television shows that we want to keep, participate in, or watch. Losing track of this information is one of the first things that occurs when memory becomes impaired.

There are, of course, many different types of calendars that can be used. Early in the disease course (e.g., in mild cognitive impairment or very mild Alzheimer's disease) any of these would be fine, as a certain amount of new learning is possible. However, the best approach—and the only approach that works as the disease progresses—is to use a calendar system that can easily become a habit to the patient as described earlier

In general, we recommend a large desk or wall calendar that always stays in one place. In this way it will not become lost, and the patient with memory loss will be able to get into the habit of going there to look at it. It is important that the previous days are "crossed off," so that the patient will automatically know what the current date is.

Special Places

In the same way that the patient with memory loss can get into the habit of going to look at the calendar, they can get into the habit of going to other places as well. For example, shoes can be kept in a special place in the front hall so that there is never a search for them. Shopping lists can be kept on the left side of the refrigerator. Microwave dinners can be kept on the right-hand side of the freezer. Clothes for the next day can be laid out on a certain chair such that the patient never needs to ask what they should wear for the day. And even the order of the clothes, laid out in the same way each day, helps the patient to get dressed properly (e.g., underpants first, then pants).

At a more general level we discourage caregivers from rearranging closets or the kitchen drawers or any other organizational system with which the patient is familiar. We have even heard reports from caregivers that rearranging furniture can be a disorienting experience for the patient. Alzheimer's patients can continue to function in long-standing environments because they can rely upon their intact habits and remote memories.

Bulletin Boards and Whiteboards

Just like the calendar and special places, bulletin boards and whiteboards mounted in a fixed location can provide a way to help the patient with memory loss know what is happening.

Let's return to the patient and his wife described in the section on Habits. Several years have passed, and he is more impaired, now in the moderate stage of Alzheimer's disease. He is too impaired to read. And the calendar is now too complicated for him to figure out, even with the dates crossed off. But with the help of their daughter, they have found a new system that works. In place of the calendar, in the same spot in which it had hung, they have a magnetic board. Here they put up pictures that let the patient know what is going on that day. Using the camera on her cell phone, the daughter has taken pictures of many of the common friends and family members that they see, common places they visit, such as the post office, bank, grocery store, and a favorite restaurant, as well as activities such as walking and gardening. Each morning his wife puts up the people, places, and activities that they will be seeing, visiting, and doing that day. She tells us that she isn't sure that he can remember the things on the board for more than a minute or two, but now he simply goes and looks—sometimes 10 or 20 times in an hour—rather than asking her every time.

POWER OF PICTURES

It is said that a picture is worth a thousand words (Fig. 22.1). For patients with Alzheimer's disease, this is certainly true. Some of our research, in fact, has shown that although memory is enhanced by pictures relative to words for young adults, this effect of pictures is greater for healthy older adults, greater still for patients with mild cognitive impairment, and is the greatest for patients with Alzheimer's disease (Ally, Gold, & Budson, 2009). This enhancement of memory for pictures versus words in Alzheimer's disease is likely due to a number of things. We all tend to pay more attention to pictures. Pictures are more

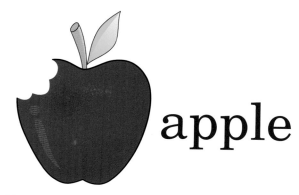

Fig. 22.1 A picture is worth a thousand words.

distinctive and therefore easier to remember. When we see a picture, we may store the information twice: once as an image and once as its meaning. And patients with Alzheimer's disease develop difficulty processing written words as the disease progresses.

The simple take-home message is this: using pictures is one way to help the patient with Alzheimer's disease remember information (Lancioni et al., 2014). So instead of simply telling the patient that his granddaughter will be visiting today, show him her picture.

MAGIC OF MUSIC

There is a magic of music that can seemingly transform a patient with even severe dementia into the younger, more vibrant individual they were when the oldies they are listening to first hit the radio waves. Patients who typically need to be cajoled to get out of their chair for any reason spontaneously rise and move to the music or even start to dance. Those who usually appear vacant are suddenly present and smiling. Others tap their feet or hands to the beat.

These well-documented effects of music, both from anecdotal reports and from published studies (Guetin et al., 2013), are probably multifactorial. They likely relate to the brain structures that music activates and the fact that songs and tunes with these effects have often been learned as a teenager and young adult. Structures activated by music include the basal ganglia and cerebellum (Rauschecker, 2014), which are relatively unaffected by Alzheimer's disease. Music learned in one's youth has been well consolidated over time, no longer depends upon the hippocampus and other medial temporal lobe structures, and is therefore relatively resistant to the effects of Alzheimer's disease (see Appendix C for more on these ideas). Lastly, our research and others' has shown that patients with mild Alzheimer's disease are more likely to remember information if it is sung to them rather than being spoken, although there is a limitation on how much specific information can be conveyed in the lyrics (Lancioni et al., 2014; Leggieri et al., 2019; Simmons-Stern, Budson, & Ally, 2010; Simmons-Stern et al., 2012).

MEDITERRANEAN-STYLE DIETS

There is now clear evidence that Mediterranean-style diets are beneficial for brain health (Boxes 22.1 and 22.2). Studies have shown, for example, that middle-aged adults are less likely to show progression of Alzheimer's disease biomarkers when they follow a Mediterranean-style diet (Berti et al., 2018) and that the MIND (Mediterranean-DASH [Dietary Approaches to Stop Hypertension] Intervention for Neurodegenerative Delay) diet slows cognitive decline (Morris et al., 2015a) and reduces the incidence of Alzheimer's disease (Morris et al., 2015b). Other studies have shown that Mediterranean-style diets are beneficial for cognition in general, and that eating fish, in particular, is key (Keenan et al., 2020). Less clear, however, is whether such benefits extend to those who already have cognitive impairment, with some studies showing benefit (de la Rubia Ortí et al., 2018), and others not (Calil et al., 2018). From these and other studies, we recommend that individuals at risk for dementia (including those with mild cognitive impairment) consider following a Mediterranean-style diet. For those who already have Alzheimer's disease or another dementia, we would not recommend that patients change their diets to something they do not like with the hope that it will slow down the progression of their dementia.

SOCIAL AND COGNITIVELY STIMULATING ACTIVITIES

A 79-year-old patient with mild Alzheimer's disease, socially isolated and living alone, comes to see us with her daughter in the clinic. She is forgetting to take her medications, and only thinks about eating when she is reminded. She scores 21 out of 30 on the Mini-Mental State Examination (MMSE). She is clearly failing at

---

BOX 22.1   Mediterranean Diet

- Fish
- Olive oil
- Avocadoes
- Fruits
- Vegetables
- Nuts
- Beans
- Whole grains

BOX 22.2   MIND (Mediterranean-DASH [Dietary Approaches to Stop Hypertension] Intervention for Neurodegenerative Delay) Diet

- Olive oil daily
- Green leafy vegetables daily
- Other vegetables daily
- Whole grains daily
- Nuts and beans every other day
- Berries 2× a week
- Poultry 2× a week
- Fish 1× a week

---

home, and the decision is made to move her to assisted living. After several weeks of acclimating in the facility, a seemingly miraculous change comes about. She is the "life" of her unit, has many friends, and now appears to have little or no difficulty in navigating her routines. In fact, she seems better than when she entered the facility over a month ago. A routine follow-up of her MMSE confirms this: she now scores 25 out of 30!

The scenario outlined is very common. Why it occurs is not exactly clear. Certainly, some of the change may be due to improvements in mood, apathy, or both. We know, however, that there are other positive psychological and neurophysiological changes that occur (Nithianantharajah & Hannan, 2009). Whatever the mechanism, when patients move from an isolated to an enriched environment, we typically see clinically relevant improvements in function.

Even if there is no change in living, it has also been proven that leisure activities, particularly those that are socially and cognitively stimulating, can be helpful in slowing memory loss, reducing the risk of mild cognitive impairment and Alzheimer's disease, reducing neuropsychiatric symptoms, and improving function (Akbaraly et al., 2009; Boyke et al., 2008; Krell-Roesch et al., 2019; Leung et al., 2010; Petersen et al., 2018).

AEROBIC EXERCISE

Probably the most important nonpharmacological activity to retard memory loss, reduce the risk of Alzheimer's disease, and actually improve memory is to participate in aerobic exercise (Scarmeas et al., 2009). It has been known for many years that in rodents aerobic exercise leads to hippocampal neurogenesis—new brain cells growing in the hippocampus. Evidence has also been found in older adults that aerobic exercise can increase brain volume (Colcombe et al., 2006; Erickson et al., 2011; Gordon et al., 2008). Most importantly, exercise has been shown to improve cognitive function (Erickson et al., 2011; Weuve et al., 2004). In addition to its benefit in healthy older adults, exercise is recommended for those with mild cognitive impairment (Petersen et al., 2018). And this benefit of exercise is in addition to the benefits to cardiovascular health and mood. Thus despite literature suggesting that exercise does not improve cognition for those who already have dementia (Lamb et al., 2018), we advocate for all of our patients to participate in aerobic exercise, such as walking or swimming. And because the studies in rodents show a linear relationship between the amount of exercise and the increase in hippocampal neurogenesis, we tell our patients and families that some exercise is good, and more is better—just as long as their heart, lungs, bones, and joints can tolerate it.

REFERENCES

Akbaraly, T. N., Portet, F., Fustinoni, S., et al. (2009). Leisure activities and the risk of dementia in the elderly: Results from the Three-City Study. *Neurology, 73*, 854–861.

Ally, B. A., Gold, C. A., & Budson, A. E. (2009). The picture superiority effect in patients with Alzheimer's disease and mild cognitive impairment. *Neuropsychologia, 47*, 595–598.

Berti, V., Walters, M., Sterling, J., et al. (2018). Mediterranean diet and 3-year Alzheimer brain biomarker changes in middle-aged adults. *Neurology, 90*(20), e1789–e1798.

Boyke, J., Driemeyer, J., Gaser, C., et al. (2008). Training-induced brain structure changes in the elderly. *The Journal of Neuroscience, 28*, 7031–7035.

Budson, A. E., & O'Connor, M. K. (2017). *Seven Steps to Managing your Memory: What's Normal, What's Not, and What To Do About it*. New York: Oxford University Press.

Burgener, S. C., Buettner, L. L., Beattie, E., et al. (2009). Effectiveness of community-based, nonpharmacological interventions for early-stage dementia: Conclusions and recommendations. *Journal of Gerontological Nursing, 35*, 50–57.

Calil, S. R. B., Brucki, S. M. D., Nitrini, R., et al. (2018). Adherence to the Mediterranean and MIND diets is associated with better cognition in healthy seniors but not in MCI or AD. *Clinical Nutrition ESPEN, 28*, 201–207.

Colcombe, S. J., Erickson, K. I., Scalf, P. E., et al. (2006). Aerobic exercise training increases brain volume in aging humans. *The Journals of Gerontology. Series A, Biological Sciences and Medical Sciences, 61*, 1166–1170.

de la Rubia Ortí, J. E., García-Pardo, M. P., Drehmer, E., et al. (2018). Improvement of main cognitive functions in patients with Alzheimer's disease after treatment with coconut oil enriched Mediterranean diet: A pilot study. *Journal of Alzheimer's Disease: JAD, 65*(2), 577–587.

Erickson, K. I., Voss, M. W., Prakash, R. S., et al. (2011). Exercise training increases size of hippocampus and improves memory. *Proceedings of the National Academy of Sciences of the United States of America, 108*(7), 3017–3022.

Gordon, B. A., Rykhlevskaia, E. I., Brumback, C. R., et al. (2008). Neuroanatomical correlates of aging, cardiopulmonary fitness level, and education. *Psychophysiology, 45*, 825–838.

Guetin, S., Charras, K., Berard, A., et al. (2013). An overview of the use of music therapy in the context of Alzheimer's disease: A report of a French expert group. *Dementia (London), 12*, 619–634.

Keenan, T. D., Agrón, E., Mares, J. A., et al. (2020). Adherence to a Mediterranean diet and cognitive function in the Age-Related Eye Disease Studies 1 & 2. *Alzheimer's & Dementia: The Journal of the Alzheimer's Association, 16*(6), 831–842.

Krell-Roesch, J., Syrjanen, J. A., Vassilaki, M., et al. (2019). Quantity and quality of mental activities and the risk of incident mild cognitive impairment. *Neurology, 93*(6), e548–e558.

Lamb, S. E., Sheehan, B., Atherton, N., et al. (2018). Dementia And Physical Activity (DAPA) trial of moderate to high intensity exercise training for people with dementia: Randomised controlled trial. *British Medical Journal, 361*, k1675.

Lancioni, G. E., Singh, N. N., O'Reilly, M. F., et al. (2014). Persons with moderate Alzheimer's disease use simple technology aids to manage daily activities and leisure occupation. *Research in Developmental Disabilities, 35*, 2117–2128.

Leggieri, M., Thaut, M. H., Fornazzari, L., et al. (2019). Music intervention approaches for Alzheimer's disease: A review of the literature. *Frontiers in Neuroscience, 13*, 132.

Leung, G. T., Fung, A. W., Tam, C. W., et al. (2010). Examining the association between participation in late-life leisure activities and cognitive function in community-dwelling elderly Chinese in Hong Kong. *International Psychogeriatrics, 22*, 2–13.

Morris, M. C., Tangney, C. C., Wang, Y., et al. (2015a). MIND diet slows cognitive decline with aging. *Alzheimer's & Dementia: The Journal of the Alzheimer's Association, 11*(9), 1015–1022.

Morris, M. C., Tangney, C. C., Wang, Y., et al. (2015b). MIND diet associated with reduced incidence of Alzheimer's disease. *Alzheimer's & Dementia: The Journal of the Alzheimer's Association, 11*(9), 1007–1014.

Nithiananantharajah, J., & Hannan, A. J. (2009). The neurobiology of brain and cognitive reserve: Mental and physical activity as modulators of brain disorders. *Progress in Neurobiology, 89*, 369–382.

Petersen, R. C., Lopez, O., Armstrong, M. J., et al. (2018). Practice guideline update summary: Mild cognitive impairment: Report of the Guideline Development, Dissemination, and Implementation Subcommittee of the American Academy of Neurology. *Neurology, 90*(3), 126–135.

Rauschecker, J. P. (2014). Is there a tape recorder in your head? How the brain stores and retrieves musical melodies. *Frontiers in Systems Neuroscience, 8*, 149.

Scarmeas, N., Luchsinger, J. A., Schupf, N., et al. (2009). Physical activity, diet, and risk of Alzheimer disease. *The Journal of the American Medical Association, 302*, 627–637.

Simmons-Stern, N. R., Budson, A. E., & Ally, B. A. (2010). Music as a memory enhancer in patients with Alzheimer's disease. *Neuropsychologia, 48*, 3164–3167.

Simmons-Stern, N. R., Deason, R. G., Brandler, B. J., et al. (2012). Music-based memory enhancement in Alzheimer's disease: Promise and limitations. *Neuropsychologia, 50*, 3295–3303.

Weuve, J., Kang, J. H., Manson, J. E., et al. (2004). Physical activity, including walking, and cognitive function in older women. *The Journal of the American Medical Association, 292*, 1454–1461.

23

Future Treatments of Memory Loss, Alzheimer's Disease, and Dementia

QUICK START: FUTURE TREATMENTS OF MEMORY LOSS, ALZHEIMER'S DISEASE, AND DEMENTIA

Symptomatic and disease-modifying treatment	• Alzheimer's disease can be treated either to improve symptoms and function or to slow disease progression. • Symptomatic treatments work by altering neurotransmitter function. • Disease-modifying treatments are aimed at slowing the loss of neurons.
Disease-modifying treatments: amyloid plaques	• The amyloid cascade hypothesis describes how a build-up of β-amyloid can lead directly to amyloid plaques, neurofibrillary tangles, neurotransmitter disruption, and dementia. • Approaches to decrease β-amyloid have included active immunotherapy; passive immunotherapy; reducing the formation, accumulation, or oligomerization of β-amyloid; and blocking the enzymes that cleave β-amyloid from amyloid precursor protein. • No anti-amyloid treatments have yet proven efficacious. • Many disease-modifying treatments are currently in clinical trials.
Disease-modifying treatments: neurofibrillary tangles	• As tangles are further downstream in the cascade that leads to clinical symptoms, treatments directed against tangles may be more efficacious in patients who have already developed clinical Alzheimer's disease than treatments directed against β-amyloid. • Tangle formation may be the final common pathway in many degenerative diseases and thus treatments directed against tangles may also be efficacious against other dementias such as frontotemporal dementia and chronic traumatic encephalopathy.
Beyond amyloid and tau	• Although the preponderance of clinical trials continues to focus on amyloid and tau, there is now the recognition that other avenues of treatment must be pursued. • There are currently many trials ongoing or planned. These approaches include treatments that can enhance neuroprotection, reduce inflammation, induce neuronal growth factors, or involve lifestyle changes. • It is now also recognized that a successful disease modifying approach may require a combination of approaches to be successful.

Because of the rapid aging of the population and the accompanying increase in the prevalence of Alzheimer's disease, there is enormous interest from both the federal government and private industry in developing new and better treatments. In general, these treatments are aimed at two targets: treating the symptoms of Alzheimer's disease and attempting to slow the progression of the disease.

STRATEGIES TO TREAT THE SYMPTOMS OF ALZHEIMER'S DISEASE

Patients for whom we prescribe a cholinesterase inhibitor, memantine, or a combination of the two often ask how these medications work and what else can be done. After explaining the mechanism of these standard of care, U.S Food and Drug Administration (FDA)-approved medications, we often have a discussion of some of the types of treatment that are currently being developed. There are two basic reasons why we discuss future treatments. One is to give patients (and their children who are often worried about developing Alzheimer's disease when they are older) hope for the future. The second is that some patients may be interested in participating in one of the numerous clinical trials of novel medications that are being developed for Alzheimer's disease, available in many large medical centers and Alzheimer's disease specialty clinics/clinical research centers.

Additional Symptomatic Treatments

One strategy to further help patients with Alzheimer's disease is to facilitate neuronal transmission, that is, communication between brain cells. The cholinesterase inhibitors and memantine improve the function of neurons that use acetylcholine, glutamate, and dopamine as their neurotransmitters. There are, however, other neurotransmitter systems in addition to these that can be augmented. It is now well documented that Alzheimer's disease affects many neurotransmitter systems. Table 23.1 summarizes these transmitter systems. At some point we might envision a drug cocktail that will boost the level of multiple neurotransmitter systems, thereby facilitating cognition. We are now at the beginning of this type of strategy when we combine memantine with a cholinesterase inhibitor. We may eventually become sufficiently sophisticated to tailor the cocktail based on the specific symptoms that the patient is experiencing or even the patient's genotype.

There continues to be research ongoing aimed at developing additional symptomatic treatments. Recent trials include drugs to affect acetylcholine, *N*-methyl-D-aspartic and serotonin activity as well as trials to examine the effect of anti-inflammatory, metabolic, and hormonal treatments. Many of these trials are evaluating the effects of adding drugs to the current standard of care (cholinesterase inhibitors) (Cummings, Tong, & Ballard, 2019). Additionally, in a recent clinical trial, suvorexant showed a modest improvement in Alzheimer's disease patients with sleep disorder and based on this was approved by the FDA for treatment of insomnia in Alzheimer's disease dementia and can now be prescribed (Herring et al., 2020).

DISEASE-MODIFYING TREATMENTS

Development of symptomatic treatments notwithstanding, the major focus of new drug development for Alzheimer's disease is on disease-modifying drugs. That is, drugs that address the underlying cause of the disease and in doing so prevent cell death. If this strategy is successful, then the progression of the disease could theoretically be slowed and perhaps even be halted (Fig. 23.1).

TABLE 23.1 Neurotransmitters Depleted in Alzheimer's Disease

Transmitter System	Degree of Involvement in Alzheimer's Disease	Approved Medications	Clinical Trials Ongoing?
Acetylcholine	✓✓✓	donepezil (Aricept), rivastigmine (Excelon), galantamine (Razadyne)	✓✓
Glutamate	✓✓✓	memantine (Namenda)	✓
Serotonin	✓✓	—	✓✓
Norepinephrine	✓✓	—	✓
Dopamine	✓	memantine (Namenda)	✓
GABA	✓	—	✓
Peptides	✓	—	✓

GABA, Gamma-aminobutyric acid.

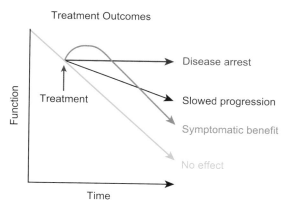

Fig. 23.1 Possible treatment outcomes.

If this strategy could be combined with both early diagnosis—or even preclinical diagnosis—and the use of symptomatic drugs, we could be on the pathway of successfully managing Alzheimer's disease.

Although the cause of Alzheimer's disease is unknown, there are a number of promising hypotheses regarding the pathogenesis of the disease, and these hypotheses have led to the development of potential disease-modifying treatments.

Alzheimer's Initial Observations

When Alois Alzheimer had the opportunity to examine the brain of his first patient, Auguste D, in 1906, he characterized the two forms of pathology that are the neuropathological hallmarks of the disease that now bears his name: senile plaques and neurofibrillary tangles.

Senile plaques appear to have a fluffy central core surrounded by thick irregular processes (Fig. 23.2). The central core is made up of a sticky protein called amyloid, and the surrounding material is a combination of dystrophic processes (axons and dendrites) and astrocytes. These plaques are primarily found in the association areas of the frontal, parietal, and temporal cortices and the piriform cortex, hippocampus, and amygdala (Fig. 2.1). Neurofibrillary tangles are intraneuronal cytoplasmic structures that are composed of paired filaments. Under the microscope they look like skeins of yarn (see Fig. 23.2). These tangles appear to consist primarily of a hyperphosphorylated form of the microtubule-associated protein *tau*. Microtubules are one of three major constituents of the neuronal cytoskeleton;

neurofilaments and microfilaments are the other two. All of these can be thought of as infrastructural elements of neurons that participate in functions such as axonal transport and maintenance of the structural integrity of the cell. In Alzheimer's disease, neurofibrillary tangles are present in the cortex, hippocampus, amygdala, nucleus basalis of Meynert, dorsal raphe, other brainstem nuclei, and ultimately in many other brain regions (see Chapter 4 for additional information on senile plaques and neurofibrillary tangles).

Baptists Versus Tauists?

For many years there was an ongoing debate regarding which form of pathology, senile plaques or neurofibrillary tangles, is the primary culprit in Alzheimer's disease. The debate became known as the "baptists" versus the "tauists." The baptists favored the view that β-amyloid protein and β-amyloid plaques are the culprits that start an inexorable cascade that ultimately destroys neurons. They are referred to as baptists because β-amyloid protein (or amyloid plaque) can be shortened to βAP but is now more commonly known as β-amyloid or βA. The tauists put forth the view that neurofibrillary tangles are the primary cause of cell death. They were called tauists because of the role of hyperphosphorylated tau in forming the tangles.

As with many scientific debates, there is often a synthesis of the two competing views and this is now the case in the baptist-tauist debate. The current view is that the earliest pathological event is the formation of amyloid. There is now evidence that the accumulation of brain amyloid precedes the emergence of cognitive symptoms by at least and perhaps up to 20 years (Bateman et al., 2012). There is also evidence that β-amyloid is toxic to neurons, but the primary culprit in cell death is now believed to hyperphosphorylated tau. Hyperphosphorylated tau breaks down the infrastructure of the neuron and in doing so leads to neuronal death. The current view further hypothesizes that through mechanisms that are not fully understood, β-amyloid promotes the emergence of hyperphosphorylated tau and that once tau invades a neuron it can spread throughout the brain from neuron to neuron (Pooler et al., 2013). It is important to realize that although amyloid plaques are unique to Alzheimer's disease, neurofibrillary tangles are present in other neurodegenerative diseases and are generally considered markers of cell death.

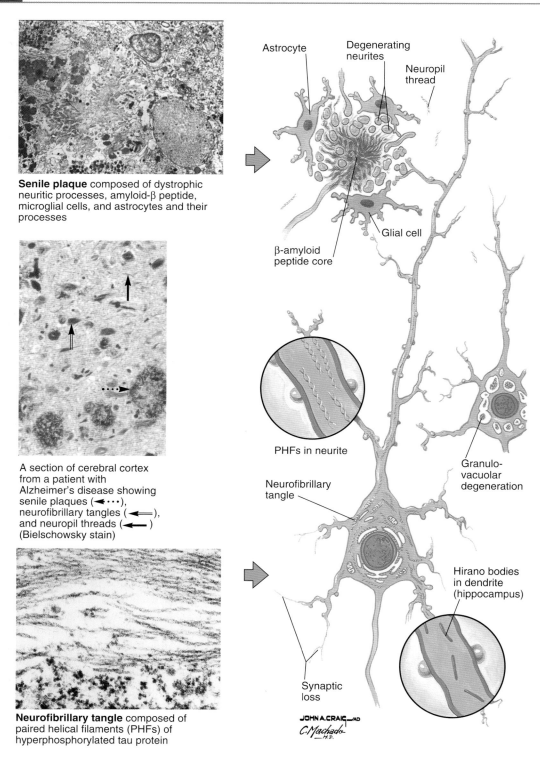

Senile plaque composed of dystrophic neuritic processes, amyloid-β peptide, microglial cells, and astrocytes and their processes

A section of cerebral cortex from a patient with Alzheimer's disease showing senile plaques (◄···), neurofibrillary tangles (⇐⇐), and neuropil threads (◄━━) (Bielschowsky stain)

Neurofibrillary tangle composed of paired helical filaments (PHFs) of hyperphosphorylated tau protein

Astrocyte

Degenerating neurites

Neuropil thread

β-amyloid peptide core

Glial cell

PHFs in neurite

Granulo-vacuolar degeneration

Neurofibrillary tangle

Hirano bodies in dendrite (hippocampus)

Synaptic loss

JOHN A. CRAIG—MD
C. Machado—M.D.

Fig. 23.2 Microscopic pathology in Alzheimer's disease. (Netter illustration from www.netterimages.com. Copyright Elsevier Inc. All rights reserved.)

The Amyloid Cascade Hypothesis

The amyloid cascade hypothesis has been the dominant heuristic driving effort to produce disease modifying treatments. Although most of the effort to date has been focused on βA, more recently in addition to the continuing work related to amyloid, there are also now increasing efforts to address the role of tau and other downstream effects of amyloid in the progression of Alzheimer's disease (Longo & Massa, 2020).

The hypothesis starts with the premise that the earliest sign of the pathogenesis of Alzheimer's disease is the accumulation of toxic forms of amyloid. It then follows that the focus of treatment of disease-modifying drugs is to slow and eventually stop the accumulation of amyloid.

Fig. 4.10 summarizes the amyloid cascade hypothesis (Hardy & Selkoe, 2002; Selkoe, 2011). As Fig. 4.10 shows, the initial assumption is that different gene defects can lead, either directly or indirectly, to an increase in toxic forms of β-amyloid. This increase may be because of either overproduction of or failure to clear these toxic forms of amyloid. Gradual accumulation of aggregated β-amyloid protein leads to a multistep cascade that includes inflammation, neuritic and synaptic changes, neurofibrillary tangles, neurotransmitter loss, and gliosis, and ultimately results in cell death and dementia.

β-Amyloid is a small piece of a much larger protein called the amyloid precursor protein (APP). The APP is a transmembrane protein that, when activated, is cut into smaller segments which operate either inside or outside the neuron. There are several ways that the APP can be cut, one of which leads to the production of β-amyloid (see Figs. 23.3 and 4.11).

There is considerable evidence to support the amyloid cascade hypothesis, for example:

- In a few hundred extended families worldwide, researchers have discovered mutations in genes that virtually guarantee an individual will develop Alzheimer's disease at a young age. Each of these abnormal genes increases β-amyloid production (those in the APP, presenilin 1, or presenilin 2).
- All Alzheimer's disease patients have amyloid plaque counts that far exceed those found in normal aging.
- Down's syndrome patients, who invariably develop Alzheimer's disease pathology by age 50 years,

produce too much β-amyloid protein from birth (presumably because they have a third copy of the gene coding for the APP, found on chromosome 21).
- β-Amyloid fibrils damage neurons in culture and activate brain inflammatory cells (microglia).
- It is hypothesized, with increasing supportive evidence, that β-amyloid can also induce hyperphosphorylated tau which leads to the formation of neurofibrillary tangles and that these tangles can spread from neuron to neuron throughout the brain.

Despite this evidence, the amyloid cascade hypothesis is still a hypothesis, and as with all hypotheses there are unanswered questions. Nevertheless, the amyloid cascade hypothesis continues to be the most widely accepted view of the pathogenesis of Alzheimer's disease and as such amyloid has been and continues to be a major therapeutic target.

Amyloid-Directed Treatments

Considerable research is now ongoing in an attempt to develop treatments that will intervene in the amyloid cascade and in doing so slow (or perhaps even stop) the progression of the disease. Some of these treatments act to directly modulate β-amyloid whereas others are aimed at the downstream effects of β-amyloid plaques such as activation of tau and microglia-induced inflammation. As discussed in the following sections, with the recognition that amyloid may be present in the brain 10 to 20 years before the onset of symptoms, the strong trend in anti-amyloid disease modifying clinical trials is to push these therapies earlier and earlier in the disease.

There are three major ongoing approaches to intervening in the amyloid cascade (Figs. 4.10, 4.11, 23.3 and 23.4). The first, secretase inhibitors, involves blocking the formation of β-amyloid by interfering with the enzymes that cleave the amyloid precursor protein in a manner that yields the toxic form of β-amyloid. The second approach, anti-aggregants, is aimed at preventing the aggregation of single strands of β-amyloid (monomers) into units containing multiple strands (oligomers) of β-amyloid. There is some evidence that, although monomers are not neurotoxic, as few as two aggregated strands (dimers) may be (Long & Holtzman, 2019; Selkoe, 2011). The third strategy, vaccines, involves removing the neuronal plaques, which consist of an

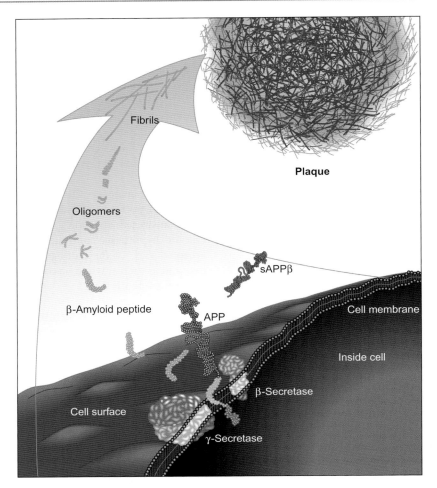

Fig. 23.3 **Plaque formation.** *APP*, Amyloid precursor protein. (From: NIA/NIH, 2008. Alzheimer's disease: Unraveling the mystery. NIH Publication 08-3782, 23.)

aggregated β-amyloid core surrounded by parts of dying neurons.

Active Immunotherapy

Also known as the Alzheimer's disease active vaccine, the basic strategy here is to mobilize the immune system to produce antibodies to recognize and attack β-amyloid. The role of these antibodies is to remove existing plaques and to block the formation of subsequent plaques. To accomplish this goal patients are injected with a fragment of the β-amyloid protein.

Initial studies in mice that were genetically engineered to produce pathological forms of β-amyloid, and experienced difficulty in maze learning and other learning and memory tasks, benefited from β-amyloid vaccination. Vaccinated mice had both fewer plaques and enhanced learning and memory compared with nonvaccinated mice.

The first large-scale clinical trial in humans conducted by Elan Pharmaceuticals was with the entire 42 amino acid β-amyloid protein (compound AN1792) or a placebo infused into volunteers (Gilman et al., 2005). The trial received enormous publicity and was enrolled quickly with 300 volunteers with Alzheimer's disease. The trial, however, was stopped prematurely because of side effects. The goal of AN1792

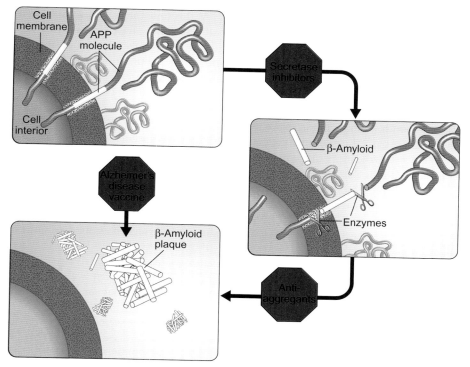

Fig. 23.4 Possible points of intervention for anti-amyloid treatments. *APP,* Amyloid precursor protein.

infusions was to produce an immune response to β-amyloid, but approximately 6% of patients in the trial experienced an inflammatory response (i.e., encephalitis). On the positive side, many of the patients in the study were followed for several years after their vaccinations in 1999. Several cases have come to autopsy and the results indicated substantially less plaque in the brain of patients from the study who received active vaccine as opposed to placebo (Holmes et al., 2008; Nicoll et al., 2003). Additionally, some of these patients received follow-up at 1 and 4.5 years after vaccination. After one year, vaccinated antibody responders (those with increased titers) did better on a cognitive test battery. A subset of these patients was again evaluated 4.5 years after their initial vaccination. These 17 patients all continued to show increased titers of antibody against β-amyloid compared with placebo controls. Additionally, compared with placebo controls, the vaccinated patients showed significantly less functional decline on measures of activities of daily living and dependence on a caregiver. These patients also did not show any additional episodes of brain inflammation

(encephalitis) (Vellas et al., 2009). Because of the potential side effects of treatment with an active vaccine, however, the major current emphasis is on evaluating passive immunotherapy

Passive Immunotherapy

The basic strategy here is to administer either laboratory-produced antibodies to β-amyloid or harvesting anti-amyloid antibodies from humans who have lived to an old age and not developed Alzheimer's disease. The idea is that a passive vaccine would be safer because antibodies are produced in a manner that does not mobilize the body's immune system. Laboratory-produced antibodies and those harvested from human blood can be given like any other drug in fixed doses, and unlike an active vaccine do not persist in the body after the dosing stops.

The first passive vaccine to be extensively evaluated was bapineuzumab. Two large-scale (2000 patients each), phase III, 18-month, randomized, placebo-controlled clinical trials conducted over a five-year period failed to show sufficient differences between placebo and bapineuzumab-treated patients to warrant further development of the vaccine. These trials were conducted in patients with mild to moderate stage Alzheimer's disease (MMSE scores 16–26) (Salloway, Sperling, & Fox, 2014).

A second passive vaccine developed by Lilly (solanezumab) was evaluated in two large-scale (1000 patients each), phase III, 18-month, randomized, placebo-controlled clinical trials. These trials also examined patients with mild to moderate stage Alzheimer's disease (Mini-Mental State Examination [MMSE] scores 16–26). Both trials demonstrated a good safety profile for the vaccine. They did not, however, demonstrate sufficient efficacy to meet FDA guidelines for approval (Doody, Thomas, & Farlow, 2014). However, when the data for the two trials were combined to increase power, and the patients with mild disease (MMSE 20–26) were analyzed separately, the results were within the range of what the FDA requires for efficacy to approve a drug. Based upon these findings a third large scale was undertaken in patients with mild Alzheimer's disease (MMSE 21–26). As noted earlier, the hope was that intervention earlier in course of Alzheimer's disease would be more beneficial. Unfortunately, the results of this trial also did not show sufficient efficacy for FDA approval.

Since the completion of these early efforts there have been multiple clinical trials completed with anti-amyloid passive vaccines, but none yet have produced positive results (i.e., results that would lead to approval by the FDA (Aisen et al., 2020). As with many endeavors of this complex nature, researchers have gleaned valuable information from each trial that has led to common themes in the design of most ongoing recent trials. These changes include using vaccines that are more potent in removing amyloid, only including patients with confirmed amyloid deposition via positron emission tomography (PET) scans, including patients who are earlier and earlier in the disease, and using outcome measures (e.g., neuropsychological tests and clinical interviews with patients and caregivers) that are more sensitive to change early in the disease. At this time the patients in various ongoing trials include those with diagnoses of very early Alzheimer's disease and mild cognitive impairment (MCI) due to Alzheimer's disease. Other trials include patients who do not meet clinical criteria for a diagnosis of MCI or Alzheimer's disease, but have risk factors, including genotype (homozygous e4), family history, and positive amyloid PET scans.

At this time there are several trials ongoing that have had promising phase II trials; that is, have shown that they remove amyloid plaques and slow the cognitive and functional progression of the disease based on both cognitive measures and study partner reports. These treatments have now moved on to large-scale, registration quality, phase III trials that, if successful, could be submitted to the FDA for approval. One recent example is a passive vaccine developed by Biogen called aducanumab. Biogen has announced that based upon the results of two large-scale trials with more than 3000 participants, they will be submitting their results to the FDA for approval sometime in 2020. Of note is that the Biogen vaccine is derived from human as opposed to laboratory produced antibodies. Other passive vaccines with encouraging phase II data that are currently being evaluated in large scale phase III trials include gantenerumab (Roche) that is also is using human derived antibodies, and a trial conducted by Eisai using laboratory produced amyloid antibodies (BAN2401).

Pushing the envelope back even further to earlier in the disease process is the "A4" study (AntiAmyloid Treatment in Asymptomatic Alzheimer's Disease) sponsored by the National Institute on Aging (NIA). This study has been following patients since 2014 who are at risk for Alzheimer's disease but have no outward symptoms of the disease. A positive PET scan for amyloid determines the risk for the disease and is the entry criteria to enter the study. Subjects in this ongoing study are randomized to either receive the solanezumab vaccine, at a considerably higher dose than used in previous trials, or a placebo (Sperling et al., 2014, see https://www.clinicaltrials.gov/ct2/show/NCT02008357). Similarly, another NIA sponsored trial that commenced in mid 2020, AHEAD, also aims at treating patients who have no symptoms but are at risk for Alzheimer's disease based on positive PET scan for amyloid or genetic predisposition (Aisen et al., 2020). The study will use the Eisai vaccine BAN2401.

Blocking the Formation of β-Amyloid

Recall that β-amyloid is cleaved from the larger amyloid precursor protein (APP) (Figs. 4.11 and 23.3). The cleaving is accomplished in a two-step process by enzymes called secretases. APP is one of many proteins that are associated with the neuronal cell membrane. As it is being produced in the cell it penetrates through the cell membrane and eventually resides inside, through, and outside the neuron. There are three enzymes that cut or cleave APP and, depending upon which enzyme is involved and where the cleaving occurs, APP can follow one of two pathways.

In normal processing, the amyloid precursor protein (695–770 amino acids long) is first cleaved by α-secretase and then by γ-secretase to form harmless soluble fragments called sAPP α. sAPP α has beneficial properties related to neuronal growth and survival. In abnormal processing, however, the amyloid precursor protein is first cut by β-secretase and then by γ-secretase to form the toxic β-amyloid proteins (42 amino acids sometimes known as $A\beta_{1-42}$) that self-aggregate to first form oligomers and then fibrils and then plaques. The plaques are clearly toxic to neurons, but there is also evidence that even oligomers may be toxic (Haass & Selkoe, 2007; Moreno et al., 2009; Selkoe, 2011).

Changing the behavior of either β-secretase or γ-secretase could reduce or prevent the formation of harmful β-amyloid. Drugs that can block or alter the clipping action of these secretases are called *secretase inhibitors*. There are a number of secretase inhibitors in development, but to date there have been no positive clinical trial results,

The initial trials evaluated results from a γ-secretase inhibitor (Lilly, LY450139, semagacestat) has led to questions regarding this approach. Results from two large-scale (>2600 patients) phase III trials demonstrated that the drug not only failed to slow cognitive decline in people with mild to moderate Alzheimer's disease, but that it actually worsened cognition. Based upon this, both trials were immediately halted and no other trials with γ-secretase inhibitors have been conducted.

Multiple trials evaluating β-secretase inhibitors (BACE inhibitors) have been conducted. In 2017 Merck announced that their BACE inhibitor, verubecestat, failed to slow progression of mild to moderate Alzheimer's disease. Moreover, they suggested that based on subgroup analysis there might be a worsening of cognition. Additional disappointing news for verubecestat came in 2018 when Merck announced that the drug also failed to slow progression in patients with prodromal Alzheimer's disease. More recently several other pharmaceutical companies have reported similar results for their BACE inhibitors.

Why a secretase inhibitor would disrupt cognition in patients with Alzheimer's disease is unclear. One widely shared hypothesis is that BACE inhibitors decrease β-amyloid by too much. There is support for

this view in animal models. Several recent studies in mice have shown that high doses of BACE inhibitors not only reduce β-amyloid production, but they also dampened synaptic function. By lowering the dose of the BACE inhibitor, however, β-amyloid production was still reduced by a lesser degree, but there was no corresponding decline in synaptic dysfunction. Because of the potential of BACE inhibitors to slow disease progression and the possibility that they could be combined with anti-amyloid vaccines, it is possible that we will see additional trials with lower doses and careful monitoring for cognitive decline.

Blocking Accumulation of β-Amyloid

Because β-amyloid exists in many forms in the human brain, one important question becomes which form is most toxic. As Figs. 23.3 and 4.11 show, when β-amyloid is initially cleaved it forms single pieces or monomers. The monomers are soluble and may not yet be toxic. The monomers are then thought to combine into clusters to form β-amyloid oligomers, and finally the oligomers form insoluble fibrils also known as β-sheets. This process is collectively known as aggregation. These β-sheets further accumulate and become deposited as plaques. It is not clear how long this entire process takes, but some researchers hypothesize that it occurs over many years (see an online animation of this process at http://www.youtube.com/watch?v=73PRA7wUqS0).

The importance of fully understanding this amyloid cascade is that it provides the opportunity to develop interventions. When researchers initially hypothesized that the β-amyloid did not become toxic until the stage of insoluble beta sheets, they proposed that interventions that blocked this stage could be therapeutic. The more recent view, as mentioned above, however, is that β-amyloid may be toxic as early as formation of oligomers and perhaps as early as a cluster of two monomers (dimers) (Haass & Selkoe, 2007).

The first anti-aggregation drug to be tested in patients was Alzhemed (3-amino-1-propanosulfonic acid, 3APS), which is in development by the Canadian pharmaceutical company Neurochem. Alzhemed binds to soluble β-amyloid and in doing so is hypothesized to block the chain of events leading to the formation of toxic beta sheets. Studies in cell culture and in animals lent support to this hypothesis.

In a small phase II clinical trial (Aisen et al., 2006), 58 patients with Alzheimer's disease were randomized to receive either placebo or one of three doses of Alzhemed over a three-month double-blind period. The results of the study indicated that the drug was generally safe and well tolerated. Analyses of cerebrospinal fluid (CSF) also showed that there was a reduction of β-amyloid. Unfortunately, neither this phase II nor two large phase III studies showed any efficacy of Alzhemed in reducing cognitive decline in patients with Alzheimer's disease (Aisen, 2011).

More recently, there has been increased interest in this approach following additional analysis of the phase II and phase III data showing that the drug had slowed cognitive decline in patients who were ApoE4 homozygotes (Abushakra et al., 2017). In 2013 a start-up company, Alzeon, licensed a prolog version of Alzhemed, and after several preliminary studies has announced that they plan to start a phase III trial in 2020 (Tolar, Abushakra, & Sabbagh, 2020).

Targeting the Neurofibrillary Tangle: Tau and Neurofibrillary Degeneration

So far, we have been discussing emerging therapies that target β-amyloid, but as mentioned earlier there is also a school of thought that argues therapeutic approaches for disease progression should target the neurofibrillary tangle. Neurofibrillary lesions, made up from aggregated hyperphosphorylated forms of the microtubule-associated protein tau, represent the second defining pathology in Alzheimer's disease (Fig. 23.5). While in the early stages of disease-modifying trials β-amyloid was the preferred target. As more information has been gathered regarding the role of tau in Alzheimer's disease progression it has become clear that anti-tau approaches to treatment are equally important. As discussed earlier in this chapter, amyloid is believed to be instrumental in initiating a process that leads to hyperphosphorylated tau, which in turn destroys the infrastructure of the neuron, eventually killing the cell. More recently there is convincing evidence that this hyperphosphorylated tau can seep out of the cell and into the synaptic space, be taken up into the postsynaptic neuron, and initiate events that lead to cell death. It is now generally accepted that this process is the primary factor leading to the spread of cell death throughout the brain, and the progression of the disease (see Fig. 23.6).

The primary role of tau is to stabilize microtubules in the neuron, much like railroad ties stabilize the rails of the track. These microtubules normally serve in axonal transport of cellular nutrients and precursors of neural transmitters. When abnormal phosphorylation occurs, the microtubule network breaks down, there is a disruption of axonal transport, and eventually there is neurodegeneration (Mandelkow & Mandelkow, 1998). Additionally, there is evidence that certain forms of tau may have direct neurotoxic properties (Gauthier et al., 2020; Klafki et al., 2006).

Although the preponderance of evidence is that the senile plaque is an initiating event in Alzheimer's disease and that the neurofibrillary tangle is part of the chain (the amyloid cascade) that eventually leads to neuronal degeneration and dementia, there is also evidence that, at least for some causes of dementia, the neurofibrillary tangle may be the primary cause of cell death.

One example of this is the neurodegenerative disease known as familial frontotemporal with parkinsonism (FDP-17), which has been linked to chromosome 17 (see Chapter 10). In this form of dementia, dysregulation of tau alone can cause neurodegeneration. Similarly, as discussed in Chapter 15, in chronic traumatic encephalopathy the cause of dementia is due to dysregulation of tau producing neuronal death. Tauopathies have also been linked to progressive supranuclear palsy (see Chapter 12), and primary age-related tauopathy (PART, see Chapter 5). In these examples, neurodegeneration occurs in the absence of β-amyloid. Because of the potential role of tau in neurodegeneration, a number of therapeutic strategies are now being pursued that influence the regulation of this toxic protein including blocking tau aggregation and blocking tau from spreading from cell to cell (Congdon & Sigurdsson, 2018).

The TauRx compound LMTB was the first anti-tau treatment to be evaluated in clinical trials. This treatment is hypothesized to reduce tau by blocking aggregation. This drug has been used in three phase III trials in mild to moderate Alzheimer's disease and one trial in behavioral variant frontotemporal dementia. Each of these trials reported negative results. The drug is currently being tested in another phase III trial in early Alzheimer's disease.

More recently, phase II trials have been initiated and are ongoing evaluating the effects of anti-tau antibodies on the progression of Alzheimer's disease. In general, these trials are designed much like the anti-amyloid trials in that they are evaluating patients with MCI or early

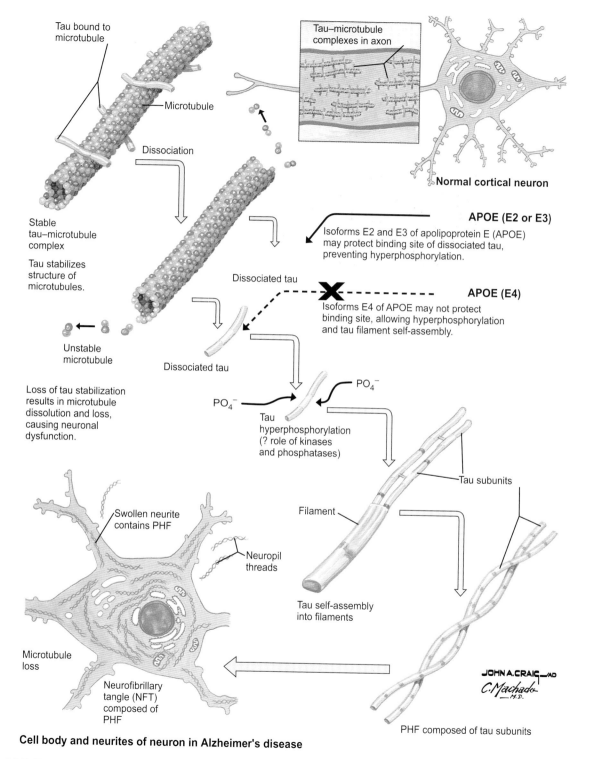

Tau bound to microtubule

Microtubule

Tau–microtubule complexes in axon

Dissociation

Normal cortical neuron

Stable tau–microtubule complex

Tau stabilizes structure of microtubules.

APOE (E2 or E3)
Isoforms E2 and E3 of apolipoprotein E (APOE) may protect binding site of dissociated tau, preventing hyperphosphorylation.

Dissociated tau

APOE (E4)
Isoforms E4 of APOE may not protect binding site, allowing hyperphosphorylation and tau filament self-assembly.

Unstable microtubule

Dissociated tau

Loss of tau stabilization results in microtubule dissolution and loss, causing neuronal dysfunction.

PO_4^-

PO_4^-

Tau hyperphosphorylation (? role of kinases and phosphatases)

Tau subunits

Filament

Swollen neurite contains PHF

Neuropil threads

Tau self-assembly into filaments

Microtubule loss

Neurofibrillary tangle (NFT) composed of PHF

PHF composed of tau subunits

Cell body and neurites of neuron in Alzheimer's disease

JOHN A. CRAIG—AD
C. Machado
—M.D.

Fig. 23.5 Tangle formation in Alzheimer's disease. *PHF,* Paired helical filaments. (Netter illustration from www. netterimages.com. Copyright Elsevier Inc. All rights reserved.)

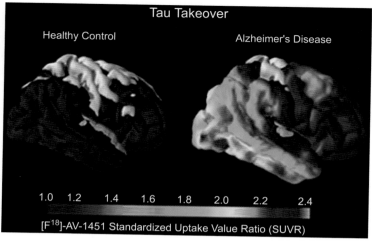

Fig. 23.6 Hyperphosphorylated tau spreading throughout the brain.

Alzheimer's disease, using PET scans for β-amyloid and tau to assure the presence of disease in the brain, and evaluating both change in cognition and function over 18- to 24-month periods. Two of the earliest studies were initiated in 2019 by Biogen (gosuranemab) and Lilly (zagotenemab). Both of these trials target extracellular tau with the goal of stopping the spread tau from cell to cell. As of the writing of this book, both of these phase II trials were in the double-blind stage. Since the initiation of these trials, multiple other anti-tau studies have been commenced using both drugs and biologics (Cummings, Tong, & Ballard, 2019; Cummings et al., 2019).

In summary, there is now general agreement that Aβ accumulation begins 15 to 20 years before the onset of symptoms of Alzheimer's disease. Moreover, amyloid can now be imaged in the human brain using markers that can be seen in PET scans. This presents a remarkable opportunity to intervene in patients at risk long before the onset of symptoms. To date, lowering amyloid burden in patients with moderate disease for whom the disease progression has been underway for years has not produced beneficial effects. Based on these early studies, the approach is to now intervene with anti-amyloid treatments in the very earliest stages of the disease and perhaps even before cognitive symptoms are noted. Research is also now underway to develop anti-tau therapies with the goal of slowing or preventing the spread of tau pathology from cell to cell throughout the brain, and additional symptomatic drugs that may be beneficial to patients who already are showing cognitive decline.

Beyond Amyloid and Tau

Although the preponderance of research, about 60%, continues to be aimed at removing amyloid and tau, many if not most researchers in the field are coming to the conclusion that although removing amyloid and tau are important in arriving at a disease modifying treatment, there are other mechanisms and pathways that need to be pursued. Over the past few years, and in light of the difficulties of obtaining successful results with anti-amyloid treatments, many researchers, both in academia and the pharmaceutical industry, have turned their attention to other approaches. These approaches range from developing treatments that can enhance neuroprotection, reduce inflammation or induce neuronal growth factors, to approaches that involve lifestyle changes. This raises the possibility that some of these therapies in combination with anti-amyloid and tau will lead to the most efficacious results. It is well beyond the scope of this chapter to cover the many approaches underway (see Long & Holtzman, 2019, for a comprehensive recent review), but we would like to briefly discuss some of the treatments which have moved out or are about to move out of the laboratory and into clinical trials.

Regulating Inflammation

When the brains of Alzheimer's disease patients that have been donated to brain banks are studied, a common finding is that they rarely contain only plaques and tangles. The much more common finding is that along with the plaques and tangles comes evidence of inflammation. This may explain why the donors of some of the brains that do have only plaques and tangles did not have symptom of dementia before they died. These findings have prompted researchers to consider the possibility that anti-inflammatory treatments may be a useful therapeutic agent. Recently, Alector and Abbvie pharmaceuticals have launched a joint effort targeting inflammation in the brain that is regulated by microglial cells.

In donated human brains there are increased tau tangles clustered around amyloid plaques when people have a mutation of the TREM2 microglial receptor. This finding has prompted Alector and Abbvie pharmaceuticals to develop an antibody that increases signaling in the TREM2 receptor that in turn leads to better regulation of microglia. The outcome in mice treated with this antibody was that microglia expressed more pro-inflammatory and repair genes, and nearby amyloid deposits were nearly cut in half. Alector completed a phase I safety study in humans and started a phase II trial that measures both safety and efficacy in-2020.

This type of treatment in this and other similar recent trials has been called the "Deep Biology Approach" (Longo & Massa, 2020) and recognizes the important recent contributions made in the field of molecular neurobiology that will likely be critical in making further advances in disease modifying treatments.

Is Alzheimer's Disease a Bacterial Infection?

More than century ago Alzheimer raised the possibility that amyloid plaques might be a response to "microorganisms." Since that time the idea that Alzheimer's disease is caused by a bacterial infection has been discussed as an alternative idea. More recently this idea has moved to the forefront, in part because of the finding that the germ that causes periodontal disease has been found in brain tissue from patients with Alzheimer's disease. The theory behind this hypothesis is that the initial event in Alzheimer's disease is a bacterium (*Porphyromonas gingivalis*) entering the brain, perhaps owing to a leakier blood–brain barrier that accompanies aging. This bacterium then induces an immune response characterized by activation of microglia leading to neuroinflammation and neurodegeneration.

In this view of the neurobiology of Alzheimer's disease, the initiating factor is a bacterial infection leading to chronic activation of the immune system and

leading to the production of amyloid plaques. The bacterial infection is hypothesized to be caused by keystone bacterium *P. gingivalis*. This is the same bacterium that causes gum disease and interestingly people with gum disease (gingivitis) are somewhat more likely to develop Alzheimer's disease.

P. gingivalis is hypothesized to enter the blood stream and gain access to the brain because of increased permeability of the blood–brain barrier related to aging and genetic factors. Once inside the brain, *P. gingivalis* survives by secreting proteases called gingipains while also replicating and spreading from neuron to neuron. Gingipains digest neuronal proteins and eventually kill the neuron by destroying its infrastructure. This process then leads to activation of the brain's natural defense systems including inflammation and the production of Aβ plaques that surround and sequester the bacterium (Dominy et al., 2019). From a therapeutic standpoint, this raises the possibility of using antibacterial treatments to stop the progression of Alzheimer's disease. Supporting this idea is the finding that patients with Alzheimer's disease have increased levels of the bacterial protease gingipain in their brains.

Researchers at Cortexyme have produced a drug, CORE 388, that is a gingipain inhibitor. They have reported that CORE 388 reduces inflammation in mice and protects neurons from gingipain toxicity. Cortexyme has completed a phase I safety study in humans and initiated a phase II/III trial in early 2020 in 500 subjects with mild to moderate Alzheimer's disease.

Can Brain Stimulation Reduce Amyloid?

Memory TEMT is an investigational technology that applies Transcranial Electromagnetic Treatment (TEMT) to the brain. The technology uses a cap to deliver specialized electromagnetic waves to the brain. The company reported the results of a small clinical trial consisting of eight patients with mild to moderate Alzheimer's disease in September 2019. The trial used an open label design in which all patients were treated with the investigational procedure (i.e., no placebo controls). Subjects were treated at home by wearing a specialized cap that delivered the stimulation as they went about day-to-day activities for two one-hour periods each day for two months. Results of the study showed that seven of the eight patients had improved cognition. There were no significant sideeffects reported (Arendash et al., 2019). It will be interesting to see if this study can be replicated in a randomized, placebo-controlled trial, and if the effects persist after daily treatment stops.

A second approach to using external stimulation involves using sights and sounds to produce a particular pattern of naturally occurring brain waves. Gamma waves are the high frequency brain waves that have been associated with cognitive processes such as working memory, sensory processing, and spatial navigation. Recent work by Massachusetts Institute of Technology (MIT) researchers has now indicated that gamma waves may also play a role in treating Alzheimer's disease. The MIT group conducting this work has reported that stimulating the brains of mice with patterned light pulses has not only boosted the preponderance of gamma waves, but has also removed amyloid in Alzheimer's disease mice (mice genetically engineered to produce amyloid) and improved learning and memory. In other experiments, similar results for specific sound patterns were reported (Martorell et al., 2019). Based upon this work, Cognito Therapeutics has undertaken two clinical trials that are currently ongoing to evaluate the possibility that patients with Alzheimer's disease exposed to patterned flashes of light and sound would experience both a reduction in Aβ and enhanced cognitive functioning. In these studies, all participants wore headgear that included opaque glasses that delivered a pattern of light pulses and headphones that delivered a pattern of sound that was shown in mice to increase gamma waves and remove Aβ plaques. A control group underwent the same procedure but with a pattern of light and sound that did not induce gamma waves. The patients underwent this procedure daily for either six or 12 months. They also underwent periodic amyloid PET scans to measure density of amyloid plaques as well as cognitive testing. The results of this study are being analzyed, and if it is successful, the apparatus to deliver the stimulation could become available for home use.

Lifestyle Changes

Patients and caregivers often ask us about whether lifestyle changes can slow the progression or prevent the onset of Alzheimer's disease. The short answer is perhaps, but not yet. There are a number of recently completed and ongoing clinical trials to address this question, but as yet no conclusive evidence.

The FINGER (Finnish Geriatric Intervention Study to Prevent Cognitive Impairment and Disability) trial enrolled 1250 participants aged 60 to 77 years who were at risk for cognitive decline. Participants were randomly assigned to a group that received a two-year multidomain intervention consisting of diet, exercise, cognitive training, and vascular risk monitoring while the control group received general medical advice. The interpretation of results stated that a multidomain intervention could improve or maintain cognitive functioning in an elderly at-risk population (Rosenberg et al., 2018). Although promising, it is difficult to extrapolate from this study any information about whether similar effects would be found in a trial with Alzheimer's disease patients. Nevertheless, we recommend to our patients that they do their best to maintain a lifestyle that promotes good overall brain health by including regular physical activity, a healthy diet, and keeping cognitively active by engaging in lifetime learning and social stimulation. Multiple trials are currently ongoing to investigate the contribution of each of these factors.

THE FUTURE OF ALZHEIMER'S DISEASE THERAPY

Alzheimer's disease is a devastating neurodegenerative disease for patients, their families, and society. The difficulty of managing this disease for all concerned will grow dramatically over the next 30 to 40 years, as the number of cases increases 4- to 5-fold and the total cost of care increases to a trillion dollars. As with all major illnesses, early detection and treatment will continue to be critical factors in the successful management of Alzheimer's disease. We have suggested that there are three major areas in which substantial progress needs to be made to successfully treat Alzheimer's disease: (1) continued progress in early detection and diagnosis, (2) further development of symptomatic medications and by recognizing that combinations of symptomatic therapies may be required, and (3) continued advances in the development of disease-modifying treatments. These treatments will continue to include addressing amyloid and tau, but will clearly need to recognize that non-amyloid and -tau approaches will lead to a more diverse approach to treatment (Fig. 23.7). This progress will be facilitated by the rapid advances in molecular biology that can elucidate mechanisms that are either upstream or downstream to amyloid. This strategy, which has recently been dubbed the "Deep Biology Strategy," will hopefully lead to progress over the next ten years that will eclipse the considerable progress of the past 20 years.

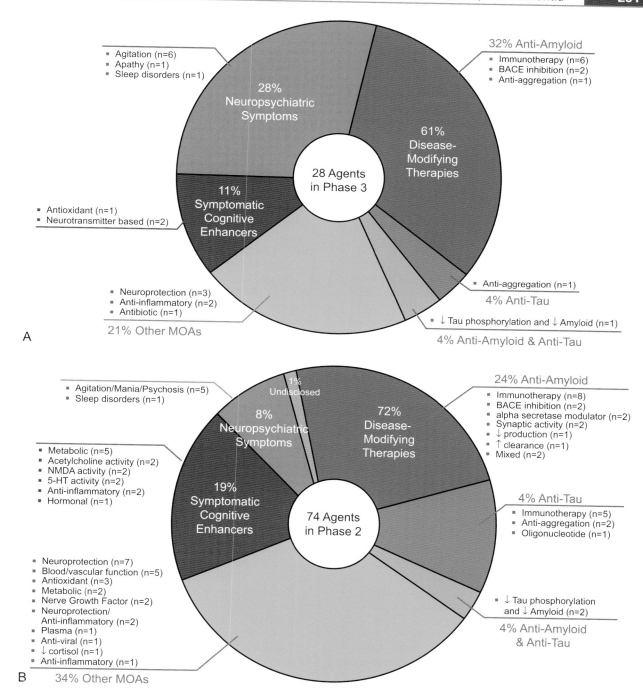

Fig. 23.7 Mechanisms of action (*MOA*) of agents in phase III **(A)**. Mechanisms of action of agents in phase II **(B)**.

REFERENCES

Abushakra, S., Porsteinsson, A., Scheltens, P., et al. (2017). Clinical effects of tramiprosate in APOE4/4 homozygous patients with mild Alzheimer's disease suggest disease modification potential. *The Journal of Prevention of Alzheimer's Disease, 4*(3), 149–156.

Aisen, P. S. (2011). Clinical trial methodologies for disease-modifying therapeutic approaches. *Neurobiology of Aging, 32*(Suppl 1), S64–S66. https://doi.org/10.1016/j.neurobiolaging.2011.09.008.

Aisen, P. S., Cummings, J., Doody, R., et al. (2020). The future of anti-amyloid trials. *The Journal of Prevention of Alzheimer's Disease, 7*(3), 146–151.

Aisen, P. S., Saumier, D., Briand, R., et al. (2006). A phase II study targeting amyloid-beta with 3APS in mild-to-moderate Alzheimer disease. *Neurology, 67*, 1757–1763.

Arendash, G., Cao, C., Abulaban, H., et al. (2019). A clinical trial of transcranial electromagnetic treatment in Alzheimer's disease: Cognitive enhancement and associated changes in cerebrospinal fluid, blood, and brain imaging. *Journal of Alzheimer's disease: JAD, 71*(1), 57–82.

Bateman, R. J., Xiong, C., Benzinger, T. L. S., et al. (2012). Clinical and biomarker changes in dominantly inherited Alzheimer's disease. *The New England Journal of Medicine, 367*, 795–804.

Congdon, E. E., & Sigurdsson, E. M. (2018). Tau-targeting therapies for Alzheimer disease. *Nature Reviews Neurology, 14*(7), 399–415.

Cummings, J., Lee, G., Ritter, A., et al. (2019). Alzheimer's disease drug development pipeline: 2019. *Alzheimer's & Dementia (New York, NY), 5*, 272–293.

Cummings, J. L., Tong, G., & Ballard, C. (2019). Treatment combinations for Alzheimer's disease: Current and future pharmacotherapy options. *Journal of Alzheimer's Disease: JAD, 67*(3), 779–794.

Dominy, S. S., Lynch, C., Ermini, F., et al. (2019). *Porphyromonas gingivalis* in Alzheimer's disease brains: Evidence for disease causation and treatment with small-molecule inhibitors. *Science Advances, 5*(1), eaau3333.

Doody, R., Thomas, R. G., Farlow, M., et al. (2014). Phase 3 trials of solanezumab in mild-to-moderate Alzheimer's disease. *The New England Journal of Medicine, 370*, 311–321.

Gauthier, S., Aisen, P. S., Cummings, J., et al. (2020). Non-amyloid approaches to disease modification for Alzheimer's disease: An EU/US CTAD Task Force Report. *The Journal of Prevention of Alzheimer's Disease, 6*, 1–6.

Gilman, S., Koller, M., Black, R. S., et al. (2005). Clinical effects of Abeta immunization (AN1792) in patients with Alzheimer's disease in an interrupted trial. *Neurology, 64*, 1553–1562.

Haass, C., & Selkoe, D. J. (2007). Soluble protein oligomers in neurodegeneration: Lessons from the Alzheimer's amyloid beta-peptide. *Nature Reviews Molecular Cell Biology, 8*, 101–112.

Hardy, J., & Selkoe, D. J. (2002). The amyloid hypothesis of Alzheimer's disease: Progress and problems on the road to therapeutics. *Science, 297*, 353–356.

Herring, W. J., Ceesay, P., Snyder, E., et al. (2020). Polysomnographic assessment of suvorexant in patients with probable Alzheimer's disease dementia and insomnia: A randomized trial. *Alzheimer's & Dementia: The Journal of the Alzheimer's Association, 16*(3), 541–551.

Holmes, C., Boche, D., Wilkinson, D., et al. (2008). Long-term effects of Abeta42 immunisation in Alzheimer's disease: Follow-up of a randomised, placebo-controlled phase I trial. *Lancet, 372*, 216–223.

Klafki, H. W., Staufenbiel, M., Kornhuber, J., et al. (2006). Therapeutic approaches to Alzheimer's disease. *Brain, 129*, 2840–2855.

Long, J. M., & Holtzman, D. M. (2019). Alzheimer disease: an update on pathobiology and treatment strategies. *Cell, 179*(2), 312–339.

Longo, F. M., & Massa, S. M. (2020). Editorial: Next-generation Alzheimer's therapeutics: leveraging deep biology. *The Journal of Prevention of Alzheimer's Disease, 7*(3), 138–139.

Mandelkow, E. M., & Mandelkow, E. (1998). Tau in Alzheimer's disease. *Trends in Cell Biology, 8*, 425–427.

Martorell, A. J., Paulson, A. L., Suk, H. J., et al. (2019). Multi-sensory gamma stimulation ameliorates Alzheimer's-associated pathology and improves cognition. *Cell, 177*(2), 256–271. e22. https://doi.org/10.1016/j.cell.2019.02.014.

Moreno, H., Yu, E., Pigino, G., et al. (2009). Synaptic transmission block by presynaptic injection of oligomeric amyloid beta. *Proceedings of the National Academy of Sciences of the United States of America, 106*, 5901–5906.

Nicoll, J. A., Wilkinson, D., Holmes, C., et al. (2003). Neuropathology of human Alzheimer disease after immunization with amyloid-beta peptide: A case report. *Nature Medicine, 9*, 448–452.

Pooler, A. M., Polydoro, M., Wegman, S., et al. (2013). Propagation of tau pathology in Alzheimer's disease: Identification of novel therapeutic targets. (5), 49. *Alzheimer's Research & Therapy, 5*(5), 49. https://doi.org/10.1186/alzrt214.

Rosenberg, A., Ngandu, T., Rusanen, M., et al. (2018). Multidomain lifestyle intervention benefits a large elderly population at risk for cognitive decline and dementia regardless of baseline characteristics: The FINGER trial. *Alzheimer's & Dementia: The Journal of the Alzheimer's Association, 14*(3), 263–270.

Salloway, S., Sperling, R., Fox, N. C., et al. (2014). Two phase III trials of bapineuzumab in mild-to-moderate Alzheimer's disease. *The New England Journal of Medicine, 370,* 322–333.

Selkoe, D. J. (2011). Resolving controversies on the path to Alzheimer's therapeutics. *Nature Medicine, 17,* 1060–1065.

Sperling, R. A., Rentz, D. M., Johnson, K. A., et al. (2014). The A4 study: Stopping AD before symptoms begin. *Science Translational Medicine, 6*(228), 228fs13.

Tolar, M., Abushakra, S., & Sabbagh, M. (2020). The path forward in Alzheimer's disease therapeutics: Reevaluating the amyloid cascade hypothesis. *Alzheimer's & Dementia: The Journal of the Alzheimer's Association, 16*(11), 1553–1560.

Vellas, B., Black, R., Thal, L. J., et al. (2009). Long-term follow-up of patients immunized with AN1792: Reduced functional decline in antibody responders. *Current Alzheimer Research, 6,* 144–151.

24

Evaluating the Behavioral and Psychological Symptoms of Dementia

---

QUICK START: EVALUATING THE BEHAVIORAL AND PSYCHOLOGICAL SYMPTOMS OF DEMENTIA

The behavioral and psychological symptoms of dementia	• The behavioral and psychological symptoms of dementia are usually the most difficult symptoms for patients and caregivers to manage. • Symptoms usually assessed on the basis of interviews with patients and relatives include apathy, anxiety, depression, hallucinations, and delusions. • Symptoms usually identified on the basis of observation of patient behavior include aggression, screaming, restlessness, agitation, wandering, culturally inappropriate behaviors, sexual disinhibition, hoarding, cursing, and shadowing.
Benefits of treatment	• Improves quality of life for patients and caregivers. • Reduces caregiver stress. • Reduces the likelihood of institutionalization. • Decreases the patient's dependence upon the caregiver. • May improve cognition and function.

Evaluating behavioral and psychological symptoms of dementia	• It is important for the clinician to evaluate:
	  • Apathy
	  • Mood
	    • Depression
	    • Anxiety
	  • Behavior
	    • Agitation
	    • Disinhibition
	  • Psychosis
	    • Hallucinations
	    • Delusions

Formulating a treatment plan	• Caring for and educating the caregiver (see Chapter 25) • Nonpharmacological treatment of the patient (see Chapter 26) • Pharmacological treatment of the patient (see Chapter 27)

Patient EB is an 84-year-old woman who is living with her two nieces. She moved to the United States at age 22, never married, and worked in the fashion industry in New York, retiring at age 65 years. She has memory problems (denies having conversations, repeats questions), problems with executive functioning (difficulty managing finances and inappropriately gave away money), and visuospatial functioning (becomes lost walking in her neighborhood). She denies any cognitive deficits and does not understand why she needs to live with her nieces. She is agitated, expressed by constantly berating her nieces, denying her problems, and attempting to wander in the neighborhood. Her nieces are extremely frustrated in attempting to care for her. We diagnosed her with Alzheimer's disease and then had a discussion with the patient and her nieces regarding treatments.

Recall the case of EB from Chapter 18. Until now we have been discussing treatments for the cognitive aspects of Alzheimer's disease. But, as case EB demonstrates, changes in cognition and the problems that ensue because of it are only part of the problem in Alzheimer's disease (as well as other dementing illnesses). There are accompanying behavioral symptoms as well, which have significant management consequences. To wit, we have learned from our families that, in many respects, the stresses and demands of caring for a patient with behavioral problems is often the primary challenge. As one caregiver succinctly characterized the challenges in dealing with the behavioral and psychological symptoms of dementia:

When my wife would forget to buy my favorite foods at the supermarket I was upset, but when she started screaming at me to get out of our bed because she did not sleep with strangers, I knew the disease had reached a whole different level.

There has been considerable effort in recent years to develop both behavioral and pharmacological treatments for what has become known as "the behavioral and psychological signs and symptoms of dementia" (Finkel et al., 1996; Reisberg et al., 2014; Scales, Zimmerman, & Miller, 2018). Clinicians now realize that caring for these symptoms is a central part of caring for the patient with Alzheimer's disease and other dementias (Table 24.1).

WHAT CONSTITUTES BEHAVIORAL AND PSYCHOLOGICAL SYMPTOMS OF DEMENTIA?

There are many symptoms that can be classified in the category of behavioral and psychological symptoms of dementia, and considerable effort has been devoted to

TABLE 24.1   Dementias and Selected Neurodegenerative Disorders That Commonly Manifest Behavioral and Psychological Symptoms

Behavioral/ Psychological Symptom	Dementia
Apathy	• Alzheimer's disease • Vascular dementia • Behavioral variant frontotemporal dementia • Dementia with Lewy bodies • Corticobasal degeneration
Depression	• Alzheimer's disease • Parkinson's disease • Vascular dementia • Corticobasal degeneration • Dementia with Lewy bodies
Hallucinations	• Dementia with Lewy bodies • Parkinson's disease (following treatment with dopaminergic agonists) • Vascular dementia (if infarcts involve the visual system)
Delusions	• Alzheimer's disease • Dementia with Lewy bodies • Parkinson's disease (following treatment with dopaminergic agonists)
Agitation/ aggression	• Alzheimer's disease • Dementia with Lewy bodies • Behavioral variant frontotemporal dementia
Disinhibition	• Behavioral variant frontotemporal dementia

From Cummings, J. L. (2003). *The neuropsychiatry of Alzheimer's disease and related dementias* (Ch. 2, p. 32). London: Martin Dunitz Ltd.

arriving at a classification scheme. One such scheme that was presented at the first consensus conference for these symptoms in 1996 (Finkel et al., 1996) suggests that two general categories of symptoms can be evaluated:

Symptoms usually assessed on the basis of interviews with patients and relatives. These symptoms include anxiety, depressive mood, hallucinations, and delusions.

Symptoms usually identified on the basis of observation of patient behavior including aggression, screaming, restlessness, agitation, wandering, culturally inappropriate behaviors, sexual disinhibition, hoarding, cursing, and shadowing.

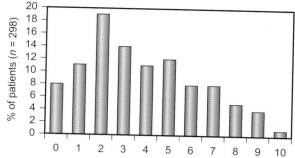

Fig. 24.1 Neuropsychiatric symptoms in Alzheimer's disease. Percentage of patients with Alzheimer's disease who exhibited 0, 1, 2, 3, and so on, neuropsychiatric symptoms elicited with the 10-item Neuropsychiatric Inventory. Note that 92% showed at least one symptom, and 51% had four or more symptoms. (From Cummings, J. L. (2003). *The neuropsychiatry of Alzheimer's disease and related dementias* (Ch. 1, p. 7). London: Martin Dunitz Ltd.)

THE BENEFITS OF TREATING BEHAVIORAL AND PSYCHOLOGICAL SYMPTOMS OF DEMENTIA

Treating these symptoms has many potential benefits for patients and caregivers. Both patients and caregivers report experiencing considerable distress when patients display these symptoms (Hiyoshi-Taniguchi et al., 2018). As noted above, it has been our experience that little is more distressing to caregivers than these symptoms. Treating these symptoms can help reduce stress in the family setting. By reducing stress, treating behavioral and psychological symptoms of dementia can improve the quality of life for patients and caregivers and may reduce the risk of institutionalization. Additionally, treating these symptoms may improve cognition and functional ability and decrease the patient's dependence on the caregiver.

MEASURING BEHAVIORAL AND PSYCHOLOGICAL SYMPTOMS OF DEMENTIA

There are now a variety of methods of measuring behavioral and psychological symptoms of dementia, ranging from informant interviews to validated scales. Some scales focus on a single symptom (e.g., depression) whereas others rate multiple symptoms. The Geriatric Depression Scale (Yesavage et al., 1983)

and the Cornell Scale for Depression (Alexopoulos et al., 1988) are commonly used to rate depression, and the Cohen-Mansfield Agitation Inventory is widely used to measure agitation (Cohen-Mansfield, 1986). The BEHAVE-AD (Reisberg et al., 2014) is an example of a multisymptom rating scale, as is the widely used Neuropsychiatric Inventory (Cummings et al., 1994).

The Neuropsychiatric Inventory is designed to provide a multidimensional profile of the behavioral and psychological symptoms that accompany dementia (Cummings et al., 1994). It is predicated on three assumptions that have been supported by research findings:

- As cognition worsens, behavioral changes become more likely.
- Multiple, simultaneous symptoms are the rule in patients with Alzheimer's disease (Fig. 24.1). For example, patients commonly exhibit agitation, psychosis, and depression.
- Once symptoms occur, they tend to persist.

The behavioral and psychological symptoms that are included in the Neuropsychiatric Inventory provide both a summary of what clinicians might expect to encounter and a framework for measuring/evaluating these symptoms (Table 24.2).

TABLE 24.2 **Neuropsychiatric Screening Questions**

Behavioral/ Psychological Symptom	Probe From the Neuropsychiatric Inventory
Delusions	Does the patient have beliefs that you know are not true (for example, insisting that people are trying to harm him/her or steal from him/her)? Has he/she said that family members are not who they say they are or that the house is not their home? I'm not asking about mere suspiciousness; I am interested if the patient is convinced that these things are happening to him/her.
Hallucinations	Does the patient have hallucinations, such as seeing false visions or hearing imaginary voices? Does he/she seem to see, hear, or experience things that are not present? By this question, we do not mean just mistaken beliefs such as stating that someone who has died is still alive; rather, we are asking if the patient actually has abnormal experiences of sounds or visions.
Agitation/ aggression	Does the patient have periods when he/she refuses to cooperate or won't let people help him/her? Is he/she hard to handle?
Depression	Does the patient seem sad or depressed? Does he/she say that he/she feels sad or depressed?
Anxiety	Is the patient very nervous, worried, or frightened for no apparent reason? Does he/she seem very tense or fidgety? Is the patient afraid to be apart from you?
Elation/euphoria	Does the patient seem too cheerful or too happy for no reason? I don't mean the normal happiness that comes from seeing friends, receiving presents, or spending time with family members. I am asking if the patient has a persistent and *abnormally* good mood or finds humor where others do not.
Apathy/ indifference	Has the patient lost interest in the world around him/her? Has he/she lost interest in doing things or does he/she lack motivation for starting new activities? Is he/she more difficult to engage in conversation or in doing chores? Is the patient apathetic or indifferent?
Disinhibition	Does the patient seem to act impulsively without thinking? Does he/she do or say things that are not usually done or said in public? Does he/she do things that are embarrassing to you or others?
Irritability	Does the patient get irritated and easily disturbed? Are his/her moods very changeable? Is he/she abnormally impatient? We do not mean frustration over memory loss or inability to perform usual tasks; we are interested to know if the patient has *abnormal* irritability, impatience, or rapid emotional changes different from his/her usual self.
Aberrant motor behavior	Does the patient pace, do things over and over such as opening closets or drawers, or repeatedly pick at things or wind string or threads?
Sleep and night-time behavior disorders	Does the patient have difficulty sleeping? (Do not count as present if the patient simply gets up once or twice per night only to go to the bathroom and falls back asleep immediately.) Is he/she up at night? Does he/she wander at night, get dressed in the middle of the night, or disturb your sleep?
Appetite and eating disorders	Has he/she had any change in appetite, weight, or eating habits? (Count as N/A if the patient is incapacitated or has to be fed.) Has there been any change in the type of food he/she prefers?

EVALUATING BEHAVIORAL AND PSYCHOLOGICAL SYMPTOMS OF DEMENTIA: PRAGMATIC GUIDELINES FOR THE CLINICIAN

An important part of any diagnostic and treatment plan of the demented patient is evaluating behavioral and psychological symptoms. In general, we have found that discussing four areas with the patient and caregiver in the course of either the initial or a follow-up interview will generally provide information regarding these symptoms.

We generally probe:

- Apathy
- Mood (anxiety, depression)

- Behavior (agitation, disinhibition)
- Psychosis (hallucinations, delusions)

The clinician may wish to address these areas using the screening questions from the Neuropsychiatric Inventory (see Table 24.2).

Apathy

Apathy is among the most common and earliest symptoms of Alzheimer's disease and other dementias (Kumfor et al., 2018; Fig. 24.2).
- Probe: lack of interest in usual activities, pursuits, and hobbies.
- Probe: loss of interest in social engagements including meeting friends or engaging with family members.
- Probe: loss of emotional engagement including reduced affect and intimacy.

Mood (Anxiety and Depression)

- Probe: patients must exhibit either a depressed mood or a decreased positive affect or pleasure.
- Probe: has there been anxiety, nervousness, or tension?
- Probe: has there been increased irritability?
- Probe: has the patient had manifestations of sadness, helplessness, or hopelessness?

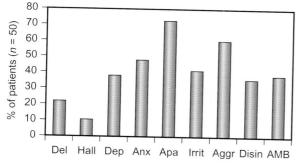

Fig. 24.2 Percentage of patients (*n* = 50) with specific symptoms on the Neuropsychiatric Inventory. *Aggr,* Aggression/agitation; *AMB,* aberrant motor behavior; *Anx,* anxiety; *Apa,* apathy; *Del,* delusions; *Dep,* depression; *Disin,* disinhibition; *Hall,* hallucinations; *Irrit,* irritability. (From Cummings, J. L. (2003). *The neuropsychiatry of Alzheimer's disease and related dementias* (Ch. 1, p. 7). London: Martin Dunitz Ltd.)

Note: Depression and anxiety occur in greater than 50% of patients with Alzheimer's disease (Sepehry et al., 2017).

Behavior (Agitation and Disinhibition)
Agitation

Note: Agitation is among the most common symptoms of dementia, occurring in about 70% of patients at some point in the course of the disease (Palm et al., 2018).
- Probe: has the patient exhibited aggressive, disruptive, and resistive behaviors such as threats, hitting, shouting, or cursing?
- Probe: has the patient exhibited less severe behaviors including pacing and frequent repetition of questions?

Disinhibition

Note: Disinhibition is characterized by inappropriate social and interpersonal interactions. This is not typical in Alzheimer's disease, but may occur and can be prominent in behavioral variant frontotemporal dementia.
- Probe: has the patient exhibited impulsive behavior including tactless and lewd comments?
- Probe: has the patient disregarded usual social conventions, for example, inappropriately touching someone?
- Probe: has the patient exhibited behaviors that have been embarrassing to his/her family?

Psychosis (Hallucinations and Delusions)

Note: The prevalence of delusions is almost 30% in Alzheimer's disease patients (Lai et al., 2019).
- Probe: presence of hallucinations or delusions that occur after the onset of dementia symptoms?

Note: Hallucinations or delusions must have been present at least intermittently for one month or longer, must not be as a result of delirium, and must be severe enough to disrupt patient function.

Note: Visual hallucinations that occur as presenting or early symptoms of a dementia syndrome are suggestive of dementia with Lewy bodies.

FORMULATING A TREATMENT PLAN FOR BEHAVIORAL AND PSYCHOLOGICAL SYMPTOMS: PRAGMATIC GUIDELINES FOR THE CLINICIAN

In our experience, treatment of behavioral and psychological symptoms can be approached in three ways.

- Caring for and educating the caregiver (see Chapter 25)
- Nonpharmacological treatment of the patient (see Chapter 26)
- Pharmacological treatment of the patient (see Chapter 27)

These approaches are by no means mutually exclusive; it is best, in fact, when approaches are used together. For example, nonpharmacological (e.g., behavioral treatments) are typically instituted by the caregiver based on a plan from the education provided by the clinician. Similarly, in many cases, combinations of pharmacological and nonpharmacological interventions produce the best outcome. In the following chapters we will provide specific pharmacological and nonpharmacological strategies for different behavioral and psychological symptoms. Before doing so, however, it may be useful to provide a general discussion of caring for and educating the caregiver.

REFERENCES

Alexopoulos, G. S., Abrams, R. C., Young, R. C., et al. (1988). Cornell scale for depression in dementia. *Biological Psychiatry, 23*, 271–284.

Cohen-Mansfield, J. (1986). Agitated behaviors in the elderly. II. Preliminary results in the cognitively deteriorated. *Journal of the American Geriatrics Society, 34*, 722–727.

Cummings, J. L., Mega, M., Gray, K., et al. (1994). The Neuropsychiatric Inventory: Comprehensive assessment of psychopathology in dementia. *Neurology, 44*, 2308–2314.

Finkel, S. I., Costae Silva, G., Cohen, G., et al. (1996). Behavioral and psychological signs and symptoms of dementia: A consensus statement on current knowledge and implications for research and treatment. *International Psychogeriatrics, 8*(Suppl. 3), 497–500.

Hiyoshi-Taniguchi, K., Becker, C. B., & Kinoshita, A. (2018). What behavioral and psychological symptoms of dementia affect caregiver burnout? *Clinical Gerontologist, 41*(3), 249–254.

Kumfor, F., Zhen, A., Hodges, J. R., et al. (2018). Apathy in Alzheimer's disease and frontotemporal dementia: Distinct clinical profiles and neural correlates. *Cortex, 103*, 350–359.

Lai, L., Lee, P. E., Chan, P., et al. (2019). Prevalence of delusions in drug-naïve Alzheimer disease patients: A meta-analysis. *International Journal of Geriatric Psychiatry, 34*(9), 1287–1293.

Palm, R., Sorg, C. G. G., Ströbel, A., et al. (2018). Severe agitation in dementia: An explorative secondary data analysis on the prevalence and associated factors in nursing home residents. *Journal of Alzheimer's Disease: JAD, 66*(4), 1463–1470.

Reisberg, B., Monteiro, I., Torossian, C., et al. (2014). The BEHAVE-AD assessment system: A perspective, a commentary on new findings, and a historical review. *Dementia and Geriatric Cognitive Disorders, 38*, 89–146.

Scales, K., Zimmerman, S., & Miller, S. J. (2018). Evidence-based nonpharmacological practices to address behavioral and psychological symptoms of dementia. *The Gerontologist, 58*(Suppl_1), S88–S102.

Sepehry, A. A., Lee, P. E., Hsiung, G. R., et al. (2017). The 2002 NIMH provisional diagnostic criteria for depression of Alzheimer's disease (PDC-dAD): Gauging their validity over a decade later. *Journal of Alzheimer's Disease: JAD, 58*(2), 449–462.

Yesavage, J. A., Brink, T. L., Rose, T. L., et al. (1983). Development and validation of a geriatric depression screening scale: A preliminary report. *Journal of Psychiatric Research, 17*, 37–49.

25

Caring for and Educating the Caregiver

QUICK START: CARING FOR AND EDUCATING THE CAREGIVER

- Alzheimer's is a disease that affects the entire family.
- Approximately 70% of patients with Alzheimer's disease are cared for at home by a family member.
- Supporting the caregiver is vitally important.
  - Listen to the caregiver.
  - Educate the caregiver.
  - Make sure the caregiver is taking care of his or her own health.
    - Does the caregiver have a primary care provider?
    - Would the caregiver benefit from referral to a psychotherapist?
- Helpful books for caregivers include:
  - *Six Steps to Managing Alzheimer's Disease and Dementia* (Budson & O'Connor, 2021)
  - *The 36-Hour Day* (Mace & Rabins, 2017)
- Three predictable transition points where the caregiver needs help:
  - Coping with the diagnosis—understanding the nature of the disease:
    - Understanding the stage of disease
    - Prognosis: What is the disease progression?
    - Familial/genetic implications?
    - Treatment options
    - Is there resistance to the diagnosis?
    - Financial and legal planning
  - Disease progression:
    - Accepting outside help (e.g., home health aide, homemaker, social worker)
    - The Alzheimer's Association (www.alz.org) in the United States and similar organizations in other countries have many resources.
    - Support groups can provide caregivers with great benefit.
  - Late-stage decisions
    - The decision to seek 24-hour care is not a selfish decision but one that is almost always in the best interest of the patient.
    - There is no absolute right or wrong time to make this move.
    - Because the decision to institute 24-hour care can come about with little warning, a plan should be in place.
    - Relinquishing primary caregiving does not mean the caregiver will not be involved.
    - We encourage caregivers to begin to consider how they will fill the void when they are no longer spending considerable time caregiving.

Alzheimer's is a disease that has effects on many more individuals than just those with the dementia. The effect of the disease on families and other caregivers is staggering.

- Approximately 70% of patients with Alzheimer's disease are cared for at home, typically by a family member.

- In 2019 caregivers spent an average of 1139 hours/year (21.9 hours/week) providing direct care—an impressive figure when compared with the average of 2000 hours/year that constitutes a full-time, 40-hour/week job (Alzheimer's Association, 2020).

- In 2019, 16.3 million American family members and other unpaid caregivers provided an estimated 18.6 billion hours of care, an economic contribution valued at nearly $244 billion annually (Alzheimer's Association, 2020).

To help the families of our newly diagnosed patients we often recommend that they read a book for caregivers such as *Six Steps to Managing Alzheimer's Disease and Dementia: A Guide for Families* (Budson & O'Connor, 2021) or *The 36-Hour Day* (Mace & Rabins, 2017). In *Six Steps to Managing Alzheimer's Disease and Dementia*, Andrew Budson, a neurologist (yes, same author) and Maureen O'Connor, a neuropsychologist, review a number of important topics including how to manage behavioral problems, build a care team, and plan for the future. In *The 36-Hour Day*, a classic now in its sixth edition, the authors, Nancy Mace, a social worker, and Peter Rabins, a psychiatrist, take a straightforward approach to many of the problems faced by Alzheimer's disease patients and their families. In both of these books, there are topics that range from diagnosis and medical care to dealing with problems of mood and behavior. Introducing these books also allows us to discuss with the caregiver our understanding of what is perhaps one of the most difficult jobs: caring for the patient with Alzheimer's disease or other dementia. Our goal in this conversation is 4-fold:

1. To let caregivers know that we fully understand the difficult job they are undertaking.
2. To help them understand that Alzheimer's is a disease that affects the whole family.
3. To introduce the concept that this disease is best treated as a partnership between the patient, the caregiver, and the clinician.
4. To let caregivers know that the treatment of this disease involves treating, supporting, and educating them along with their loved one. We often tell caregivers:

Once the diagnosis and treatment plan are in place, it is likely that our staff and we will spend more time with you than with the patient. This is because we recognize that the single most important aspect of how the patient does throughout the disease is how the caregiver does.

We encourage and try to help everyone become a "four-star caregiver." Having said this, we also recognize that some individuals are more suited to being caregivers than others. This is never presented as a criticism, but simply that individuals each have their own strengths and weaknesses. Later in this chapter we will discuss strategies for recognizing and handling this situation. If we as clinicians have learned one thing in the more than 25 years we have been caring for Alzheimer's disease patients and their families, it is to do our best not to be judgmental.

As is common in the typical medical model, caregivers often feel that, although they are provided with adequate information and support when the diagnosis is given, support in the subsequent care may be lacking (Park et al., 2018). In our roles as health professionals we work to try to help the patient and caregiver throughout the entire disease process.

CARING FOR THE CAREGIVER

Caregivers, simply by virtue of being caregivers, are at increased risk for a variety of medical and psychological problems. Caregivers have many more illnesses than noncaregiving older adults (Oliveira, Sousa, & Orrell, 2019). These are primarily stress-related illnesses such as headache and chronic fatigue, as well as psychological illnesses, particularly anxiety and depression. One study found that mood disorders, anxiety disorders, insomnia, substance abuse or dependence, cardiovascular disease, and rheumatoid arthritis were more common in household members of persons with Alzheimer's disease than controls who did not live with someone with Alzheimer's disease (Suehs et al., 2014). Caregivers frequently indicate that they feel captive, burdened, and distressed. There are several things the treating clinician can do to help, but often the most important and helpful one is simply acknowledging that the caregiver may be experiencing these emotions.

- In the course of a follow-up, simply asking the question of the caregiver, "How are you doing?" and listening to their response may be the single most important part of the visit. Although we often cannot solve the problems they are facing, letting them know we are aware and concerned can do a world of good.
- Referral to psychological services may be appropriate. When possible, we will take part in the initial visit between the caregiver and the therapist.
- Being sure that the caregiver has a primary care provider. We have been struck by the number of

caregivers who are so busy taking care of the patient that they neglect their own health. They frequently either ignore or try to self-treat their own medical illnesses.

THREE PREDICTABLE TRANSITION POINTS WHERE THE CAREGIVER NEEDS HELP

In our experience there are three points in the course of caring for the Alzheimer's disease patient that pose particular difficulty for the caregiver: (1) diagnosis, (2) disease progression—the onset of increasingly debilitating declines in function and/or the onset of the behavioral and psychological symptoms—and (3) the transition to 24-hour care.

Coping With the Diagnosis

The diagnosis of any major illness, including Alzheimer's disease, poses challenges for both the patient and family (Box 25.1).

Among the issues that need to be discussed during the visit when the diagnosis is made include:

The Nature of the Disease

We discuss Alzheimer's as a brain disease in which cells in the brain are slowly, but surely, dying. As these cells die, abilities are lost. Most families and patients resonate to this discussion because they have recognized the progressive nature of their cognitive decline, and because

---

BOX 25.1   Issues to be Discussed With the Caregiver When the Diagnosis is Disclosed

- The nature of the disease.
  - Brain cells are dying, causing a decline in cognition and memory.
  - Changes also occur in personality and behavior.
- There are different stages of Alzheimer's disease, each with its own challenges.
- The disease progresses over time.
- As in most other major illnesses, family members are at higher risk of developing the disease.
- There are a number of treatment options available.
- Financial and legal planning will be needed at some time.

---

they are fearful that Alzheimer's disease "means they are crazy," something of which they are both fearful and embarrassed. Explaining that Alzheimer's disease is a medical disorder and specifically a brain disease can thus be helpful.

We also explain that the brain not only enables cognition and memory but it also regulates personality and behavior. This fact means that, as the disease progresses, behavior and personality will change—sometimes only subtly, sometimes dramatically. So, for example, when the wife finds that her husband with Alzheimer's disease is acting in an irritable, aggressive, or inappropriate manner, it does not mean that he is being "a jerk." It means that the disease has affected his personality and behavior.

Stage of Disease

It is important to present Alzheimer's as a long-lasting disease (an average of 8–12 years) that is very different in different stages. We usually discuss three stages—early/mild, middle/moderate, and late/severe—noting that about 3 to 4 years are spent in each (Table 25.1). We then discuss with the patient and caregiver which stage the patient falls into, and the level of care that is likely to be necessary in each stage.

Progression

Patients and families typically want to know how quickly the disease will progress. We begin by noting that progression is quite variable in Alzheimer's disease. We also indicate that making predictions beyond the next year is difficult (an analogy that helps is to point out that they would have little faith in a weather forecast that predicted more than two weeks in advance). With this in mind, we discuss the changes in activities and living situation that we might foresee in the next year.

Genetic Implications

Most families ask about this early on. At initial diagnosis we usually briefly state that like any other major illness, if a first-degree relative has the disease, family members are at greater risk. Later, we may discuss more fully what is known about the genetic risks. Of course, in the rare cases of autosomal dominant familial disease, we have a different discussion. See Chapter 30 for more on this important topic.

TABLE 25.1   Three Stages of Alzheimer's Disease

Stage	Mini-Mental State Examination (MMSE) Range	Montreal Cognitive Assessment (MoCA) Range	Description
I (Early/Mild)	18–26	15–26	Subtle changes in cognition; patient can often live alone with supervision that must increase as the patient progresses throughout this stage.
II (Middle/Moderate)	10–18	7–15	Patient now needs supervision/help with most activities. Living alone is now impossible.
III (Late/Severe)	<10	<7	24-hour care is present or imminent.

Treatment

Patients and families are always anxious to discuss treatment options. Please see Section III: *Treatment of Memory Loss, Alzheimer's Disease, and Dementia* (see Chapters 18–23).

Resistance to Diagnosis

Resistance can come from the patient (most common), the caregiver/family, or both. Resistance from the patient usually goes hand-in-hand with resistance to being at the evaluation and often manifests as "there is nothing wrong with my memory." It is our experience that there is little the clinician can do at that point to persuade the patient that there is a problem. The goal in this situation is not to argue the point, but to convince him or her to begin treatment. Over time, as a relationship begins to form between the clinician, patient, and caregiver, we usually find that the patient's resistance softens. Resistance from the caregiver usually reflects underlying discomfort with the diagnosis, typically because of fear. There may be fear over the loss of the loved one, fear of being left alone (emotionally and physically), or fear of a prolonged illness that they have observed in another family member. It is our view that to successfully treat the patient, the patient and caregiver must be accepting of the diagnosis. See Carpenter and Dave (2004) for a review on the important topic of disclosing the diagnosis.

Financial and Legal Planning

We feel that a lengthy discussion of financial and legal ramifications of the disease at the first or second visit is perhaps too much for a family to deal with and digest. But planting the seed that these are important issues can be helpful. We then go over these points again at a later visit, typically by encouraging caregivers to discuss these issues with their family lawyer and/or financial planner.

Disease Progression

It can be surmised from the complexity described already, that, in many respects, Alzheimer's disease is not a single uniform illness. As the disease progresses, the symptoms of the patient and consequent demands on the caregiver can change significantly (Hiyoshi-Taniguchi, Becker, & Kinoshita, 2018). At a talk we gave to a group of caregivers, one of the caregivers noted the following:

> *The most difficult part of being a caregiver is dealing with the progressive nature of the disease. Just when I think I have the situation in control, just when I think the programs and structure I have created are working, something changes and it is back to the drawing board.*

This caregiver, of course, is referring to both declines in cognition and/or the onset of behavioral and psychological symptoms. In these instances, families need help in accepting the changes and implementing strategies to cope.

Accepting Outside Help

Many caregivers are reluctant to accept any outside help. This may stem from the caregiver's belief that caring for their spouse or parent is their job, or from not wanting "strangers" in their home. It also may stem from the patient's reluctance to having anyone other than the caregiver help them. This situation can be potentially disastrous because it greatly exacerbates caregiver stress, leading to the exact situation that the clinician and both the patient and caregiver are trying to avoid: a debilitated caregiver leading to a crisis which requires immediate large amounts of outside help or earlier 24-hour care than would otherwise be necessary. Further complicating the situation is that individuals under stress are poor decision-makers.

We have found several approaches help in defusing the situation of the caregiver who refuses outside help:

- A discussion with the caregiver that they are the single most important factor in the prognosis for the patient and it is therefore essential that they remain healthy. An important part of remaining healthy is to reduce stress. Accepting outside help is an important part of stress reduction.
- Enlisting the services of a social worker, elder care services, or the Alzheimer's Association in the United States (www.alz.org 800-272-3900) and Australia (https://www.alz.org/au/dementia-alzheimers-australia.asp), Alzheimer Society in Canada (https://alzheimer.ca/en 800-616-8816), and the Alzheimer's Society in England, Wales, and Northern Ireland (www.alzheimers.org.uk 0300 222 1122) can be helpful.
- Encouraging the caregiver to attend a support group to learn how other caregivers handle stressful situations can be very beneficial.
- Asking the caregiver to consider counseling.

Late-Stage Decisions

Almost inevitably, patients with Alzheimer's disease will reach a point when a single caregiver can no longer adequately care for them. At this time caregivers must seek placement in a facility where caregiving is a shared responsibility. This usually means placement in an assisted living or a nursing home facility. In a small minority of cases, families attempt to arrange for round-the-clock help to come into the home. Although on the surface this seems like a desirable plan, we have rarely seen it accomplished successfully. There are, unfortunately, a number of challenging obstacles that make this a difficult path. To begin, round-the-clock care is very expensive; by estimates of some of the families we have worked with who have done this successfully,

round-the-clock care can cost up to $100,000 annually. Few families have these resources. Even when financial resources are available, it is difficult to find skilled and reliable caregivers. As we point out to families who propose this, "Whenever a caregiver does not show up, you are the backup."

In some cases, as the disease progresses, there is a stepwise transition from living at home, to assisted living, to nursing homes. In all cases these transitions are difficult for the caregiver—sometimes more so than for the patient. For our patients whom we follow on a regular basis, we will often initiate the conversation in anticipation of these transitions.

The decision to move a loved one from the home is always a very difficult and emotionally laden decision (Müller et al., 2017). It is important to start to plant the seed early that a move from the home will be necessary at some time, and to continue that discussion as the disease progresses. When we recognize that the caregiver can no longer successfully care for the patient at home we continue this conversation with a discussion that includes the following points that may ease the transition for the caregiver:

- *The decision to seek 24-hour care is not a selfish decision but one that is almost always in the best interest of the patient.* We usually begin by praising the caregiver's efforts to date, and reviewing all the wonderful things they have done over the past year (caregivers rarely get such outside praise). We then discuss how inevitably, in all cases of Alzheimer's disease (or other dementia), there comes a time that no single person can care for the patient. Moreover, attempting to do so may actually not be in the best interest of the patient. This leads to a discussion of the concept of "caregiving shared by professionals," and a discussion of ways in which this can be accomplished, including help in the home through homemakers and home health aides, adult day care, assisted living, and nursing homes.
- *There is no absolute right or wrong time to make this move.* We emphasize that all caregivers and patients are different and that the time to implement a move to assisted living or nursing home is when the caregiver—with guidance from the clinician—thinks it is appropriate and will be best for both patient and caregiver together. We also take this as an opportunity to tell the caregiver that, in our experience, the time for the move may come on suddenly.

- *Because the decision to institute 24-hour care can come about with little warning, a plan should be in place.* Because the time to start 24-hour care often comes at a time of crisis, we urge caregivers to begin to visit facilities during the middle stage of the disease (Mini-Mental State Examination 10–18, Montreal Cognitive Assessment 7–15) to identify a facility in which they would feel comfortable having their loved one. When they find a facility, we urge them to complete the necessary paperwork to the degree that they can, so that, when the time comes, they can initiate placement with just a phone call. We also explain that there may be a delay until a place in the facility becomes available.

- *Relinquishing primary caregiving does not mean they will not be involved.* We let caregivers know that, once the move is made, how much or little they are involved in care will be up to them, again indicating that there is no right amount, but rather it is an individual decision.

- *We encourage them to begin to consider how they will fill the void when they are no longer spending considerable time caregiving.* Lastly, we encourage them to consider the things they liked to do before they became a caregiver. Work (paid or volunteer), travel, hobbies, and time with family and friends should all be considered.

REFERENCES

Alzheimer's Association. (2020). Alzheimer's disease facts and figures. *Alzheimer's & Dementia, 16*(3), 391+.

Budson, A. E., & O'Connor, M. K. (2021). *Six steps to managing Alzheimer's disease and dementia: A guide for families.* New York: Oxford University Press.

Carpenter, B., & Dave, J. (2004). Disclosing a dementia diagnosis: A review of opinion and practice, and a proposed research agenda. *The Gerontologist, 44,* 149–158.

Hiyoshi-Taniguchi, K., Becker, C. B., & Kinoshita, A. (2018). What behavioral and psychological symptoms of dementia affect caregiver burnout? *Clinical Gerontologist, 41*(3), 249–254.

Mace, N. L., & Rabins, P. V. (2017). *The 36-hour day: A family guide to caring for people who have Alzheimer disease, related dementias, and memory loss.* Baltimore: Johns Hopkins University Press.

Müller, C., Lautenschläger, S., Meyer, G., et al. (2017). Interventions to support people with dementia and their caregivers during the transition from home care to nursing home care: A systematic review. *International Journal of Nursing Studies, 71,* 139–152.

Oliveira, D., Sousa, L., & Orrell, M. (2019). Improving health-promoting self-care in family carers of people with dementia: A review of interventions. *Clinical Interventions in Aging, 14,* 515–523.

Park, M., Choi, S., Lee, S. J., et al. (2018). The roles of unmet needs and formal support in the caregiving satisfaction and caregiving burden of family caregivers for persons with dementia. *International Psychogeriatrics, 30*(4), 557–567.

Suehs, B. T., Shah, S. N., Davis, C. D., et al. (2014). Household members of persons with Alzheimer's disease: Health conditions, healthcare resource use, and healthcare costs. *Journal of the American Geriatrics Society, 62,* 435–441.

See also Chapter 28 for additional discussion of these important topics.

26

Nonpharmacological Treatment of the Behavioral and Psychological Symptoms of Dementia

QUICK START: NONPHARMACOLOGICAL TREATMENT OF THE BEHAVIORAL AND PSYCHOLOGICAL SYMPTOMS OF DEMENTIA

Important Principles for Treating Behavioral and Psychological Symptoms of Dementia—The 3Rs:
- Reassure
  - Let patients know that they will be cared for and their wishes will be respected.
- Reconsider
  - Consider how things look from the patient's point of view.
- Redirect
  - Do not confront patients when they are wrong, frustrating, or delusional.
  - Distract them by moving to a different activity or topic of conversation.

General Behavioral Strategies for Managing Behavioral and Psychological Symptoms of Dementia
- Manage the environment
  - Keep routines and other things as constant as possible.
  - Use pictures liberally in signs and other written communication.
  - Use night-lights and other lighting at night.
- Keep the patient safe
  - Alzheimer's Association/Medic Alert "Safe Return" bracelet
  - GPS tracking system for the watch or car
  - Locks on doors, gates, and cabinets
  - Disconnect the stove
  - Remove or lock up weapons and power tools.
- Redirect the patient
  - Change the topic of conversation

- Participate in safe and familiar activities
  - Listen to old music
  - Watch old movies
  - Look at photo albums
  - Discuss past events
  - Fold laundry.
  - Walk or drive with the patient.
- Care for the caregiver (see also Chapter 25)
  - Support groups
  - Counseling/therapy—individual and family
  - Educational activities
  - Respite care
  - Online chat rooms, blogs, and message boards.

Dealing With Specific Behavioral and Psychological Symptoms of Dementia
- Apathy
  - Involve the patient in preferred activities.
  - Simplify the activities if needed.
  - Do not trade apathy for agitation.
- Depression
  - Avoid asking the patient to "snap out of it."
  - Encourage social interaction.
  - Seek counseling/therapy.
- Psychosis: delusions and hallucinations
  - Delusions are common.
    - Stealing possessions
    - Infidelity
    - House is not their home
    - Spouse is not their spouse.

(Continued)

- Hallucinations
  - Visual hallucinations are common early in dementia with Lewy bodies.
  - Some hallucinations require medical investigation.
- Behavioral interventions

- React calmly.
- Help the caregiver to understand the patient's experience.
- Avoid denying the patient's experience or confronting the patient regarding the experience.

When caregivers report behavioral and psychological symptoms, we begin with an evaluation of the nature of the symptoms, level of distress they are causing the patient, and level of distress they are causing the caregiver. Based upon this evaluation, the initial decision is made whether or not to treat the symptoms. For example, a commonly reported repetitive hallucination is one of a child playing in a corner. In some instances, this hallucination may have a delusional quality, that is, the patient believes it is really happening; in other instances, the patient may realize at some level that it is not real. In either case most patients are not disturbed by this hallucination, nor are caregivers. In these situations, we will typically not suggest any treatment. By contrast, if the repetitive hallucination is of a man breaking into the house, it may be terrifying for the patient and upsetting for the caregiver, and therefore warrants treatment.

In most cases we first try to treat behavioral and psychological symptoms of dementia using behavioral (nonpharmacological) techniques. If this approach is not successful we then move on to supplementation with drugs (see Chapter 27).

Before discussing techniques for the treatment of specific behavioral and psychological symptoms, we would like to discuss some general principles.

SOME GENERAL PRINCIPLES FOR TREATING BEHAVIORAL AND PSYCHOLOGICAL SYMPTOMS IN DEMENTIA: THE 3RS

Caregivers often experience difficulty when attempting to determine if, when, and how to intervene when behavioral and psychological symptoms occur. They struggle between trying to accommodate two basic needs that are often in conflict:

1. The need for the patient to be safe, and
2. The need for the patient to be content (happy).

For example, at some point, patients will need to stop driving to prevent significant risk of endangering themselves and others. However, patients are often reluctant to do so, and even a discussion of the possibility of not driving can lead to stress and agitation. It is clear that such a situation needs intervention.

One general approach to managing behavioral and psychological symptoms of dementia has become commonly known as the 3Rs: reassure, reconsider, redirect.

Reassure

One reason the person may be unwilling to give up a particular activity—driving, for example—is that he or she is fearful of the loss of the ability to do the things they find necessary (going to the supermarket) or enjoyable (visiting a friend). In any discussion where a loss of an important activity may be involved, it is important for the caregiver to reassure the patient that there will be alternative ways in which the patient can continue doing what they need and like to do.

CASE STUDY: Reassuring the Veteran Driver

One of the most contentious discussions we have ever had about driving was with a patient who was a World War II veteran. Despite several minor accidents, becoming so lost he had to be brought home by the police, and losing his car in a parking lot, he would not even entertain the possibility of not driving. His family could not even broach the subject with him without significant agitation, including yelling and throwing objects. The family asked for our help and, after several frustrating meetings, we made no progress. We finally decided to ask him to keep a daily log of where he drove. He was willing to do this task, and what emerged was that there was one place he went to nearly every day: the American Legion Post that was only a few miles from his home, but too far to walk. Other use of the car was sporadic. When we discussed with him a plan for getting him to the American Legion Post on a daily basis, his resistance to quitting driving disappeared. What we did here was to let the patient know (reassure him) that he was in a loving environment where people cared for him, respected his needs, and would do what was necessary to meet these needs.

Reconsider

Ask, "How do things look from the patient's point of view?"

In many cases simply trying to understand how the patient with diminished cognitive capacity might perceive the situation can be used to remediate the behavioral problem.

> ### CASE STUDY: Reconsidering the Touchy Patient
>
> Several years ago, we encountered a patient who was exhibiting inappropriate sexual behavior toward a female caregiver who visited to help with his care three times a week. His wife was quite upset when the patient would inappropriately touch the caregiver during the course of the day. The patient's wife was also surprised because this type of behavior was entirely uncharacteristic for the patient. After considerable discussion with the patient and caregiver, we all came to realize that the genesis of this troublesome behavior was that one of the responsibilities of the caregiver was to help the patient bathe. The patient interpreted touching during bathing as sexual touching and thus in his view his touching the caregiver during the day was reciprocal and entirely appropriate. We rearranged the bathing schedule so that he was no longer bathed by a woman, which resolved the behavior.

Redirect

Perhaps the single most important piece of advice we can provide to a caregiver is not to be confrontational. And while this advice is easy to give, in many cases it may not be so easy to follow.

> ### CASE STUDY: Redirecting the Gourmet Cook
>
> We follow a patient who was once an excellent cook, but now has great difficulty in the kitchen. As such, her husband, the primary caregiver, has taken over the duties in the kitchen. Although he has become a competent cook, his main challenge is now to keep his wife out of the kitchen. The patient understandably continues to want to be engaged in activities in which she was once quite accomplished. The problem is that she would often cause difficult and potentially dangerous situations, such as putting a metal bowl in the microwave or putting a dish towel on the burner. These difficulties led to many confrontations and arguments. Her husband solved this problem by getting the patient her own oven—in this case a toy oven—and giving her a specific job during meal preparation that she cheerfully carries out.

Interacting with a demented patient—even when the patient is a spouse or parent—can be quite frustrating for the caregiver. The caregiver needs to strike a balance between what the patient wants to do and what is safe. When these needs conflict, there can be frustration and agitation for both patient and caregiver.

In general, we advise caregivers to carefully pick their battles. When a patient asks a caregiver for the tenth time in 15 minutes where they are going for lunch that day, it is tempting—and probably cathartic—for the caregiver to say, "Don't ask me again! I have already told you the answer 10 times in the last 15 minutes!" Unfortunately, this response will likely lead to the patient experiencing either anger and agitation or sadness and depression. A better solution is to redirect the patient to another activity that they can accomplish independently and that will distract them from focusing on lunch. In the case above, the astute caregiver took a situation that was potentially confrontational and turned it into a positive activity.

Of course, there are instances in which the caregiver must intervene more directly. These are generally cases in which safety is an imminent issue. For example, when a patient who is known to become lost in the neighborhood and cannot safely cross streets is walking out the front door, a direct approach may be necessary.

Other general strategies for dealing with behavioral and psychological symptoms in dementia using behavioral techniques are summarized in Boxes 26.1 and 26.2 (for reviews see Scales, Zimmerman, & Miller, 2018; Trahan et al., 2014). Note that the positive benefit of music for patients has become increasingly recognized, and these benefits can improve caregiver well-being and their coping capacity (Lewis et al., 2015; for reviews see Blackburn & Bradshaw, 2014; Ekra & Dale, 2020).

DEALING WITH SPECIFIC BEHAVIORAL AND PSYCHOLOGICAL SYMPTOMS OF DEMENTIA: BEHAVIORAL TECHNIQUES

Apathy

One of the most common complaints that we hear from caregivers is that the patient does not want to do anything. Caregivers comment that patients frequently just want to sit in their chairs, often falling asleep. They further comment that it is difficult to

---

BOX 26.1   **General Behavioral Strategies for Managing Behavioral and Psychological Symptoms in Dementia**

Manage the Environment

As dementia progresses, patients become more confused and disoriented. A highly structured and consistent environment, both in terms of the physical environment and temporal routine, can be helpful. (See "External Memory Aids" in Chapter 22 for elaboration and additional suggestions.)

- Keep the daily routine as constant as possible.
- Keep a calendar of daily events in a prominent place that the patient will check frequently.
- Try not to rearrange the contents of cabinets, drawers, or even the location of furniture.
- Use signs to direct and identify places in the home, such as the bathroom.
- In signs and written communication, use pictures, rather than words, whenever possible.
- Use night-lights and other lighting at night.

Keep the Patient Safe

- Obtain an Alzheimer's Association/Medic Alert "Safe Return" bracelet for the patient (www.alz.org/safereturn)
- If the patient goes out independently, consider a GPS tracking system, often as part of a watch or attached to the car (www.alz.org/comfortzone)
- If the person wanders, also consider locks on doors and gates
- Disconnect the stove from the power or gas

- Use "child-proof" locks on cabinets that house knives and dangerous chemicals
- Remove or lock up power tools and weapons

Redirect the Patient

- Change the topic of conversation
- Listen to familiar music, e.g., show tunes
- Watch old and familiar movies
- Look at family albums and discuss *prior remote* events
- Walk or drive with the patient
- Perform safe and routine activities, such as folding laundry

Care for the Caregiver (See Also Chapter 25)

- Have the family contact the local Alzheimer's Association (or the equivalent) in their community (www.alz.org 800-272-3900) Australia (https://www.alz.org/au/dementia-alzheimers-australia.asp), Alzheimer Society in Canada (https://alzheimer.ca/en 800-616-8816), or the Alzheimer's Society in England, Wales, and Northern Ireland (www.alzheimers.org.uk 0300 222 1122)
- Support groups
- Counseling/therapy—individual and family
- Educational activities
- Respite care
- Online chat rooms, blogs, and message boards (www.alzconnected.org in the United States; forum.alzheimers.org.uk in England, Wales, and Northern Ireland; similar programs in other countries.)

---

keep them busy and to find appropriate activities to do with them.

As discussed earlier, apathy is perhaps the most common behavioral symptom in Alzheimer's disease (Kumfor et al., 2018). It is tempting to consider apathy as a form of depression, but the two are separable. Although apathy and depression commonly co-occur, there can be apathy without depression and depression without apathy (Nakaaki et al., 2008; Tagariello, Girardi, & Amore, 2009). It is also tempting not to bother treating apathy because it is certainly easier to care for apathetic patients than those who are agitated and upset.

It is, however, vitally important to treat the apathetic patient.

Behavioral Treatments for Apathy

Some strategies to suggest for caregivers to help with the apathetic patient include:

- Try to get the patient involved in activities they once enjoyed.
- Simplify and organize what you ask the patient to do. Be careful, however; you don't want to trade apathy for agitation. For a review of apathy in dementia, including management, see Cipriani et al. (2014).

CASE STUDY: A Plan for the Garden

One of our caregivers tried to get her husband up from his chair (where he would sit most of the day and not interact with anyone) and go out to their garden—a garden they planted and cared for together for many years. She would take him outside and suggest several things that he might do, including planting, weeding, and watering. Within a few minutes she would find him back in his chair, much to the frustration of the caregiver. We realized that part of the problem was that the patient had lost the ability to organize and sequence the necessary gardening steps. We suggested that the caregiver try to find time to go out to the garden to work with him and then plan, organize, and supervise a very single specific task for him, such as weeding a small part of the garden that she would delineate with some string. The reports back from the garden were that this worked well and we even reaped the fruits in the form of wonderful tomatoes.

CASE STUDY: The Puzzler—Apathetic or Agitated?

One of our patients was an avid crossword puzzler. But he stopped doing these puzzles and became quite withdrawn and apathetic. His wife read that keeping the mind active could slow the progression of Alzheimer's disease and so she began to insist that he not sit around all day and that he complete crossword puzzles. This insistence led to significant agitation. He would uncharacteristically throw the puzzles, break his pencil, and scream at his wife. His wife had traded one manifestation of behavioral and psychological symptoms in dementia for another. We suggested that perhaps a simpler form of word game might be more successful. She substituted "word search" (a puzzle in which the person finds words in mixes of letters and circles them) for the crossword puzzle with great success.

BOX 26.2 Evidence-Based Nonpharmacological Practices for Managing Behavioral and Psychological Symptoms in Dementia

Sensory Practices

- Aromatherapy: Administration of scented oils via diffusion, patches, or skin cream to induce calm and positive effect (try lavender or lemon).
- Massage: Therapeutic touch applied to back, shoulder, neck, hands, or feet by qualified massage therapist, trained staff, or family to induce calm and positive effect.
- Multisensory stimulation: Combined light effects, calming sounds, smells, and tactile stimulation to overcome apathy or induce calm.
- Bright light therapy: Exposure to simulated natural light designed to help promote synchronization of circadian rhythms with environmental light–dark cycles.

Psychosocial Practices

- Validation therapy: Individual or group practice designed to validate the perceived reality and emotional experience of the individual.
- Reminiscence therapy: Individual or group practice designed to induce a positive effect through a focus on happy memories, often using photographs or other prompts.
- Music therapy: Receptive or participatory activities designed to promote well-being, foster sociability, create familiarity, and reduce anxiety.
- Pet therapy: Structured or unstructured time with animals, primarily dogs, to promote well-being, socialization and emotional support, and sensory stimulation.
- Meaningful activities: Activities designed to enhance quality of life through engagement, social interaction, and opportunities for self-expression and self-determination.

Structured Care Protocols

- Mouth care: Providing mouth care using protocols that include person-centered communication and interaction strategies as well as technical skills.
- Bathing: Providing bathing care using protocols that include person-centered communication and interaction strategies as well as technical skills.

Modified from Scales, K., Zimmerman, S., & Miller, S. J. (2018). Evidence-based nonpharmacological practices to address behavioral and psychological symptoms of dementia. *Gerontologist*, *58*(Suppl 1), S88–S102.

Depression

Although we know that many patients with Alzheimer's disease also show symptoms of depression, the relationship between Alzheimer's disease and depression is complex and controversial (for review see Bazin & Bratu, 2014). There are well-done studies to suggest the following:

- A history of depression earlier in life is a risk factor for Alzheimer's disease.
- Symptoms of depression are common in the few years preceding the diagnosis of Alzheimer's disease, prompting some researchers to hypothesize that it is an early symptom of Alzheimer's disease, especially in individuals with no lifetime history of depression.
- Depression is common early in the course of Alzheimer's disease and the incidence increases as the disease progresses until all insight is lost (Kuring, Mathias, & Ward, 2018).

Because both Alzheimer's disease and depression can produce memory dysfunction (see Chapter 17), we often see patients referred by their primary care providers who are already treated with an antidepressant. In some cases (but rarely in our experience) treating the depression eliminates the cognitive deficits. Much more commonly, the referred patient is experiencing both Alzheimer's disease and depression, and both are contributing to their cognitive deficits, and both need to be treated. To help sort out the contribution of the depression, when we evaluate these patients we ask ourselves two questions:

1. If the depression completely resolved tomorrow, would this individual's memory problems also be resolved?
2. Is the current level of depression sufficient to account for the current level of cognitive deficits?
   In almost all cases, the answer to both questions is no.

Behavioral Treatments for Depression

Some strategies and tips to suggest for caregivers to help with the depressed patient include the following:
- Avoid asking the patient to "snap out of it"
  - This type of message conveys that the caregiver does not understand what the depressed individual is experiencing, which may lead to frustration and may exacerbate the depression.
- Encourage social interaction
  - This may best be accomplished in small groups, (e.g., dinner at home with one or two close friends).

- When the interactions are in larger groups, which can be confusing to patients, encourage the patient to talk just with one or two people there.
- Seek counseling/therapy
  - Psychotherapy is most likely to be successful in patients who have relatively mild disease, so that they can understand and remember what has transpired in the session.
  - It is important to refer to a therapist who has knowledge of and experience with Alzheimer's disease.
  - Because emotional memory involves different brain structures than remembering facts, patients can benefit from talk therapy emotionally even if they do not remember the specific content of the sessions.

Psychosis: Delusions and Hallucinations

Delusions are very common in all dementias, but particularly in patients with Alzheimer's disease (usually related to their memory impairment). Delusions are false beliefs, and in dementia often take on a paranoid flavor. Hallucinations and misperceptions also occur in dementia, particularly in patients with dementia with Lewy bodies but also in patients with Alzheimer's disease in the middle stage of the disease and beyond (roughly Mini-Mental State Examination [MMSE] <16, Montreal Cognitive Assessment <11). In dementia with Lewy bodies, the hallucinations occur as an early symptom and are usually visual. In Alzheimer's disease these symptoms are more likely to be misperceptions or false memories than true hallucinations (see Chapter 2). Hallucinations and misperceptions may or may not have a delusional quality. For example, a patient may report seeing children playing in the yard and be able to describe them in great detail. Yet, when questioned, they realize that the children are not really there. In contrast, another patient may have the same report, but have the firm belief (from which they will not be dissuaded) that the children are real; these hallucinations have a delusional quality.

> A father and son were looking at the moon. The father told his son there were two moons. The son replied, you must be seeing double. No, said the father, if I were seeing double, there would be four.

People with memory problems can become suspicious to the point of paranoia. This suspiciousness can range from a mild annoyance to the patient and family, for example, "the cleaning person is stealing my loose change," to events that produce palpable fear and lead to destructive behaviors, for example., "the mailman, delivery person, and so on, is coming to take me from my home or to steal my furniture," leading to locking doors, resisting all help and visitors, and perhaps calling the police. More mild delusions can often be ignored, but the disruptive or dangerous delusions need to be treated.

CASE STUDY: Sitting With a Shotgun

We had a patient in the middle stages of dementia who believed that anyone coming to his door (e.g., the mailman, the UPS delivery person) was there to take him from his home and take all his possessions. Initially, he simply commented upon this. But, as he became more confused and forgetful, he began to perseverate on this idea. One morning his brother came to visit, as he often did, and found the door locked. He knocked but there was no answer. When he looked in the window, he saw his brother sitting with a shotgun (that we later determined was loaded) in his lap. It was clear that it was now time to treat these paranoid delusions.

Delusions

Delusions in Alzheimer's disease and other dementias can vary, but certain delusions seem to prevail, including the following:

- A relative or neighbor is stealing the patient's possessions
  - This often stems from patients misplacing or even hiding items, and when they cannot find them they assume others have stolen them.
  - This delusion can often lead to contention and distress when the patient confronts the family member or neighbor.
- Delusion of infidelity
  - These delusions can be especially troublesome when the patient accuses his or her spouse of many years of an extramarital relationship and asks the spouse to leave the home.
- Their house is not their home

- This delusion can lead to very agitated behavior in which the person constantly states that they want to go home, even when they are at home.
- This delusion frequently occurs because the patient remembers an earlier home (often the home of their childhood), and thinks that they live there.
- Their spouse is not their spouse
  - This delusion is obviously very distressing to the spouse, making it that much more difficult to care for the patient.
  - Often the patient will be remembering a past time, either expecting the spouse to look 40 years younger or expecting their previous husband or wife.

We would, however, offer one caution when evaluating delusions, whether of infidelity, stealing, or other matters. Some stories—even though they seem unlikely and fit the pattern of delusions seen in Alzheimer's disease—are actually true; see the two case studies below. In general, delusions are important to treat because they can lead to agitation, aggression, anxiety, and purposeless behavior. They are frequently stressful to the patient and the caregiver.

CASE STUDY: Just Because You're Paranoid Doesn't Mean They Aren't Out to Get You

We followed a patient who had been married to his wife for 48 years. In talking with him at one visit, he confided to me (P.R.S.) that he felt his wife was having an affair with a younger man in Boston. He told me that on several recent occasions his wife had left him with a caregiver and gone to Boston for several days. He also was sure that this person was calling his wife at home. We discussed this at some length and it was clear that this was understandably extremely troublesome to him. He had not discussed this with his wife. I asked if I might first talk to his wife about this and perhaps then we could all discuss his feelings. He agreed. I then talked with his wife and told her that I thought her husband was having delusions and conveyed the conversation that the patient and I had. I then noticed a "deer in the headlights" look come over her face and I immediately knew her husband was not having a delusion. The patient's wife then told me that his beliefs were true and we discussed how we might manage this difficult situation.

CASE STUDY: The Helpful Neighbors

Another of our patients was living alone in his own home. He was in the early stages of Alzheimer's disease (MMSE 24) and his daughter was his primary caregiver. They spoke on the phone daily and she saw him about once a week. He also was receiving help from three young women who lived next door to him. He had good retirement benefits and social security, yet he reported that he never had any money. His daughter found that his bank account was dwindling and no one could understand how he was spending the money. The patient felt that someone in the bank must be stealing his money. What we eventually learned was that the "helpful neighbors" were not only helping him get to the supermarket and drug store, but also to the cash machine, several times a week. Our patient did not recall these episodes.

Hallucinations

A person with a dementing illness may hear, see, smell, or feel stimuli that are not present. Visual hallucinations are often an early symptom of dementia with Lewy bodies. In Alzheimer's disease misperceptions and false memories are more likely. As in the case of delusions, hallucinations can range from being entertaining to the patient—seeing children playing in the back yard—to being terrifying—seeing snakes in the bed. As with delusions, the amount of distress that the delusions cause the patient determines the nature of the treatment.

One hallucination deserves particular mention: that of feeling bugs crawling on one's arm. This hallucination is not uncommon, and can result from a number of causes. It may be as a result of medication toxicity, infection or infestation (e.g., scabies, bed bugs), or another medical problem, particularly one that causes itching (e.g., morphine use, renal failure). It may also be from ordinary causes of itching, such as poison ivy or even simply dry skin. The first sign of this hallucination may be raw skin on the patient's arm from "scratching the bugs." This hallucination, almost always very disturbing to the patient and caregiver, warrants medical investigation and treatment.

Behavioral Treatments for Hallucinations and Delusions

Some strategies and tips to suggest for caregivers to help with patients with hallucinations and delusions include the following:

- *React calmly*
  - The initial occurrence of a hallucination or delusion can be disconcerting and frightening to the patient and/or family. The tendency is to treat the situation as an emergency. An emergency attitude and action can be alarming to the patient as well and may contribute to agitation, further complicating an already difficult situation.
  - As long as the hallucination or delusion is not posing a danger to the patient or others, the caregiver can simply reassure the patient and seek a medical evaluation and assistance in the usual way.
  - In many cases the combination of reassurance that this symptom is typical of the disease and a discussion of strategies to manage the symptom will handle the situation.
- *Help the caregiver understand the patient's experience*
  - Perhaps the most difficult aspect of hallucinations and delusions for the caregiver to embrace is that the experience for the patient is as real as any experience that the caregiver is having.
  - We often ask our caregivers, "If I tried to convince you that the chair sitting in the corner was not there, would you believe me?"
  - Once the caregiver appreciates what the patient is experiencing, discussing management strategies becomes easier.
- *Avoid denying the patient's experience or confronting the patient regarding the experience.*
  - Although we do not recommend denying the experience, neither do we recommend endorsing it.
  - A simple statement, such as "I understand that you believe people are stealing from you, but I think your wallet is simply misplaced," may be helpful.
  - Redirecting the patient to other topics is usually the best approach.

CASE STUDY: Sitting in the Living Room

A mid-stage dementia patient (MMSE 17) came in with her daughter and told us about seeing her dead husband sitting on the living room couch on several occasions. Although the patient was remarkably calm about the events, her daughter was not. Her daughter corrected the patient, reminded her that her husband was dead, and an argument between mother and daughter ensued.

Because the experience is real for the patient, denial, confrontation, and getting upset on the part of the daughter only served to agitate the patient. Although we did not recommend endorsing this hallucination, we suggested that she simply state to her mother: "I understand that you saw dad, but I did not. I am sure this is frightening for you." We then recommended that she change the conversation and exit the situation.

REFERENCES

Bazin, N., & Bratu, L. (2014). Depression in the elderly: Prodroma or risk factor for dementia? A critical review of the literature. *Geriatrie et Psychologie Neuropsychiatrie du Vieillissement, 12,* 289–297.

Blackburn, R., & Bradshaw, T. (2014). Music therapy for service users with dementia: A critical review of the literature. *Journal of Psychiatric and Mental Health Nursing, 21,* 879–888.

Cipriani, G., Lucetti, C., Danti, S., et al. (2014). Apathy and dementia. Nosology, assessment and management. *The Journal of Nervous and Mental Disease, 202,* 718–724.

Ekra, E. M. R., & Dale, B. (2020). Systematic use of song and music in dementia care: Health care providers' experiences. *The Journal of Multidisciplinary Healthcare, 13,* 143–151. https://doi.org/10.2147/JMDH.S231440.

Kumfor, F., Zhen, A., Hodges, J. R., et al. (2018). Apathy in Alzheimer's disease and frontotemporal dementia: Distinct clinical profiles and neural correlates. *Cortex, 103,* 350–359. https://doi.org/10.1016/j.cortex.2018.03.019.

Kuring, J. K., Mathias, J. L., & Ward, L. (2018). Prevalence of depression, anxiety and PTSD in people with dementia: A systematic review and meta-analysis. *Neuropsychology Review, 28*(4), 393–416. https://doi.org/10.1007/s11065-018-9396-2.

Lewis, V., Bauer, M., Winbolt, M., et al. (2015). A study of the effectiveness of MP3 players to support family carers of people living with dementia at home. *International Psychogeriatric, 27,* 471–479.

Nakaaki, S., Murata, Y., Sato, J., et al. (2008). Association between apathy/depression and executive function in patients with Alzheimer's disease. *International Psychogeriatric, 20,* 964–975.

Scales, K., Zimmerman, S., & Miller, S. J. (2018). Evidence-based nonpharmacological practices to address behavioral and psychological symptoms of dementia. *Gerontologist, 58*(Suppl 1), S88–S102. https://doi.org/10.1093/geront/gnx167.

Tagariello, P., Girardi, P., & Amore, M. (2009). Depression and apathy in dementia: Same syndrome or different constructs? A critical review. *Archives of Gerontology and Geriatrics, 49,* 246–249.

Trahan, M. A., Kuo, J., Carlson, M. C., et al. (2014). A systematic review of strategies to foster activity engagement in persons with dementia. *Health Education & Behavior, 41*(Suppl 1), 70S–83S.

27

Pharmacological Treatment of the Behavioral and Psychological Symptoms of Dementia

QUICK START: PHARMACOLOGICAL TREATMENT OF THE BEHAVIORAL AND PSYCHOLOGICAL SYMPTOMS OF DEMENTIA

- Pharmacological treatment of the behavioral and psychological symptoms of dementia should only be undertaken when one of the following situations is present:
  - The symptoms are causing distress to the patient or caregiver.
  - The symptoms are dangerous to the patient or others.
  - There is a specific condition for which there is a known treatment that is both efficacious and safe.
  - Nonpharmacological approaches have been tried (see Chapter 26).
- Medications to treat cognition, cholinesterase inhibitors (see Chapter 19), and memantine (see Chapter 20), are helpful in treating the behavioral and psychological symptoms of dementia and, in general, should be used first.
- Medical illnesses should always be looked for and treated.
- General principles of pharmacotherapy for behavioral and psychological symptoms of dementia:
  - Accurately diagnose the underlying dementia.
  - Identify and measure specific target symptoms.
  - Start low, go slow—but go.
  - Instruct the caregiver and patient both verbally and in writing.
  - Remove unneeded medications.
  - Change only one medication at a time.
- Pharmacotherapy for depression

- The selective serotonin reuptake inhibitors (SSRIs) sertraline (Zoloft) and escitalopram (Lexapro) are first-line therapy.
  - Bupropion (Wellbutrin) and venlafaxine (Effexor) can also be used.
- Pharmacotherapy for anxiety
  - The SSRIs sertraline (Zoloft) and escitalopram (Lexapro) are first-line therapy.
- Pharmacotherapy for pseudobulbar affect
  - Dextromethorphan/quinidine (Nuedexta) may be used.
- Pharmacotherapy for insomnia
  - Address sleep hygiene and cycle issues.
  - Try nonpharmacological treatments.
  - Treat any underlying sleep disorder.
  - Treat minor aches and pains with acetaminophen (paracetamol).
  - Treat any underlying depression or anxiety.
  - Can try a small dose of a long-acting stimulant medication to keep patient awake and alert during the day (see text).
  - Can try melatonin to regulate sleep cycle.
- Pharmacotherapy for psychosis
  - Accurately diagnose the cause of the dementia.
  - The SSRIs sertraline (Zoloft) and escitalopram (Lexapro) can reduce the fear and anxiety associated with delusions and hallucinations.
  - Atypical antipsychotics are sometimes needed.
- Pharmacotherapy for agitation

(Continued)

QUICK START: PHARMACOLOGICAL TREATMENT OF THE BEHAVIORAL AND PSYCHOLOGICAL SYMPTOMS OF DEMENTIA (*Continued*)

- Characterize and diagnose the nature of the agitation and any underlying or comorbid condition(s) present.
- Treat pains from known etiology with acetaminophen (paracetamol).
- Always start with education of the caregiver (see Chapter 25) and nonpharmacologic treatments (see Chapter 26).
- Make sure the patient is on standard pharmacologic therapy for dementia, if appropriate, including cholinesterase inhibitors (see Chapter 19) and memantine (see Chapter 20).
- If depression or anxiety is present, start with an SSRI.
- If anger or angry outbursts are the most prominent symptom, prazosin can be tried.

- Treat insomnia and other sleep disturbances, if present.
- If psychosis (hallucinations or delusions) is present, consider an atypical antipsychotic after SSRIs, cholinesterase inhibitors, and memantine.
- Dextromethorphan/quinidine (Nuedexta) can be tried.
- If no specific cause for the agitation can be determined, start with an atypical antipsychotic if rapid treatment is necessary; start with an SSRI if treatment may be initiated more slowly.
- Behavioral and psychiatric crises
  - Psychiatric hospitalizations allow medications to quickly be withdrawn and added in a safe setting.

Note that the medications discussed in this chapter are powerful drugs with dangerous side effects and adverse reactions and are not approved by the U.S. Food and Drug Administration for use in patients with dementia. See CAUTION in text.

In some cases, nonpharmacological treatment of the behavioral and psychological symptoms of dementia is not sufficient. In these instances, the judicious use of appropriate medications can be beneficial. Our rule of thumb in introducing pharmacological treatment for the behavioral and psychological symptoms of dementia is that we only do so when one of the following situations is present:

- The symptoms are causing distress to the patient or caregiver.
- The symptoms are dangerous to the patient or others.
- There is a specific condition for which there is a known treatment that is both efficacious and safe.

CAUTION: Note that the medications discussed in this chapter are powerful drugs with dangerous side effects and adverse reactions and are not approved by the U.S. Food and Drug Administration (FDA) for use in patients with dementia. All recommendations in this chapter are based upon the combination of published research studies, clinical experience, and use in non-demented patients. The physician (or other provider) must use appropriate clinical judgment as to whether the potential benefit of prescribing one of these medications

"off-label" outweighs the risks to the patient. In addition to reviewing side effects and adverse reactions, the physician (or other provider) must review the FDA-approved package insert, including black box warnings, contraindications and cautions, drug interactions, and safety and monitoring, before prescribing. The authors take no responsibility in the prescribing of one or more of these medications by the physician (or other provider) to his or her patients.

In general, pharmacotherapy for patients with behavioral and psychological symptoms of dementia falls into three general categories.

1. Drugs to treat cognition. Treating the underlying dementing disorder may also treat behavioral and psychological symptoms of dementia. Treatment with cholinesterase inhibitors and memantine has been shown to decrease the symptoms in patients with Alzheimer's disease, dementia with Lewy bodies, and vascular dementia (for review, see Desmidt et al., 2016). Note, however, that in some patients with frontotemporal dementia cholinesterase inhibitors will sometimes worsen the behavioral and psychological symptoms of dementia.

Consider three of the most common delusions in dementia:

- Possessions are being stolen
- House is not their home
- Spouse is not their spouse.

These delusions are all caused in part by impaired memory. The patient who thinks people are stealing her jewelry typically put it away for safekeeping, then forgot that she moved it (and where she put it). The patient who does not believe that his house is his home is usually remembering an earlier home—most often the home of his childhood—and thinks that is where he still lives, and perhaps that his mother is waiting for him! The patient who does not believe that her husband is her spouse is likely remembering when the husband looked younger (or perhaps is remembering a previous husband). Because memory dysfunction contributes to these delusions, it should not be surprising that improving patients' memories can reduce or eliminate these types of delusions. For this reason, when we believe that the patient's delusions are caused by memory problems, we always start by making sure that the memory medication—that is, the cholinesterase inhibitor—is maximized.

2. Drugs to treat comorbid illnesses. Although it may seem obvious, it is well worth reiterating that patients with dementing disorders often have comorbid illnesses that, although not the cause of their dementia, may be contributing to their poor cognition and their behavioral and psychological symptoms. For example, whenever we detect a change in cognition over a matter of days in one of our patients we always suspect an infection (such as a urinary tract infection or pneumonia) or another medical cause. Treating the medical illness should correct the sudden deterioration in behavior and cognition.

3. Drugs to treat specific symptoms of behavioral and psychological symptoms of dementia. Depression, anxiety, insomnia, hallucinations, delusions, and agitation are all common in dementing illnesses. These conditions also all have specific pharmacological treatment that can be helpful when implemented skillfully and judiciously.

GENERAL PRINCIPLES OF PHARMACOTHERAPY FOR THE BEHAVIORAL AND PSYCHOLOGICAL SYMPTOMS OF DEMENTIA

- Accurately diagnose the underlying dementia. Treatment of behavioral and psychological symptoms of dementia will vary depending upon the underlying dementing disorder. For example, as we saw in Chapter 8, although patients with dementia with Lewy bodies experience visual hallucinations, one must be very cautious in treating them because many antipsychotic drugs exacerbate their parkinsonian symptoms. Knowing that the patient has dementia with Lewy bodies will lead to the use of donepezil (Aricept) (or another cholinesterase inhibitor) as first-line therapy, a selective serotonin reuptake inhibitors (SSRI) such as sertraline (Zoloft) as second-line therapy, quetiapine (Seroquel) as third-line therapy, and risperidone (Risperdal) as fourth-line therapy, because donepezil and sertraline should not exacerbate parkinsonism at all, and quetiapine is less likely to exacerbate parkinsonism than risperidone.

- Identify and measure specific target symptoms. The clinician and caregiver should identify specific symptoms and behaviors that they wish to reduce, such as depression, wandering, or aggression. Each symptom should be measured at baseline such that, when a treatment is prescribed, the treatment effect on that symptom can be quantified. One common way to measure these symptoms and behaviors is to count how many times specific events occur in a period of time. (For example, the patient attempted to wander out of the house six times over a two-week period, or ask the caregiver if this is happening multiple times a day, once a day, several times a week, once a week, or once a month.)

- Start low, go slow—but go. Older adults are often more sensitive to medications. As such, doses in older individuals should start at one-third to one-half the standard adult dose. Titrations should be slower than in younger adults. Importantly, however, the drugs should be titrated until the desired response is achieved or until intolerable side effects emerge. We have too often seen patients treated for long periods on sub-therapeutic doses of drugs that are not having the desired effect. In many cases, when the doses were increased to therapeutic levels, the patients did better.

- Instruct the caregiver and patient both verbally and in writing. We have been surprised how often we will have a conversation with a patient and caregiver regarding medications only to realize they misunderstood what we said when we revisit the topic later.

Because of the frequency of misunderstanding, we now provide information regarding medications both verbally and in clear, written directions. These instructions include how and when to take the medication, what side effects may occur and how to manage them, and what to do if they run out of medication. (See Box 19.4 for example.)

- Remove unneeded medications. It is both essential and difficult to obtain an accurate list of medications in our patients with dementia. In an informal survey that we completed several years ago, we found that our average patient reported taking eight medications—and some more than 20! In many cases neither the patients nor their caregivers knew who prescribed a number of their medications or what they were for. The typical scenario was that multiple providers added medications, but medications were rarely removed. A number of the commonly prescribed medications have potential cognitive side effects or drug interactions, including anticholinergic medications, antihistamines, and others. (See Boxes 17.1 and 17.2.) We often begin by working with the patient's primary care provider to try to simplify their medication regime.
- Change only one medication at a time. This very obvious point is often overlooked and it cannot be overstated. If more than one medication is changed at once it is generally impossible to determine the cause of either beneficial or detrimental cognitive effects. We therefore recommend changing only one medication at a time.

PHARMACOTHERAPY FOR DEPRESSION

There are few things in our society today that are as depressing and anxiety provoking as realizing that one has Alzheimer's disease and is going to literally "lose one's mind." Although it rarely meets the diagnostic criteria for major depression, a significant degree of depression often occurs in patients before, during, and throughout the course of Alzheimer's disease, occurring in about half of patients (Kuring, Mathias, & Ward, 2018). Although treatment of depression in the demented patient will not resolve the cognitive deficits, successful treatment will help the mood of the patient and in doing so will improve the patient's cognition, daily function, and overall well-being (Cummings et al., 2016).

Some general guidelines for managing depression pharmacologically:

- SSRIs are generally first-line therapy. (See Box 27.1.)
- Other antidepressant classes that may be beneficial for depression:
  - Bupropion (Wellbutrin) has activating properties and can also be helpful when apathy is present; may lower the seizure threshold, particularly in doses above 300 mg per day.
  - Serotonin–norepinephrine reuptake inhibitors (SNRIs), such as venlafaxine (Effexor), are efficacious in some patients.
- Antidepressants to avoid include:
  - Tricyclic antidepressants because of anticholinergic effects
  - Mirtazapine (Remeron) because of anticholinergic effects
- Monoamine oxidase inhibitors (MAOs) because of the likelihood of dietary indiscretions in the cognitively impaired patient.

PHARMACOTHERAPY FOR ANXIETY

As mentioned, having the slightest bit of insight into knowing that one has Alzheimer's disease is quite anxiety provoking, in addition to being depressing. Consistent with this notion, one study suggested that approximately half of patients with Alzheimer's disease (48%) showed evidence of anxiety (Mega et al., 1996). Anxiety in Alzheimer's disease may improve with cholinesterase inhibitor therapy (Cummings et al., 2016), so a cholinesterase inhibitor should always be tried first (see Chapter 19). As in depression, however, the mainstay of pharmacotherapy for anxiety in dementia is the SSRIs, notably sertraline (Zoloft) and escitalopram (Lexapro) (Box 27.1). (Although citalopram [Celexa] has been extensively studied, its cardiac effects on the QTc interval make it a second-line SSRI.)

If the SSRIs are not effective in alleviating the anxiety, the class of medications which is typically tried next is the atypical antipsychotics, particularly if the anxiety is due to delusions or hallucinations. Although not as well tolerated as SSRIs, the atypical antipsychotics are helpful and sometimes necessary. Atypical antipsychotics may impair cognition and lead to sedation, falls, and cardiovascular disease. These second-line treatments should be used for as brief a period as possible, and in a situation in which the patient is regularly observed (Box 27.4).

> ### BOX 27.1 Use of Selective Serotonin Reuptake Inhibitors in Dementia
>
> - Selective serotonin reuptake inhibitors (SSRIs) are generally well tolerated in patients with cognitive impairment and dementia.
> - SSRIs are only minimally anticholinergic, are relatively non-sedating, and are therefore unlikely to worsen cognition.
> - Several SSRIs (including sertraline [Zoloft] and escitalopram [Lexapro]) are anxiolytics as well as antidepressants.
> - We generally use a low dose of:
>   - Sertraline (Zoloft) target 75–150 mg QD; general range for dementia 50–200 mg
>   - Escitalopram (Lexapro) target 10 mg QD; general range for dementia 5–10 mg.
>   - Because of its cardiac effects on the QTc interval, citalopram (Celexa) is a second line drug to be used if sertraline and escitalopram are unsuccessful. Target 20 mg QD; general range for dementia 10–20 mg.
> - If one SSRI is not effective, others may be.
> - Main side effects: gastrointestinal upset and sexual dysfunction.
> - Note that paroxetine (Paxil) may be problematic in the elderly owing to the common side effect of hyponatremia, the rapid onset of withdrawal symptoms if a dose is forgotten, and its high anticholinergic burden compared with other SSRIs.

Benzodiazepines are rarely used for anxiety in the cognitively impaired patient because they generally worsen cognition, lead to dependence, and have rebound effects.

PHARMACOTHERAPY FOR PSEUDOBULBAR AFFECT (PATHOLOGIC LAUGHTER AND CRYING)

A number of patients with Alzheimer's disease or other dementia have frequent episodes of crying or laughing—not because they are feeling very sad or happy, but because of pseudobulbar affect. Patients with pseudobulbar affect may cry or laugh with either minimal provocation or without any underlying relevant emotional state. Other terms sometimes used for this symptom include pathologic laughter and crying, emotional lability, emotional incontinence, emotional dysregulation,

labile affect, and involuntary emotional expression disorder. It is thought to result from the disruption of descending pathways from the frontal lobes to the emotional centers in the brainstem medulla—sometimes referred to as the "bulb," hence the term, "pseudobulbar." These descending pathways from the frontal lobes to the brainstem are what we typically use to inhibit crying, laughing, and other emotional states whenever we don't want to express them, such as when it would be socially inappropriate. When these pathways are disrupted the emotional centers in the brainstem can be triggered with minimal or even no discernible stimulation. (See also Box 7.4.)

Pseudobulbar affect typically comes to our attention when the patient or family reports frequent episodes of crying and concerns about depression. In talking with the patient who has pseudobulbar affect we discover that, often to our surprise and that of the family, the patient does not actually feel sad, and often has no idea why they are crying. After first carefully evaluating the patient for any other signs and symptoms of a mood disorder, we will explain that these symptoms are simply part of their brain disease, just like the memory loss. Often this explanation and reassurance are sufficient. Sometimes, however, the episodes of crying (and occasionally laughing) are sufficiently disruptive, embarrassing, and unpleasant to interfere with the patient's life. In such cases we will consider prescribing the combination medication dextromethorphan/quinidine (Nuedexta) For review see Nguyen & Matsumoto, 2019.

- Each capsule of Nuedexta contains dextromethorphan hydrobromide 20 mg and quinidine sulfate 10 mg.
- Starting dose is one capsule daily for seven days.
- Maintenance dose is one capsule twice a day.

The most common adverse reactions reported include diarrhea, dizziness, cough, vomiting, asthenia, peripheral edema, urinary tract infection, influenza, increased gamma-glutamyltransferase, and flatulence. There are many contraindications, warnings, precautions, adverse reactions, and drug interactions that can occur with this medication, most related to quinidine, a cardiac class I antiarrhythmic agent (Schoedel, Morrow, & Sellers, 2014). Please consult the comprehensive prescribing information in the package insert before prescribing this medication. Our experience is that many patients with pseudobulbar affect related to their dementia do well with this medication, although some cannot tolerate it.

PHARMACOTHERAPY FOR INSOMNIA

Sleep problems are very common in Alzheimer's disease and other dementias (Martin & Velayudhan, 2020). Pharmacological treatment for insomnia and other sleep disturbances in dementia depends upon the underlying cause. When we hear that the patient has trouble sleeping we always begin by going through the patient's day. A typical day reported by a caregiver might sound like this narrative:

> I have to wake him up around 8 AM so that I can get him on the van to the day care at 9 AM. He stays at the day care until 2:30, returning home at 3 PM. They tell me that he sleeps in the chair half of the time at day care. When he is home he generally watches TV, but he has trouble following what is going on, and so he generally naps from about 3.30 to 5.30 PM, when I wake him up for dinner. We eat from 5.30 to 6 PM, and then watch the news on the couch, followed by Jeopardy and Wheel of Fortune till 8 PM. Sometimes he falls asleep during this time as well. I start getting him ready for bed at 8, and he is generally asleep by 9 PM. I then find him wandering around the house between 3 and 6 AM. I will put him back to sleep by 6 AM if he hasn't gone back to sleep already …

This patient sleeps from 6 to 8 AM (2 hours), half the time at day care (half of 9:30 AM to 2:30 PM or 2.5 hours), 3:30 to 5:50 PM (2 hours), and half the time from 6 to 8 PM (1 hour). So, by the time he goes to sleep at 9 PM starting at 6 AM he has already slept an average of 7.5 hours. If he then sleeps from 9 PM to 3 AM he has slept an additional 6 hours and a total of 13.5 hours. It is no wonder at all that he is awake and wandering around the house from 3 to 6 AM!

In this example, the patient has poor sleep hygiene and a disrupted sleep cycle; he may or may not have other sleep problems as well. Nearly half of older adults experience difficulty in initiating and maintaining sleep (Brewster, Riegel, & Gehrman, 2018). In normal aging there is an increase in sleep problems, including:

- Restless legs syndrome; prevalence in the elderly of 8% to 20%
- Periodic limb movements of sleep; prevalence in the elderly of up to 45%

- Sleep-disordered breathing; prevalence in the elderly of 45% to 62%
- Rapid eye movement (REM) sleep behavior disorder; increased in the elderly—prevalence unclear. (Note that individuals with this disorder are at risk for Parkinson's or another Lewy body disease in the future; see Chapter 8.)

In dementia, including Alzheimer's disease and dementia with Lewy bodies, these sleep disturbances are even more common (Gabelle & Dauvilliers, 2010), and there is commonly disrupted circadian rhythm (Neikrug & Ancoli-Israel, 2010). Specific sleep disturbances should be diagnosed and treated appropriately, keeping in mind that many sleep disturbances may be side effects of medications.

Sleep problems may also be caused by depression and/or anxiety. Because depression and anxiety are common in dementia, they are also commonly causes of sleep disturbances in these patients, and can often be treated with an SSRI (Box 27.1).

The treatment for poor sleep hygiene and disrupted sleep cycle (as in our patient above) is to limit naps during the day, thereby consolidating sleep at night, as well as to follow other sleep hygiene guidelines such as not spending hours in bed doing wakeful activities (eating, talking on the phone, etc.). One or at the most two naps per day totaling 30 to 60 minutes should be the maximum if the patient is expected to sleep at night.

Sometimes we will use a small dose of a stimulant medication to help the patient stay awake during the day (Box 27.2). A small dose of a stimulant medication also has the benefit of increasing alertness and attention, which may in turn improve thinking and memory. There are many that can be used. The two we most commonly use are long-acting methylphenidate (Ritalin and other brand names) and modafinil (Provigil). Note that in dementia we generally prescribe a single dose

---

BOX 27.2 Use of Stimulant Medication in Dementia

- Methylphenidate ER (Ritalin ER) 20 mg QAM
- Modafinil (Provigil) 100 mg QAM

  Side effects and adverse reactions can include dependency, abuse, confusion, psychosis, mania, agitation, aggression, arrhythmias, hypertension, myocardial infarction, stroke, sudden death, seizures, and hypersensitivity reaction including Stevens–Johnson syndrome.

of a long-acting medication and do not increase it; in our experience if it will work for this purpose it works at a low dose, and higher doses increase side effects and adverse reactions without an increase in efficacy. If the low dose seems to be helpful without side effects we continue the stimulant; if it is unhelpful or causing side effects we discontinue it.

What about sedatives to help the patient go to sleep? We would first note that, as in the example given, having a patient take a "sleeping pill" at 9 PM is unlikely to help him stay asleep at 3 AM; most of its effects will have worn off by then. Sedatives at night may also lead to nocturnal incontinence if the patient is too sedated to get out of bed to use the bathroom. If the patient does get out of bed to use the bathroom, sedatives make it more likely that he will fall with potential injury occurring.

For all of these reasons, we do not prescribe sedative medications except in very unusual circumstances. Instead, we try to think about what is the underlying cause of the patient's difficulty sleeping (Box 27.3) and work to fix that problem.

PHARMACOTHERAPY FOR PSYCHOSIS

Psychosis (hallucinations and delusions) is common in the later stages of dementia. Visual hallucinations are also a presenting symptom of dementia with Lewy bodies, and delusions are common in Alzheimer's disease and behavioral variant frontotemporal dementia. See Chapters 24–26 for additional discussion of psychotic symptoms in dementia.

Hallucinations and delusions can manifest in a variety of ways, including agitation, anxiety, or repetitive, purposeless behavior. In general, as discussed earlier, we treat hallucinations and delusions only when they are troublesome to the patient.

Some general guidelines for managing hallucinations and delusions pharmacologically include:
- Accurate diagnosis of the underlying dementia is crucial before determining how to treat the symptoms.
- Psychotic symptoms should be sufficient to disrupt the patient's functioning before treatment is initiated.
- The psychotic symptoms should be present for at least one month and should not be due to delirium or a pre-existing psychotic disorder or substance abuse problem.

> ### BOX 27.3 Strategies for Treating Insomnia in Dementia
>
> - Are there problems with sleep hygiene or cycle?
>   - Regulate times of sleep and wake, limiting naps to no more than 1 hour/day
>   - Can try a dose of melatonin 0.5–10 mg 1 hour before bed.
> - Can non-pharmacological treatment help?
>   - Limit naps as above
>   - Limit caffeine, tobacco, and alcohol after lunch
>   - Try a glass of warm milk, soft music, soothing sounds, or a gentle back rub.
> - Is there an underlying primary sleep problem?
>   - Work-up and treat primary sleep problems when suspected.
> - Is there any pain present?
>   - Little aches and pains not noticeable during the day can interfere with sleep at night. Acetaminophen (paracetamol) 325–650 mg at bedtime can help treat insomnia (Kales et al., 2019).
> - Is the problem caused by underlying depression or anxiety?
>   - Try a selective serotonin reuptake inhibitor (SSRI) during the day, although note that SSRIs can worsen certain sleep disorders, such as periodic limb movements of sleep (Box 27.1).
> - Is the problem caused by underlying psychotic symptoms, such as delusions or hallucinations?
>   - Can try a small dose of an atypical antipsychotic, typically starting with quetiapine (Seroquel) because it tends to be sedating (a good thing here) (Box 27.4).

- The goal of treatment is not to eliminate the psychotic symptoms, but to reduce distress and improve function.
- The SSRIs sertraline (Zoloft) and escitalopram (Lexapro) can reduce the fear and anxiety associated with delusions and hallucinations.
- Atypical antipsychotics are sometimes needed (Kales et al., 2019; Box 27.4).
- Pimavanserin (Nuplazid), a selective 5-HT2A inverse agonist/antagonist, is approved in the United States for treating hallucinations and delusions associated with Parkinson's disease psychosis, and has also shown efficacy in treating these symptoms in Alzheimer's disease (Cummings et al., 2018). Note, however, that agitation was not improved in these studies.

BOX 27.4   Use of Atypical Antipsychotics in Dementia

- Non-pharmacological therapies (see Chapter 26 and for review, Scales, Zimmerman, & Miller, 2018), followed by cholinesterase inhibitors (Chapter 19), selective serotonin reuptake inhibitors (SSRIs, Box 27.1), and then other approaches, such as dextromethorphan/quinidine or prazosin, should be used first to reduce the use and/or dose of atypical antipsychotics in dementia (Kales et al., 2019).
- Atypical antipsychotics may impair cognition, be sedating, cause parkinsonism, lead to falls, cause hyperglycemia, lower the seizure threshold, cause dystonias and tardive dyskinesia, and increase the risk of heart disease, strokes, and death.
- Atypical antipsychotics should be used for as brief a period as possible, followed by a gradual taper while monitoring for symptom severity.
- Atypical antipsychotics should be used only when the patient is in a situation in which he or she can be regularly observed.
- Complications often occur with the use of atypical antipsychotics in patients with dementia; this possibility of complications should be discussed with the patient and caregiver, and consent for the use of these medications should be obtained and documented in the medical record.
- There are a number of atypical antipsychotics to choose from. Target dose is always the lowest effective dose. The ones typically used in dementia are:
  - Risperidone (Risperdal); range for dementia 0.25–1 mg QD-BID. May be best atypical antipsychotic for use in dementia (Kales et al., 2019). Available

  in tablets, oral disintegrating tablets (M-Tabs), and also 1 mg/mL solution. One of the less sedating atypical antipsychotics, ideal for use during the day when a daytime medication is needed. Also useful in liquid and oral disintegrating form when pills cannot be swallowed. Can cause prolactinemia and exacerbate osteoporosis.
  - Quetiapine (Seroquel); range for dementia 12.5–200 mg QD-BID. Somewhat sedating, recommended for use at bedtime although can be used during the day in small doses. Less likely than others to cause or worsen parkinsonism; ideal for patients with dementia with Lewy bodies. It may, however, be less effective than others.
  - Aripiprazole (Abilify); range for dementia 2.5–5 mg QD-BID. One of the least sedating atypical antipsychotics. Least effect on carbohydrate metabolism. Less likely to cause cardiac conduction abnormalities such as prolonged QTc interval.
  - Ziprasidone (Geodon); intramuscular (IM) range for dementia: 20 mg IM QD-TID. Particularly useful when an intramuscular medication is needed. Switch to PO as soon as possible.
  - Olanzapine (Zyprexa); range for dementia 1.25–10 mg QD. More sedating and higher propensity for weight gain.
- If one atypical antipsychotic is not effective, others may be.
- Atypical antipsychotics should be used with extreme caution in patients with dementia.

PHARMACOTHERAPY FOR AGITATION

Agitation is characterized by resistive verbally and sometimes physically aggressive behavior. Agitation is common in Alzheimer's disease dementia, occurring in up to 70% of cases, and is probably even more common in some other dementias, such as frontotemporal dementia. It can range from mild symptoms, such as repeating requests and demands ("When will I get dinner?"), to outbursts characterized by punching, kicking, screaming, and running. It is often troublesome to both the patient and caregiver, and sometimes can only be managed by pharmacological intervention (Box 27.5).

Agitation often comes in the form of aggressive and uncooperative behavior coupled with or perhaps

caused by other symptoms of behavioral and psychological symptoms of dementia such as hallucinations, delusions, depression, or anxiety. It is important for clinicians to be aware that agitation is a very general term and can represent a number of different behaviors and be related to multiple underlying conditions. Characterization of how the agitation is manifesting and what underlying disorder is present is most likely to lead to successful treatment. For example, the individual with underlying psychosis may do best on an atypical antipsychotic (Kales et al., 2019). A patient with underlying depression or anxiety may respond to an SSRI (Leonpacher et al., 2016). (Note that, although valproic acid [Depakote] and other anticonvulsant mood stabilizers are sometimes used, there are

---

BOX 27.5   General Guidelines for Pharmacological Management of Agitation

- Characterize and diagnose the underlying condition(s) present (see sections I and II).
- Characterize, diagnose, and treat any comorbid conditions, even if they are not thought to be contributing to the agitation.
- If pain is present from a known etiology (such as arthritis), acetaminophen (paracetamol) 325–650 mg may be helpful (Kales et al., 2019).
- Always start with education of the caregiver (see Chapter 25) and nonpharmacologic treatments (see Chapter 26). Only use pharmacologic therapies if nonpharmacologic therapies are insufficient.
- Make sure the patient is on standard pharmacologic therapy for dementia, if appropriate, including cholinesterase inhibitors (see Chapter 19) and memantine (see Chapter 20). If not, that is the first step.
- Characterize the nature of the agitation:
  - If depression or anxiety is present, start with a selective serotonin reuptake inhibitor (SSRI) (Box 27.1). If already on an SSRI, substitution of another SSRI may be appropriate.
  - If anger or angry outbursts are the most prominent symptom, prazosin can be tried. Start 1 mg QD and

titrate up to 5 mg daily in QD or BID dosing, given one hour before the time when anger is greatest. Monitor blood pressure closely (Davies et al., 2018).
- If sleep disturbance is present, see Box 27.3: Strategies for Treating Insomnia in Dementia.
- If psychosis (hallucinations or delusions) is present, consider an atypical antipsychotic (Box 27.4) after trying cholinesterase inhibitors (see Chapter 19) and SSRIs (Box 27.1).
- Dextromethorphan/quinidine (Nuedexta, see Pharmacotherapy for Pseudobulbar Affect, above) has been shown to be beneficial for agitation in Alzheimer's disease dementia and can be tried (Cummings et al., 2015).
- If no specific cause for the agitation can be determined, does it need to be treated quickly?
  - If the agitation needs to be treated rapidly because of danger to self or others, or difficulty providing care, start with an atypical antipsychotic (Box 27.4).
  - If the agitation can be treated more slowly, start with an SSRI (Box 27.1).

---

currently little or no data supporting their use and we do not recommend using valproic acid in this setting [for review see Yeh & Ouyang, 2012]. In fact, in our experience, treatment with valproic acid invariably makes things worse.)

BEHAVIORAL AND PSYCHIATRIC CRISES

Despite the best efforts of caregivers and clinicians, the behavioral and psychological symptoms of dementia lead to crises in many patients. Sometimes these crises can be managed in the home, but often management in an acute psychiatric setting is necessary. Because crises are by their nature difficult to predict, we recommend that clinicians become familiar with the different acute psychiatric facility options available in their communities so that, when the crises invariably occur, they are ready to deal with them quickly and effectively. If we believe there is a chance that a psychiatric hospitalization may be necessary for one of our patients, we try to let the family know ahead of time whenever possible. We stress that a short-term psychiatric hospitalization can be quite helpful, allowing medications to be withdrawn

or added in a safe setting and enabling changes to occur much more quickly and easily than could be accomplished at home. We reassure the family of the high likelihood of the patient then being able to return home in a more stable clinical condition.

REFERENCES

Brewster, G. S., Riegel, B., & Gehrman, P. R. (2018). Insomnia in the older adult. *Sleep Medicine Clinics*, *13*(1), 13–19.

Cummings, J., Ballard, C., Tariot, P., et al. (2018). Pimavanserin: Potential treatment for dementia-related psychosis. *Journal of Prevention of Alzheimer Disease*, *5*(4), 253–258.

Cummings, J., Lai, T. J., Hemrungrojn, S., et al. (2016). Role of donepezil in the management of neuropsychiatric symptoms in Alzheimer's disease and dementia with Lewy bodies. *CNS Neuroscience & Therapeutics*, *22*(3), 159–166.

Cummings, J. L., Lyketsos, C. G., Peskind, E. R., et al. (2015). Effect of dextromethorphan-quinidine on agitation in patients with Alzheimer disease dementia: A randomized clinical trial. *The Journal of the American Medical Association*, *314*(12), 1242–1254.

Davies, S. J., Burhan, A. M., Kim, D., et al. (2018). Sequential drug treatment algorithm for agitation and aggression in

Alzheimer's and mixed dementia. *Journal of Psychopharmacology*, *32*(5), 509–523.

Desmidt, T., Hommet, C., & Camus, V. (2016). Pharmacological treatments of behavioral and psychological symptoms of dementia in Alzheimer's disease: Role of acetylcholinesterase inhibitors and memantine. *Geriatrie et Psychologie Neuropsychiatrie du Vieillissement*, *14*(3), 300–306.

Gabelle, A., & Dauvilliers, Y. (2010). Editorial: Sleep and dementia. *The Journal of Nutrition, Health & Aging*, *14*, 201–202.

Kales, H. C., Lyketsos, C. G., Miller, E. M., et al. (2019). Management of behavioral and psychological symptoms in people with Alzheimer's disease: An international Delphi consensus. *International Psychogeriatrics*, *31*(1), 83–90.

Kuring, J. K., Mathias, J. L., & Ward, L. (2018). Prevalence of depression, anxiety and PTSD in people with dementia: A systematic review and meta-analysis. *Neuropsychology Review*, *28*(4), 393–416.

Leonpacher, A. K., Peters, M. E., Drye, L. T., et al. (2016). Effects of citalopram on neuropsychiatric symptoms in Alzheimer's dementia: Evidence from the CitAD study. *The American Journal of Psychiatry*, *173*(5), 473–480.

Martin, E., & Velayudhan, L. (2020). Neuropsychiatric symptoms in mild cognitive impairment: A literature review [published online ahead of print, 14 Apr 2020]. *Dementia and Geriatric Cognitive Disorders*, 1–13.

Mega, M. S., Cummings, J. L., Fiorello, T., et al. (1996). The spectrum of behavioral changes in Alzheimer's disease. *Neurology*, *46*, 130–135.

Neikrug, A. B., & Ancoli-Israel, S. (2010). Sleep disturbances in nursing homes. *The Journal of Nutrition, Health & Aging*, *14*, 207–211.

Nguyen, L., & Matsumoto, R. R. (2019). The psychopharmacology of pseudobulbar affect. *Handbook of Clinical Neurology*, *165*, 243–251.

Scales, K., Zimmerman, S., & Miller, S. J. (2018). Evidence-based nonpharmacological practices to address behavioral and psychological symptoms of dementia. *The Gerontologist*, *58*(Suppl 1), S88–S102.

Schoedel, K. A., Morrow, S. A., & Sellers, E. M. (2014). Evaluating the safety and efficacy of dextromethorphan/quinidine in the treatment of pseudobulbar affect. *Neuropsychiatric Disease and Treatment*, *10*, 1161–1174.

Yeh, Y. C., & Ouyang, W. C. (2012). Mood stabilizers for the treatment of behavioral and psychological symptoms of dementia: An update review. *The Kaohsiung Journal of Medical Sciences*, *28*, 185–193.

28

Life Adjustments for Memory Loss, Alzheimer's Disease, and Dementia

QUICK START: LIFE ADJUSTMENTS FOR MEMORY LOSS, ALZHEIMER'S DISEASE, AND DEMENTIA

Issues in Mild Cognitive Impairment and Alzheimer's Disease Dementia in the Very Mild and Mild Stages
- Patients with mild cognitive impairment and very mild Alzheimer's disease dementia may be able to drive.
  - A family member should ride in the passenger seat monthly while the patient is driving to help assure that the patient is driving safely.
  - Driving should stop either when the patient reaches the mild stage of Alzheimer's disease dementia or when the family member is uncomfortable riding in the car.
  - When the patient does not want to stop driving, a formal driving evaluation is available at most rehabilitation hospitals and departments of motor vehicles.
- Patients with mild cognitive impairment and Alzheimer's disease dementia at any stage need to have their financial affairs supervised.
  - Family members or legal representatives should monitor all financial matters.
  - The patient should be protected from telemarketers and other unscrupulous individuals soliciting monies and investment.
  - Independent financial investing should cease immediately.
- Patients with mild cognitive impairment and both very mild and mild Alzheimer's disease dementia may be able to continue working.
  - Working is healthy from the patient's perspective.
  - The patient will need to be in a supervised setting.
  - The job should entail no risks or dangers to the patient as well as relevant co-workers, customers, or consumers if problems in job performance were to occur.

Issues in Alzheimer's Disease Dementia in the Moderate and Severe Stages
- In general, patients with moderate to severe Alzheimer's disease dementia should not be left alone.
  - Home health aides and homemakers can provide assistance to patients and respite to caregivers.
  - Home health aides help with the patient's personal needs, such as bathing.
  - Homemakers help with household chores, such as cooking and laundry.
- Day programs provide a healthy routine for the patient and respite for the caregiver.
  - Start at least two days per week; increase as needed.
  - Call it a "club."
- Assisted living is ideal for patients who need more care than can be provided in the home when there is not a ready caregiver available. There are a large variety of assisted living facilities:
  - Some are almost independent living facilities, some are almost nursing homes, and some are in-between.
  - Unfortunately, most insurance does not pay for assisted living facilities.
- Long-term care is necessary for almost all patients with dementia at some point in their illness.
  - Encourage families to plan ahead.
  - The family should look for a facility that they like and is close to home.
  - Units that specialize in dementia care are ideal, if available.

See also Chapter 25 for additional discussion of many of these important topics.

MILD COGNITIVE IMPAIRMENT AND ALZHEIMER'S DISEASE DEMENTIA IN THE VERY MILD AND MILD STAGES

Driving

Driving is one of the most difficult issues that arises and will need to be addressed with almost every patient who has dementia. How do we know if the patient in our office is safe to drive? Cognitive assessments have, unfortunately, been disappointing in their ability to identify which patients with cognitive impairment should and should not be driving (Wernham et al., 2014). In 2000 the American Academy of Neurology published a practice parameter paper based upon a meta-analysis of the available literature. The main finding was that patients with very mild Alzheimer's disease have motor vehicle accident rates similar to 16- to 19-year-old drivers. Because we allow 16- to 19-year-olds to drive, the conclusion was (and we agree) that it is reasonable for patients with very mild Alzheimer's disease dementia to be allowed to drive as well (Dubinsky, Stein, & Lyons, 2000). (See Chapter 4 for details on distinguishing the very mild from the mild stage of Alzheimer's disease dementia.)

However, even if it is safe for patients with very mild Alzheimer's disease to drive in general, how do we know if it is safe for the particular very mild patient sitting in our office to drive? In 2010 the American Academy of Neurology published an update to their practice parameter paper which helped to identify additional risk factors for unsafe driving (Iverson et al., 2010), which has subsequently been validated (Carvalho et al., 2018) (Fig. 28.1).

This practice parameter is helpful but, even if it is safe for the patient to drive today, what about next week or next month? If it is determined that the patient with very mild Alzheimer's disease is safe to drive, we recommend that each month a family member ride as the front-seat passenger with the patient driving along his or her regular routes. Adult children are the best observers (Bixby, Davis, & Ott, 2015). For the most part, as long as the family member feels comfortable riding in the car with the patient driving, then we feel comfortable allowing the patient to continue driving. Driving should stop when either the family member no longer feels comfortable riding in the car, accidents or near accidents occur, or the patient progresses from the very mild to the mild stage of Alzheimer's disease dementia.

If there is a controversy between the patient and his or her family, we recommend a formal driving evaluation, which can be done at most rehabilitation hospitals and departments of motor vehicles. These evaluations are (unfortunately) unlikely to be covered by insurance, and cost several hundred dollars. But they are much less expensive than a single accident.

Paying Bills, Credit and ATM Cards, and Investing

Having difficulties paying bills is often one of the first signs of memory loss. Some patients will forget to pay their bills, leading to loss of important services such as heat, electricity, and telephone. Other patients will pay bills twice. Some patients will have both problems. If a patient with mild cognitive impairment or very mild Alzheimer's disease dementia is continuing to pay the household bills and do other banking duties, we recommend that their work be reviewed with a family member at least monthly to assure that no problems are developing.

In our society it is easy to have rapid access to large amounts of money or purchasing power using automatic teller machines (ATMs) and credit cards. By the time the patient is in the mild stage of Alzheimer's disease dementia it is usually prudent to remove access to these cards. As described in Chapter 26, patients with ready access to cash can be easily exploited. Solicitations from unscrupulous individuals frequently appear in the mail and by the phone. We also know of several patients who, after their car was taken away to prevent them from unsafe driving, promptly went out and purchased another one, putting the down payment on their credit card!

Even the most healthy and intelligent individual will sometimes make bad investments leading to significant financial losses. Investing is a complicated art, and depends upon being aware of the latest information along with good judgment and reasoning abilities (and of course a bit of luck). Given the complexity of investing, it is not surprising that many patients who eventually develop Alzheimer's disease or another dementia will have made poor investments in the years before

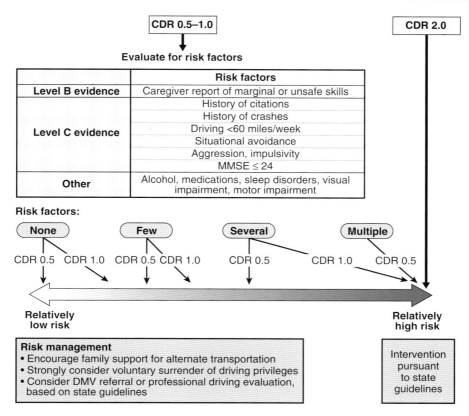

Fig. 28.1 Possible algorithm for evaluating driving competence and risk management in patients with dementia. *CDR,* Clinical Dementia Rating Scale; *DMV,* Department of Motor Vehicles; *MMSE,* Mini-Mental State Examination. (From Iverson, D. J., Gronseth, G. S., Reger, M. A., et al. (2010). Practice parameter update: evaluation and management of driving risk in dementia. Report of the Quality Standards Subcommittee of the American Academy of Neurology. *Neurology 74,* 1316–1324.)

their diagnosis. The tragedy is that sometimes lifelong savings or retirement funds are lost within a short period of time. We recommend that a patient diagnosed with mild cognitive impairment or any type of dementia immediately relinquish any form of investing (Martin et al., 2019).

Working

Should a patient with mild cognitive impairment work? As more adults work into their 70s and 80s, there are more individuals who are working at the time of their diagnosis of mild cognitive impairment (and, more occasionally, very mild Alzheimer's disease or other dementia). Whether individuals with mild cognitive impairment and very mild Alzheimer's disease dementia should continue working depends upon the individual,

their job, and how long they have been doing the work. If the individual has been doing the job for many years, it is likely that many of the manual and cognitive skills have already been consolidated in memory, and can therefore be maintained for a period of time (see Appendix C for more information on consolidation of memory).

From the patient's perspective, working is almost always good: working typically provides a healthy routine, intellectual stimulation, socialization, and other helpful qualities such as maintaining feelings of self-worth and avoiding depression. From the employer's and society's perspective, it depends upon whether the patient's cognitive impairment disrupts the performance of the job and whether there are risks or dangers involved.

For example, an individual with mild cognitive impairment could continue to work on an assembly line in which their task is procedural in nature (not requiring memory, judgment, or reasoning), is relatively circumscribed, and the person at the next stage of the assembly line will be aware of any errors made. Another example of an appropriate job to continue includes making handmade crafts such as pottery or articles of clothing; again the work depends largely on procedural memory (not affected by mild Alzheimer's disease dementia; see Appendix C), and the quality of the work will generally be readily apparent.

Inappropriate jobs to continue include those that involve supervision at almost any level, from watching children at a daycare center to managing a business. Other inappropriate jobs to continue include those that involve memory, judgment, and reasoning that affect people's lives at any level, such as a clinical or legal professional. Sales jobs may be appropriate if the work is circumscribed, the patient is already quite experienced, and the supervision of the patient is appropriate. For example, one of our patients was able to continue his job and be productive as a florist well into the mild stage of Alzheimer's disease dementia.

ALZHEIMER'S DISEASE DEMENTIA IN THE MODERATE TO SEVERE STAGES

Home Alone

One way to define the moderate stage of Alzheimer's disease dementia is when the patient is no longer able to stay home alone for more than an hour or two. As discussed in more detail in Chapter 4, problems in the moderate stage of Alzheimer's disease dementia include severe memory difficulties, poor problem-solving, wandering, and often the start of problems of incontinence and needing help with hygiene. Not surprisingly, patients in the moderate stage of Alzheimer's disease get into trouble when left alone. Even patients without incontinence who do not wander may leave the stove on. And those who do not leave the stove on may fall prey to a telemarketer or accidentally lock themselves out of the house. We therefore strongly encourage families to have round-the-clock supervision available for patients in the moderate stage of dementia.

Needing round-the-clock care is a huge task for the caregiver, and should not be done alone. Studies have shown that even caregivers who want to provide care themselves 24 hours a day/7 days a week invariably "burn out" faster than if they had shared the care of the patient. Other factors relating to family caregiver burnout include caregiver depression and patient agitation, aggression, irritability, aberrant motor behavior, and hallucinations (Hiyoshi-Taniguchi, Becker, & Kinoshita, 2018). Some families, particularly if large and/or close-knit, can do well sharing caregiving duties, giving the primary caregiver needed time alone. Note that if there are a number of different family members helping out, it is usually better for the patient if the family comes to the patient's house, rather than the patient to the family's house, although we have seen it work well both ways.

Sooner or later, most families greatly benefit from additional help taking care of the patient. Home health aides, day programs, assisted living, and long-term care are some of the commonly used options.

(See Chapter 25 for more on these important topics.)

Home Health Aides and Homemakers

Home health aides can assist caregivers with activities of daily living such as showering, shaving, and brushing the teeth of the patient. Homemakers do not provide personal care to the patient but help with laundry, cooking, light cleaning, and other tasks. Sometimes the same individual helps with both types of tasks. These individuals also provide much needed time for the caregiver to pay the bills, do household chores, go out with friends, or simply spend a few minutes by themselves.

Day Programs

Day programs can provide much needed respite for the caregiver, and also a nice routine for the patient. Many of our patients truly look forward to the "bus" (really a van) that comes to take them to their "club" (really the day program). We recommend that patients go to the day program at least two days a week to allow them to develop a routine; three or four days a week is probably ideal early on, and can be increased as the need arises and/or the caregiving duties become more difficult. Day programs provide appropriate activities for the patients, and some will also help with hygiene issues such as showering a patient when they are there. We also find that patients who attend day programs do better in the evening when they return home.

Assisted Living Facilities

Assisted living is ideal for patients who need more care than can be provided for them in their home for a number of reasons:

- Patients may be living alone without family members in the area.
- The caregiver may not be able to provide adequate care because of their own medical problems.
- Family members may be busy with their own families or jobs and unable to provide care to the patient.

Unlike long-term care services for those with more severe dementia, health insurance does not usually pay for assisted living, greatly reducing the numbers of individuals who would otherwise benefit from it. Some states (e.g., Vermont), however, have now recognized that assisted living is a less expensive and more appropriate alternative to nursing home care (which is often paid for by state-funded Medicaid programs) for many patients and will contribute substantially to the cost. The local council on aging or similar agency can often facilitate this type of placement.

There are a huge variety of services which assisted living facilities can provide, with some providing more services and some less. All will provide residents with their own room, as well as common areas for activities and dining. Most have additional services available, such as nurses to administer medications and aides to help with personal hygiene. Often these additional services are available "à la carte," with additional cost for each service. Some assisted living residences are part of a larger facility that includes long-term care residences, whereas patients in other facilities will need to move to a different long-term care residence when the severity of their dementia is more than can be handled in assisted living.

Long-Term Care Facilities

When patients can no longer be managed at home or in assisted living, a long-term care facility is necessary. Ideally the move to long-term care should be done with a certain amount of planning. Unfortunately, patients frequently end up at a long-term care facility in a time of crisis, often after a medical illness. The typical scenario is that the patient is admitted to an acute care facility after a fall, urinary tract infection, pneumonia, or even dehydration, and it is determined that they are not safe to return home. In either situation, families should look for a facility that they are comfortable with and is close to home. Some facilities accept patients with a wide range of cognitive and physical impairments, whereas others specialize in one type or severity of impairment.

If possible, we recommend considering a special unit that focuses on patients with Alzheimer's disease and other types of dementia. These units are often inside a more general nursing home, consisting of a floor or a wing. These are often referred to as Alzheimer's Special Care Units, Dementia Special Care Units, or Memory Care Units. Unfortunately, only about 15% of nursing homes have these Alzheimer's special care unit beds (Alzheimer's Association, 2020). Many states have legislation requiring such units to have special standards regarding the services provided, training of the staff, activities offered, ability of the staff to care for residents with behavioral and psychological symptoms of dementia, and also what fees they charge.

See also Chapter 25 for additional discussion of these important issues.

REFERENCES

Alzheimer's Association. (2020). Alzheimer's disease facts and figures. *Alzheimer's & Dementia, 16*(3) 391+.

Bixby, K., Davis, J. D., & Ott, B. R. (2015). Comparing caregiver and clinician predictions of fitness to drive in people with Alzheimer's disease. *The American Journal of Occupational Therapy, 69*(3), 1–7.

Carvalho, J. O., Springate, B., Bernier, R. A., et al. (2018). Psychometrics of the AAN Caregiver Driving Safety Questionnaire and contributors to caregiver concern about driving safety in older adults. *International Psychogeriatrics, 30*(3), 355–364.

Dubinsky, R. M., Stein, A. C., & Lyons, K. (2000). Practice parameter: risk of driving and Alzheimer's disease (an evidence-based review): Report of the quality standards subcommittee of the American Academy of Neurology. *Neurology, 54,* 2205–2211.

Hiyoshi-Taniguchi, K., Becker, C. B., & Kinoshita, A. (2018). What behavioral and psychological symptoms of dementia affect caregiver burnout? *Clinical Gerontologist, 41*(3), 249–254.

Iverson, D. J., Gronseth, G. S., Reger, M. A., et al. (2010). Practice parameter update: evaluation and management of driving risk in dementia. Report of the Quality Standards Subcommittee of the American Academy of Neurology. *Neurology, 74*, 1316–1324.

Martin, R. C., Gerstenecker, A., Triebel, K. L., et al. (2019). Declining financial capacity in mild cognitive impairment: A six-year longitudinal study. *Archives of Clinical Neuropsychology, 34*(2), 152–161.

Wernham, M., Jarrett, P. G., Stewart, C., et al. (2014). Comparison of the SIMARD MD to clinical impression in assessing fitness to drive in patients with cognitive impairment. *Canadian Geriatrics Journal, 17*, 63–69.

29

Legal and Financial Issues in Memory Loss, Alzheimer's Disease, and Dementia

QUICK START: LEGAL AND FINANCIAL ISSUES IN MEMORY LOSS, ALZHEIMER'S DISEASE, AND DEMENTIA

- Alzheimer's advocacy groups can provide helpful and up-to-date information for families.
  - Encourage your families to contact the Alzheimer's Association (www.alz.org, 800-272-3900) in the United States or similar organizations in other countries.
- Legal capacity is the capacity to make decisions and judgments necessary to sign legal documents, and depends upon the answers to three questions:
  - What type of deliberation needs to be undertaken to fully understand the implications and ramifications of the document, if signed?

- How impaired is the patient?
- Is everyone in the family in agreement? Or are there other family members who will likely be contesting the patient's capacity to make these decisions?
- Important legal documents are:
  - Guardianship
  - Living will
  - Power of attorney
  - Power of attorney for healthcare
- Alzheimer's disease is expensive. There are, however, a number of resources available that may assist in defraying the costs of the disease.

Many families need our assistance to know what legal and financial issues need to be addressed when their loved one develops Alzheimer's disease or another dementia. Although many social workers and some other clinicians may directly assist in these matters, knowledge of these issues is essential for all clinicians to allow us to help our families to obtain the assistance they need. A wonderful source of continuously updated information for families regarding all of these issues is the Alzheimer's Association in the United States (www.alz.org, 800-272-3900) and Australia (https://www.alz.org/au/dementia-alzheimers-australia.asp), Alzheimer Society in Canada (https://alzheimer.ca/en, 800-616-8816), and the Alzheimer's Society in England,

Wales, and Northern Ireland (www.alzheimers.org.uk, 0300 222 1122).

LEGAL PLANNING

Important issues in legal planning include the capacity to make decisions and judgments and the preparation of legal documents.

Legal Capacity: The Importance of Starting the Process Early

One issue that frequently arises in the clinic is whether it is appropriate for the patient to sign a legal document.

The issue is that of "capacity"; that is, does the patient have the capacity to make important decisions and judgments regarding who should have legal control of himself or herself. The answer depends, in turn, upon the answer to several other questions:

- What type of deliberation needs to be undertaken to fully understand the implications and ramifications of the document, if signed?
- How impaired is the patient?
- Is everyone on the same page? Or are there other family members who will likely be contesting the patient's capacity to make these decisions?

If patients are diagnosed at the earliest signs of memory loss, and these issues are brought up soon afterward, most will have the capacity to understand and sign legal documents related to who should have legal control of their affairs. In general, patients with mild cognitive impairment or Alzheimer's disease dementia in the very mild or mild stage (Clinical Dementia Rating [CDR] 0.5 or 1.0; Mini-Mental State Examination [MMSE] >20; Montreal Cognitive Assessment [MoCA] >15) have the capacity to make decisions related to the control of their own legal, financial, and health decisions. (For more on stages of Alzheimer's disease see Chapter 4.)

Note that, because different documents pertain to different issues that may involve a different level of complexity or require a different level of understanding, patients may have capacity for one document but not for another. However, the capacity required for the documents discussed here is similar for each document.

As the clinician, you can help determine whether the patient has the capacity to sign certain documents by (1) talking with the patient, (2) working with the family, and (3) using your knowledge of the patient's cognitive status to assess whether the patient is able to understand the issue raised in the document to be signed. For example, Mr. John Jones (the patient) and his wife (primary caregiver) come to the clinic today, and Mrs. Jones asks, "Is it all right for John to sign paperwork for legal and healthcare power of attorney?" We know that Mr. Jones has mild Alzheimer's disease dementia with a MMSE score of 23 (and a CDR of 1.0; see Chapter 4), and that he probably has the cognitive ability necessary to have the legal capacity to sign these documents. We ask Mr. Jones, "Do you understand what it means for you to sign these documents, the legal and healthcare power of attorney?" If he answers, "Yes, it means that Mary can make legal and medical decisions for me if I am not able

to," then this answer, coupled with his cognitive status, leads us to the conclusion that he has the capacity to sign the documents. If, on the other hand, he gives the more common answer, "I don't know … what do these documents mean?" we would then need to explain each one to him:

Clinician: Mr. Jones, the first document, the legal power of attorney, would allow your wife to make legal and financial decisions for you if you are having trouble making them, such as what investments to make with your retirement savings. Do you feel comfortable with her making those legal and financial decisions for you if you are not able to make them?

Patient: Oh yes, I would want Mary to make those decisions for us.

Clinician: The second document, the healthcare power of attorney, would allow your wife to make medical decisions for you if you are having trouble making them, such as whether you should have an elective surgery or not. Do you feel comfortable with her making those medical decisions for you if you are not able to make them?

Patient: I hope I won't need to have surgery. But if I did, I would want Mary to help me make that decision.

In this scenario the patient understands what each document means and his answers, coupled with our knowledge of his cognitive status, lead us to conclude that he has the legal capacity necessary to sign them. The question of whether a patient has the capacity to allow a family member to take control of his or her affairs is typically contentious only when there is more than one family member vying for control. When multiple family members are involved, it is best to get them all in the room together with the patient. It typically becomes readily apparent who has the patient's best interests at heart, or who will be the most responsible with financial affairs. If a family consensus can be reached, then things go smoothly. If not, it will be up to the courts to decide.

It goes without saying that the less impaired the patient is, the greater capacity the patient will have, and the easier these types of issues and decisions become. We therefore encourage the family to start the legal planning early—before the patient becomes too impaired to make these decisions and loses capacity. Note that it is important that all family discussions regarding capacity and other legal issues be well documented in the medical record.

Legal Documents

There are a number of legal documents of which the patient and family should be aware. An attorney is necessary to prepare and execute these documents. Finding the right attorney is important. If the patient has a family attorney, he or she may be able to assist the family in these matters, or refer them to an appropriate attorney. If not, one good place to start in the United States is the local Alzheimer's Association office (www.alz.org/apps/findus.asp, 800-272-3900) or the local Agency on Aging office (or contact the Eldercare locator http://www.eldercare.acl.gov/, 800-677-1116). Similar services can be found through the Alzheimer's Association in Australia (https://www.alz.org/au/dementia-alzheimers-australia.asp), Alzheimer Society in Canada (https://alzheimer.ca/en, 800-616-8816), and the Alzheimer's Society in England, Wales, and Northern Ireland (www.alzheimers.org.uk, 0300 222 1122).

- *Guardianship* (conservatorship in some U.S. states) is the court-appointed individual to make decisions on the patient's behalf regarding the patient's assets and/or healthcare. Guardianship is only given by the court when it finds that the patient is legally incompetent. Note that a diagnosis of Alzheimer's disease alone does not make a patient legally incompetent.
- A *living will* is a document that indicates the medical choices the patient would wish to make if he or she is unable to make them, such as whether cardiopulmonary resuscitation (CPR) should be performed should there be a catastrophic event and his or her heart were to stop beating.
- *Power of attorney* is the document that allows the patient to name an individual to make legal and financial decisions when he or she is unable to. A "durable" power of attorney means that the power of attorney is valid after the patient can no longer make his or her own decisions. Usually the power of attorney is "durable."
- *Power of attorney for healthcare* is the document that allows the patient to name an individual to make medical and other healthcare decisions when he or she is unable to. These decisions would include choosing between different:
  - Physicians and other healthcare providers

- Types of treatment (e.g., surgery vs. medical vs. palliative)
- Long-term care facilities.

Note that there is overlap between the living will and the power of attorney for healthcare, such that it might be possible that the living will specifies the preference for one treatment (e.g., DNR—do not resuscitate), whereas the individual with the power of attorney for healthcare specifies another (e.g., CPR when appropriate). In these circumstances there is an assumption that the power of attorney for healthcare is following what the wishes of the patient would be if he or she were able to articulate them in the particular circumstance that has arisen. Given this assumption, it would be highly unlikely that physicians or attorneys would "overrule" the power of attorney for healthcare, despite an apparent contradiction with the patient's living will.

FINANCIAL PLANNING

In Chapter 28 we discussed the importance of the patient transitioning the household finances to a family member or other caregiver, including banking, bill paying, and investing. In this chapter we touch on the issue of how to help the patient and family cover the costs of Alzheimer's disease or other dementia.

Alzheimer's disease is expensive. In addition to the continuing costs that the patient has related to ongoing medical treatment and prescription drugs, new costs will likely occur related to in-home services (home health aide, homemaker, respite, and others), day programs, and eventually long-term care services (assisted living and nursing homes). Here we list a number of programs that patients or their families may be able to take advantage of in the United States to help defray some of these costs. Most other countries have similar programs and services.

- *Medicare* is the federal health insurance program for those aged 65 years and older. Medicare covers:
  - Inpatient hospital care
  - Some outpatient care
  - Some medical items
  - Some prescription medications
  - Some home healthcare
    - Some skilled nursing care
    - Some rehabilitation care.

Medicare does not cover long-term nursing home care. See www.medicare.gov or call 800-633-4227 for more information.

- *Medigap* is additional insurance paid for out-of-pocket expenses that can fill in the "gaps" in Medicare coverage (such as co-insurance payments). There are several different options, with the more expensive policies paying for additional gaps. See www.medicare.gov/supplement-other-insurance/medigap/whats-medigap.html for more information.

- *Medicaid* will pay for medical care and long-term care for patients with very low income and asset levels. Many individuals end up qualifying for Medicaid after using up their own money and other assets (the so-called "spend down" period). Patients must be very careful, however, regarding giving away their assets to family members; state laws typically prevent this action from allowing them to qualify. As with many aspects of financial planning, beginning early is the key to success. See www.medicaid.gov for more information.

- The *Department of Veterans Affairs (VA)* provides health and long-term care services for many veterans. Through its Geriatric Research Education Clinical Centers (GRECCs), the VA has become a leader in the care of individuals with Alzheimer's disease and other dementias. See www.va.gov/GRECC/ or call 800-827-1000 and have the family contact their nearest GRECC.

- *Social Security disability income (SSDI)* are benefits for those younger than age 65 who have worked during their life to obtain additional income from social security. All patients with Alzheimer's disease or other dementia less than age 65 who have previously worked should look into this program, which is now easier to apply for (see www.alz.org/living_with_alzheimers_social_security_disability.asp). For more information contact Social Security at www.socialsecurity.gov/, or 800-772-1213.

- *Social Security income (SSI)* are benefits for those aged 65 or older who are both disabled and also have limited income and assets. For more information contact Social Security at www.socialsecurity.gov/, or 800-772-1213.

- The *Family and Medical Leave Act* is very helpful for family members who are working while caring for an individual with dementia. See www.dol.gov/whd/fmla/ for more information.

- *Tax benefits* may be available, including deductions and credits, depending upon the specific circumstance of the patient and family. Programs such as the Household and Dependent Care Credit may be applicable. See www.irs.gov or call 800-829-1040.

- *Disability insurance* provides income for a worker who can no longer work because of illness or injury. Most employer-paid disability policies provide 60% to 70% of the individual's gross income. Personal disability policies differ in the amount of benefit that they provide.

- *Long-term care insurance* will usually pay for the cost of nursing homes and other long-term care facilities. If the patient is fortunate enough to have this insurance, it should be reviewed carefully to make sure that Alzheimer's disease (or other dementia) is covered, how long the benefits will last, and other details.

- *Life insurance* policies can sometimes loan money to the patient before their death (a "viatical" loan) when the patient is not expected to live beyond 6 to 12 months.

- *Retirement accounts* can be used, including individual retirement accounts (IRAs), and employee-funded accounts such as 401(k) and 403(b).

- *Personal savings and assets* are, of course, another option. These include savings and checking accounts, money market accounts, property, and real estate.

30

Special Issues in Memory Loss, Alzheimer's Disease, and Dementia

QUICK START: SPECIAL ISSUES IN MEMORY LOSS, ALZHEIMER'S DISEASE, AND DEMENTIA

Some Patients Do Not Want to Have Their Memory Evaluated
- Help patients understand that the goal is to improve their memory and allow them to continue doing the activities that they enjoy.
- Explain that there are a number of medications available that could help them.

Some Patients Do Not Want You to Talk to Their Family
- A few patients are able to manage the disease on their own, at least for a while.
- For the majority of patients, involvement of family or friends is a critical part of the patient's care, helping him or her to deal with and manage memory loss caused by Alzheimer's disease or another dementia.

Talking to Adult Children of Patients About Their Risk of Alzheimer's Disease and What They Can Do About It
- Having one parent with the disease increases the lifetime risk of developing Alzheimer's disease by between 2-fold and 4-fold.
- We stress, however, that Alzheimer's disease is common: everyone is at risk.
- Activities shown to reduce the risk of Alzheimer's disease include:
  - Eating a Mediterranean-style diet
  - Participating in social and cognitively stimulating activities
  - Performing aerobic exercise.

THE PATIENT WHO DOES NOT WANT TO COME TO THE APPOINTMENT

Difficulty in convincing patients to come to appointments to evaluate their memory can sometimes be one of the biggest obstacles faced by families. Patients do not want to come to the appointment for a variety of reasons. Some patients may not want to come to the appointment because they are fearful of the diagnosis of Alzheimer's disease, particularly if they watched their parent, spouse, or friend suffer with this disorder. Others may not want to come to the appointment because they are afraid they

will be sent to a nursing home. And some may simply not want to come to the appointment because they do not recognize a problem and cannot be bothered with coming.

We admit that we have not been able to convince every patient to come to an appointment. We have, however, been successful with a couple of strategies. The most reliable of these is to explain to the patient (typically on the phone) that our goal is to improve their memory to allow them to continue doing the activities that they enjoy, and that there are a number of medications available to help their

297

memory, and even to delay the onset of Alzheimer's disease. Sometimes it is not even what you say, but just spending a minute and making a connection with the patient helps to make the appointment less frightening.

A number of families will grab us in the hallway before the appointment and say something like, "Please take her blood pressure … the only way I was able to get her to you was to pretend that this was for her routine blood pressure check." Although we do not condone deception as a way to bring a patient to an appointment (in part because it may lead to mistrust, in part because of the ethical implications), patients brought in this way typically do just fine. These patients discover that a memory evaluation is quite similar to other medical evaluations, not as frightening or threatening as they had feared.

THE PATIENT WHO DOES NOT WANT YOU TO TALK TO THEIR FAMILY

Sometimes it happens that patients come to the clinic and they do not want you to tell their family about their memory difficulties. Should we agree with respecting their desire for confidentiality, despite the difficulties and potential danger in which they may be placing themselves and others? Or should we insist that their family be involved? Our answer is that it depends upon the circumstances (see patient examples). For the vast majority of patients, the involvement of family or friends is a critical part of the patient's care, helping him or her to deal with and manage memory loss whether owing to Alzheimer's disease or because of another dementia. There are a few patients, however, who are able to manage the disease on their own, at least for a while.

CASE STUDY

The First Patient

A patient came to our office about 10 years ago, driving himself the 3 hours to get to our clinic, with concerns about his memory. He had noticed mild changes in his memory, and was worried that he might be at the earliest stage of Alzheimer's disease. He had watched his father go through the disease, and so he knew the signs well. After evaluating him we made a diagnosis of mild cognitive impairment, and prescribed a course of medication. He did not want us to mention anything to his children or his wife, which we thought was acceptable at the time given how mild his memory difficulties were, how responsibly he was acting, and that he was taking a medication which had the potential to improve his memory to the level which it was at the previous year.

Several years passed in this manner. His memory became worse, and he was diagnosed with very mild Alzheimer's disease dementia. At each visit we discussed the importance of letting his family know about his difficulties, but he continued to decline our suggestion. He was able to persuade us, however, that he was taking all of his medications correctly, was driving safely, not getting lost, and not running into any serious difficulties. Finally, a minor crisis occurred at home when he forgot to come home to take the dog out for a walk—a small thing, but very uncharacteristic for him—and he ended up explaining to his family about his disease and about not wanting to burden them with it. Our next visit with the patient included his wife and two anxious sons. We had

a very productive meeting and learned many things we wished we had known about earlier, such as that he used many woodworking tools in the basement and was beginning to have minor injuries associated with not using the tools correctly. Overall, however, we were pleased that we were able to provide good treatment to the patient while at the same time respecting his wishes not to tell his family about his memory problems.

The Second Patient

Another patient came to our clinic several years ago. We knew that there were going to be some issues before she came in, because she had scheduled and then canceled the appointment four times before finally coming in to see us. It had also been clear to us ahead of time that she did not want her family involved, because when our secretary scheduled the visit and mentioned to the patient that she should bring someone close to her to the appointment, such as a family member or close friend, she adamantly refused to do so.

During the appointment she was incredibly anxious. We were sympathetic to her. It was perfectly clear that she was absolutely terrified that she might have Alzheimer's disease. Her mother had recently died of the disease, and we gathered that the experience of her mother's illness and death had been quite traumatizing to her. Her mother, however, first showed symptoms in her mid-80s and died at age 91. The patient herself was only 68 years old. Even before we finished interviewing her we could tell that her memory problems were significant, and we wondered whether she was really able to cover her difficulties as well as she stated.

We took an extra 10 minutes, and spoke with her about some of what we typically save for the first follow-up visit. We discussed that, if it turned out that she did have Alzheimer's disease, there are many treatments that could help her—more than were available when her mother was diagnosed. Additionally, we discussed a number of experimental treatments that were currently in clinical trials, treatments that had the possibility to significantly slow the progression of Alzheimer's disease.

We then asked about her family and, when we learned that they were supportive, we explained the importance of having her family with her. She hesitated,

and we gently but firmly insisted that she involve her family and bring at least one family member with her to the follow-up appointment. We insisted because we were concerned that she needed the emotional support of family to effectively come to terms with her memory problems. Additionally, her memory was already poor enough such that she would be unable to hide it for long—assuming that it was not already apparent to those around her. Both her daughter and husband came with her to the next appointment, at which time we told her that she had mild Alzheimer's disease dementia. Although tears were shed, with their help she was able to accept the diagnosis, and she worked to have a positive attitude.

TALKING TO ADULT CHILDREN OF PATIENTS ABOUT THEIR RISK OF ALZHEIMER'S DISEASE AND WHAT THEY CAN DO ABOUT IT

Although their first concern is always for their parent, the second concern of almost all adult children who have parents with Alzheimer's disease is, "So what are my risks, doc? Will I develop Alzheimer's disease too?" As we discussed in Chapter 4, compared with not having a parent with the disease, having one parent with Alzheimer's disease increases the lifetime risk of developing it by between 2-fold and 4-fold (Lampert et al., 2013), and more distant family relatives with Alzheimer's also increase one's risk (Cannon-Albright et al., 2019). Knowledge of this increase in risk causes many middle-aged children of patients with Alzheimer's disease to become apprehensive that they, too, will develop this disorder. We generally point out to these family members that, although the risk of Alzheimer's disease is increased with a family history of the disorder, Alzheimer's disease is extremely common as we age, such that everyone is at risk for the disorder, with or without a family history. More importantly, if the overall risk of Alzheimer's disease is about 2.5% between ages 65 and 70 years, the risk without a family history is probably around 1.5% and the risk with a family history is probably between 3% and 6%. Thus, although the relative risk may be doubled or quadrupled, the overall risk is still quite small.

The next question asked by those at risk for Alzheimer's disease is, "So what can I do to prevent it?" Although there

is no definitive answer to this question, we emphasize the activities that have been repeatedly shown to be helpful. As discussed in Chapter 22, activities that can slow down memory loss and stave off Alzheimer's disease include eating a Mediterranean-style diet (Berti et al., 2018; Morris et al., 2015), participating in social and cognitively stimulating leisure activities (Akbaraly et al., 2009; Boyke et al., 2008; Krell-Roesch et al., 2019; Leung et al., 2010; Petersen et al., 2018), and performing aerobic exercise (Erickson et al., 2011; Scarmeas et al., 2009). These are therefore the activities and lifestyle changes that we recommend. If they ask us about vitamins, herbs, or supplements, we share with them the information discussed in Chapter 21; if there is a deficiency in vitamin D or any of the B vitamins it should certainly be remedied, but other than remedying vitamin deficiencies, none of these factors has sufficient evidence that would justify their use. Some family members are interested in reading books on this topic and, if they are, we recommend the evidence-based one we wrote, *Seven Steps to Managing Your Memory: What's Normal, What's Not, and What to Do About It* (Budson & O'Connor, 2017).

REFERENCES

Akbaraly, T. N., Portet, F., Fustinoni, S., et al. (2009). Leisure activities and the risk of dementia in the elderly: Results from the Three-City Study. *Neurology, 73*, 854–861.

Berti, V., Walters, M., Sterling, J., et al. (2018). Mediterranean diet and 3-year Alzheimer brain biomarker changes in middle-aged adults. *Neurology, 90*(20), e1789–e1798.

Boyke, J., Driemeyer, J., Gaser, C., et al. (2008). Training-induced brain structure changes in the elderly. *The Journal of Neuroscience, 28*, 7031–7035.

Budson, A. E., & O'Connor, M. K. (2017). *Seven steps to managing your memory: What's normal, what's not, and what to do about it.* New York: Oxford University Press.

Cannon-Albright, L. A., Foster, N. L., Schliep, K., et al. (2019). Relative risk for Alzheimer disease based on complete family history. *Neurology, 92*(15), e1745–e1753.

Erickson, K. I., Voss, M. W., Prakash, R. S., et al. (2011). Exercise training increases size of hippocampus and improves memory. *Proceedings of the National Academy of Sciences of the United States of America, 108*(7), 3017–3022.

Krell-Roesch, J., Syrjanen, J. A., Vassilaki, M., et al. (2019). Quantity and quality of mental activities and the risk of incident mild cognitive impairment. *Neurology, 93*(6), e548–e558.

Lampert, E. J., Roy Choudhury, K., Hostage, C. A., et al. (2013). Prevalence of Alzheimer's pathologic endophenotypes in asymptomatic and mildly impaired first-degree relatives. *PLoS One, 8*, e60747.

Leung, G. T., Fung, A. W., Tam, C. W., et al. (2010). Examining the association between participation in late-life leisure activities and cognitive function in community-dwelling elderly Chinese in Hong Kong. *International Psychogeriatrics, 22*, 2–13.

Morris, M. C., Tangney, C. C., Wang, Y., et al. (2015). MIND diet associated with reduced incidence of Alzheimer's disease. *Alzheimer's & Dementia, 11*(9), 1007–1014.

Petersen, R. C., Lopez, O., Armstrong, M. J., et al. (2018). Practice guideline update summary: Mild cognitive impairment: Report of the Guideline Development, Dissemination, and Implementation Subcommittee of the American Academy of Neurology. *Neurology, 90*(3), 126–135.

Scarmeas, N., Luchsinger, J. A., Schupf, N., et al. (2009). Physical activity, diet, and risk of Alzheimer disease. *The Journal of the American Medical Association, 302*, 627–637.

Page numbers followed by "*f*" indicate figures, "*t*" indicate tables, and "*b*" indicate boxes.